Food Is A
Wonder
Medicine

FOOD IS A WONDER MEDICINE

The Power
To Heal Is
On Your Plate

Neal Barnard, M.D.
Foreword by Dean Ornish, M.D.
With recipes and menus by Jennifer Raymond

MAGNI PUBLISHING / McKINNEY, TEXAS

Produced by arrangement with Harmony Books
A division of Crown Publishers, Inc.
Previously published as "Food For Life"

Published by Magni Group, Inc.
P.O. Box 849, McKinney, Texas 75070 USA

Manufactured in the United States of America

Library of Congress Cataloging-in-Publication Data

Barnard, Neal D., 1953-
Food Is A Wonder Medicine: The Power to Heal Is On Your Plate
by Neal Barnard.– 1st paperback ed.

ISBN 1-882330-07-2

10 9 8 7 6 5 4 3

Contents

··

Acknowledgments

....

It has been a great pleasure to work with many people in the development of this book. My collaborator, Jennifer Raymond, used her finely tuned culinary skills to turn powerful nutritional guidelines into menus and recipes that are familiar, delicious, and easy to make. Each one is a gem.

Although innumerable physicians and other experts shared their wisdom as this book was being researched, particular thanks go to Dean Ornish, M.D., T. Colin Campbell, Ph.D., Randall Lauffer, Ph.D., Denham Harman, M.D., and Victoria Moran for sharing innumerable insights and for allowing themselves to be quoted herein.

I owe a continuing debt to Virginia Messina, M.P.H., R.D., and Mark Messina, Ph.D., for their ongoing assistance on a wide variety of nutrition issues. Heartfelt thanks also go to Denis Burkitt, M.D., Oliver Alabaster, M.D., and John McDougall, M.D., for their inspiration and encouragement, and for their pioneering work unraveling mysteries of nutrition in medicine.

Particular appreciation goes to Patti Breitman, an outstanding literary agent, whose wisdom and experience guided this project along. I also owe a great debt to Peter Guzzardi, whose skillful editing and support for all aspects of the publication of this book are deeply appreciated.

Thank you to the dedicated staff of the Physicians Committee for Responsible Medicine for their autonomous and creative work while I was ensconced at the medical library.

Finally, I would like to thank my parents, Donald and Margaret Barnard, who have not only tolerated with enviable equanimity a son whose medical career uses a fork instead of a scalpel, but who are also among my best research subjects.

Foreword

For the past seventeen years, in a series of clinical investigations, my colleagues and I at the Preventive Medicine Research Institute have been conducting research which demonstrates that even severe coronary heart disease often can begin to reverse, without cholesterol-lowering drugs or surgery. Within a few days to a few weeks, most of our study participants reported marked reductions in the frequency of chest pain (angina). Many became pain-free. Within one month, many participants showed an increased blood flow to the heart and an improved ability of the heart to pump blood. Within one year, even severe coronary artery blockages began to reverse in most of our study participants. In addition, most of them were able to reduce or even discontinue their cardiac medications, under their doctors' supervision. The patients each lost an average of twenty-two pounds during the first year, even though they were eating a great quantity of food and they were eating more frequently. These improvements have given many people new hope and new choices.

The implications of our findings go beyond reversing heart disease. If heart disease can be reversed, then it may be prevented. Since more Americans die each year of heart and blood vessel diseases than all other causes combined, the potential savings in lives and economics may be enormous.

In his new book, Dr. Neal Barnard makes a powerful and persuasive case for why you may wish to change your diet. Changing your diet may decrease your risk not only of cardiovascular disease but also of breast cancer, colon cancer, prostate cancer, osteoporosis, diabetes, hypertension, and a variety of other chronic degenerative diseases that afflict our country. In this book, Dr. Barnard not only tells you *why* you may want to change your diet, he also shows you *how*. He offers detailed, practical guidance on state-of-the-art healthful eating, and a complete twenty-one-day program to help make the transition from old dietary habits to new and better ones. He will also help you start your own program of exercise and provides effective ways to manage stress.

One of the surprising findings in our study is that, for many people, it is easier to make big changes in diet and life-style than to make only moderate ones. Although this goes against conventional wisdom, we found it to be true. When people make only moderate changes in diet and life-style, they have the worst of both worlds. They have the sense of deprivation because they're not able to eat and do everything that they want, but they're not making changes big enough to make them feel much better or to have much effect on their weight, their cholesterol, or their health. On the other hand, when people make comprehensive changes in their diet and life-style, they begin to feel so much better so quickly that the choices become clear and, for many people, worth making.

Dr. Neal Barnard has been a leader in educating people about the health benefits of improving their diets. I recommend this book heartily.

Dean Ornish, M.D.
President and Director
Preventive Medicine Research Institute
University of California, San Francisco

The New Scientific Breakthroughs

In science, there are times when dramatic discoveries alter our most basic assumptions. People thought the earth was at the hub of the solar system until Copernicus found the sun at the center of our celestial ballet. Columbus's failure to fall off the earth's edge forced the map into a globe. Newtonian principles relating mass, velocity, acceleration, and energy forged the structure of physics until Einstein's theory of relativity shook its very foundation. In each case, old ideas were relegated to the history shelves, and we took in hand the power of new knowledge.

Something similar has happened in the world of nutrition. For centuries we thought of food choices as a modest force in medicine. We were wrong. In nutrition, a dynamic, new, and optimistic world has replaced the flat vista of the past.

After decades of frustrating calorie-counting diets, new weight-loss discoveries allow most people to lose weight, keep it off permanently, and never count another calorie or mix another diet drink.

Heart disease can not only be prevented; with proper diet and life-style, it can be reversed. That was something most doctors never dreamed of a few years ago. New research has yielded a program that can begin the process of reversal for most heart patients within one year.

We have new artillery in the war on cancer. More than 80 percent of cancers are attributable to factors we can potentially control. And for people with cancer, dietary factors can alter hormone levels, boost immunity, and improve survival.

When I was growing up, my father was hospitalized for ulcers and used to take antacids before and after meals. I figured that five children and a busy medical practice in the days when doctors still made house calls would give anyone ulcers. Well, ulcer treatment has been revolutionized as well. A certain kind of bacteria turns out to be responsible for ulcers, and a new two-week treatment can eliminate the problem, usually permanently.

As incredible as it sounds, using the regimen in this book adult-onset diabetes can be beaten. The majority of adult-onset diabetes patients no longer need medications when they follow this program. And according to the latest scientific evidence, childhood-onset diabetes can be prevented in many, perhaps most, cases.

There are other emerging findings. Arthritis has long been an enigma for doctors, but new dietary measures have helped many people and are included here. Many multiple sclerosis patients have benefited dramatically from dietary changes. And scientists are now asking whether foods can delay the signs of aging or even help men to keep their hair. The answer to that question is "We don't know yet," but what we do know is detailed here. Even such unlikely problems as varicose veins and hemorrhoids are being linked to foods.

There are other peculiar twists to the new dietary findings. For example, it turns out that foods influence not only our health and longevity but can also affect a man's ability to function sexually. The same sort of diet that allows the blood supply to nourish the heart also allows blood to flow unimpeded on its way to the sexual organs.

Women are dramatically affected as well. The high fat content of the customary diets of Western countries causes an artificial elevation of estrogen, the female sex hormone. Reducing the fat content of the diet not only reduces cancer risk but also makes menstrual periods much more comfortable.

There is one benefit to changing your diet that you may not have expected: You can save a substantial amount of money. A research nutritionist at the George Washington University calculated that a menu based on grains, vegetables, fruits, and beans can save a family of four about $40 per week. That adds up to $2,100 per year, or a new car every six or seven years.

This book will give you the details you need. As I drafted this guide, I aimed to do two things: give you the latest and best knowledge on using foods intelligently, and make the process of change as easy and clear-cut as possible.

Included is detailed information on how to plan meals, how to make changes in eating habits easy, and how to make them stick, plus menus and recipes—both for people who like to cook and for those who do not want to spend much time in the kitchen.

Special considerations for pregnancy and nursing, and for children, are included in Chapter 6.

Now, food is not everything. Your health is also affected by tobacco, alcohol, physical activity, and the stress of modern life. And some people will have medical problems in spite of taking very good care of themselves. No program is foolproof, including this one.

On the other hand, foods can be more powerful than I had ever imagined. When I arrived at medical school, I knew little about nutrition. I knew that red meat was not exactly a health food, but on the other hand, my family includes several cattle-raisers. In fact, they outnumbered the doctors 4 to 3. As a youngster, I even worked at McDonald's.

In my medical studies, I learned about what happens to people when they get a little older. In lectures, I saw slides of hearts damaged by heart attacks, the dead and discolored portions carefully outlined by the instructor's pointer. I assisted at autopsies of patients who had died of strokes caused by the loss of blood supply to the brain. As the pathologist took samples, he showed me holes as big as golf balls in parts of the brain that were supposed to allow a person to speak and move. I met patients whose legs had been amputated when diabetes destroyed their circulation.

I began to learn about the causes of these conditions. Scientists were pointing fingers at the foods on which these people were raised—and on which I was raised, too.

During medical school, certain patients took a permanent place in my memory. On the ward to which I was assigned, there was a room on the left in which a woman of about thirty-five years of age lay in bed. Her eyes were hollow and black. She was very thin and always wore a scarf on her head to hide the fact that her hair had fallen out from chemotherapy. She had breast cancer. Her husband and two small children frequently came to visit, and their faces were often glistening with tears.

Our job was to push chemotherapy. We also pushed morphine and Demerol, narcotic painkillers that lessened the pain of the cancer that had spread to her bones and now grew within them. We also pushed lies: "I think we've turned a corner. There are some positive signs. We're seeing a good effect from the medicine." Eventually the pretense failed. One day, we pulled the sheet over her lifeless face and went into the next room, where there was another woman of about the same age. She also had a scarf on her head, and her eyes had the same wasted look.

Breast cancer is an epidemic. It devastates families. But for us it became routine. There was nothing that could prevent it. The best that could be done was to discover it on a mammogram or physical exam, and begin treatment as early as possible. But research has started to emerge, showing that in countries with low cancer rates people ate differently from people in countries where cancer is at epidemic proportions. Investigators learned of the effect of foods on sex hormones, of the protective natural chemicals that are in vegetables and fruits, and of many other factors. A mountain of research has shown that food plays an important role in cancer of the breast, colon, prostate, and other organs, and can increase or decrease the likelihood of survival of cancer patients.

This stunned me. It suggested that the women who had died in that hospital might not have developed cancer in the first place. The painful battle need never have occurred. It was not their fault—or our fault. We could not have been sure that a different diet would have worked. But none of us had even known to try.

Time for a Change

Over the past few decades, the science of nutrition has raced ahead, giving us a good understanding of cholesterol, fat, fiber, and vitamins. But there has been almost no change in what schoolchildren are taught to eat since the four food groups were introduced in 1956—two years before the Hula-Hoop craze.

The Department of Agriculture's promotional posters used to list milk as the first group and meat as the second. Grains got a group, and fruits and vegetables had to share a group. Because livestock products were assigned two of the four groups, menus developed under this plan were often loaded with fat and cholesterol. That is how an entire generation learned to eat, and how they, in turn, raised their children.

The results are tragic. There are 4,000 heart attacks *every single day* in this country. The traditional four food groups and the eating patterns they prescribed have led to cancer and heart disease in epidemic numbers, and have killed more people than any other factor in America. More than automobile accidents, more than tobacco, more than all the wars of this century combined.

As our children grow up, heart disease awaits most of them, taking more victims than any other cause of death. The second leading cause of death will be cancer, and third will be stroke. All are strongly linked to food decisions. At this point, we know which foods are dangerous and which are safe. We can easily spot which children have eating habits that will put them at risk. But we do nothing. Often, we actually encourage bad diets. The same father who would run in front of a speeding car to push a child out of danger nods approvingly as his daughters or sons learn eating habits that will later take their lives.

A child born today has a one-in-three risk of eventually developing cancer. It might occur around age thirty or maybe forty, or maybe later. But as high as the risk of cancer is, the risk of heart disease is even higher. Children grow into adulthood with a one-in-two risk of heart disease. Americans die years earlier than their counterparts in Japan, for instance, where very different dietary habits are preferred. We send our children to the best schools we can afford, and try to equip them with moral values that will last a lifetime, but we give them food habits that, when they grow up, will cut short two lives out of every three.

The issues are not all life-threatening. Millions of Americans wrestle with expanding waistlines, frustrated by diet schemes that promise results but prove useless. Most are unaware of the new science of weight control.

If old eating habits are so destructive, why haven't we changed? One reason is force of habit, first demonstrated in the worried scowl that comes over a child's face when confronted with any new food. The other reason is politics. Livestock producers have put enormous pressure on the federal government to keep their products listed as daily requirements. Tobacco companies, with their legendary political clout, are amateurs compared to the livestock promoters. The dairy industry has managed to receive a half-billion to a billion dollars in federal support *every year*. Meat and dairy products got food groups number 1 and number 2 on the old four-food-groups posters. In classroom lessons and after-school television advertising, images of high-fat, no-fiber foods are drummed into children's heads, while cholesterol is pounded into their hearts.

This book aims to change things. It is based on a completely new nutritional plan, first proposed on April 8, 1991, by the Physicians Committee for Responsible Medicine (PCRM), along with some of the world's most respected scientists. Dr. Denis Burkitt is the medical pioneer who discovered the value of fiber. His name and work are studied by every medical student in the world. Dr. Burkitt traveled to Washington, D.C., to speak at the 1991 PCRM press conference and to ask reporters to spread the lifesaving message far and wide. Dr. T. Colin Campbell, the Cornell University biochemist who heads the prestigious China Health Study, which revealed in stark detail how differences in diet lead to dramatic differences in health, also joined our press conference announcing the New Four Food Groups. We were also honored to be joined by Dr. Oliver Alabaster, a cancer researcher and author at the George Washington University School of Medicine. To him, a change in eating habits had a personal meaning. His mother was diagnosed with breast cancer when she was only forty-one, and died a few years later. As Dr. Alabaster knows only too well, if we can change the way people eat, we can let some children know their parents a bit longer.

The plan in this book is a simple one, but it has the power to bring health and vigor to a new level, and add years to life.

The New Four Food Groups program recommends that your diet be based on grains, legumes, vegetables, and fruits. The latter two are no longer forced to share a single group, and meat and dairy lose their food-group status. Centering your diet on the New Four Food Groups will lead to a huge reduction in fat intake and an increase in fiber, complex carbohydrates, beta-carotene, and other important nutrients. This plan is not just low in cholesterol; it has *no cholesterol at all.* Evidence shows that the cumulative effect of these food choices, made three times a day, 365 times a year, is dramatic. As will be described in the following chapters, this evidence comes from scientific studies of the dietary habits of people who have stayed well and people who have become ill; comparisons of health statistics of populations following different diets; and experiments in which both patients and healthy people have tested various diets.

This book was written both for people who are healthy and want to stay that way, and for people who are struggling with health problems. It is specific in its recommendations, and includes references both to other books for the layperson and to scientific literature.

Of course, people change their diets for lots of different reasons. One advantage of a diet based on grains, vegetables, and other plant foods is that the animals that might otherwise have been eaten can all breathe a sigh of relief. About six billion chickens are fattened up yearly in the U.S. From the de-beaking process on the factory farm to the miseries of the slaughter line, their eight-week life is no treat. The same could be said for pigs, cattle, veal calves, turkeys, and other animals raised on modern farms.

A plant-based diet lets the earth breathe easier, too. The cultivation of crops for direct human consumption is much more efficient than using grains or legumes to fatten up livestock. Only a fraction of the nutrients that cattle or other animals take in are left in their muscles at the time of slaughter. The rest have been used up to power their movements, metabolism, body warmth, and other life functions. Nearly twenty years ago, *Scientific American* reported that producing a pound of bacon requires ten times as much crop land (in the form of feed grains) as is used to make the same quantity of bacon analog from soybeans. The cultivation of those feed crops requires land, water, and pesticides and other chemicals that add to our environmental problems.

Meanwhile, the U.S. imports 78 million pounds of beef from Brazil annually, according to the USDA Economic Research Service, and the destruction of the Latin American rain forest to provide grazing land is an ever-growing nightmare. You can help the environment and the animals at the same time that you are doing tremendous favors for your waistline, your coronary arteries, and your general health.

Food choices give us enormous power. The change in our eating habits has already begun. Oatmeal and whole-grain toast are pushing bacon and eggs off the American breakfast plate, and at lunch and dinner we are starting to think about what fiber and fat mean. But that is just the beginning. The program described in this book uses the full power of healthful eating. First, we explore the new facts you need to know about healthful eating. Then, in a three-week program which you can tailor to your individual needs, you begin a new menu that is delicious, easy to prepare, and designed for maximum weight control, cholesterol reduction, cancer prevention, and all-around good health. You will find delightful menus and recipes; tips for entertaining, travel, and dealing with reluctant family members; and ways to adapt favorite traditional recipes.

This book goes beyond old-fashioned "diets," calorie counts, and other shortsighted ideas; the program you find here is easier and much more powerful. The changes described in this book will give you and your children eating habits you can live with, so that you all can enjoy a long life free of heart disease, cancer, stroke, and many other serious illnesses. For many, it can mean a level of health we had not thought we could attain.

How to Use This Book

I suggest that you think short term. Rather than resolve to make any long-standing changes in your eating habits, a three-week period is all you need to consider. Why three weeks? That is how long it takes to break an old habit or start a new one.

In my medical practice I have helped many people overcome all kinds of bad habits, ranging from tobacco and alcohol use to cocaine and heroin abuse, not to mention destructive food habits of every variety. Time and again I find that it takes an average of about three weeks for a new positive habit to take root, and a few weeks more for it to become really solid.

First, familiarize yourself with the concepts in Chapters 1 through 7. Then follow the menu program or take your pick of the recipes and food items in Chapter 8. For three weeks, stick to these foods. You can add others, too, if they meet the same nutritional criteria. Try the simple exercises and stress-reduction tips on pages 299-303. At the end of three weeks, see how you feel. If you like the results, continue with the program for another three weeks.

Please note that every person has a different medical history, different genetic endowment, and different potential risks and benefits from dietary changes, so the results of dietary change will vary from one person to the next. The same is true of any medication or medical procedure.

Also, nothing in this book takes the place of medical decision making between yourself and your physician. If you have a particular medical condition, obesity, or are on medication, consult your doctor before making a substantial change in your diet. Dietary changes can sometimes change your need for medication or have other important effects. Also see your doctor before any substantial increase in physical activity if you are over forty or have any medical problem.

If you are pregnant or nursing, or if you follow this program for more than three years, please consult the guidelines in Chapter 6.

The science of nutrition is controversial and is changing gradually, so I encourage you to consult other sources of information, including the references listed in this volume.

If, for whatever reason after the three weeks, you decide to resume the average American diet, please see your doctor regularly, and reconsider changing to the powerful menu described in this book.

1

Forever Young

Some people seem to stay young forever. They never lose their hair, their skin stays youthful, and they remain slim and physically active. Others go bald before they reach twenty, develop an extra layer of fat by thirty, and have deep wrinkles by forty. The assaults of time are not entirely due to genetics. Foods can be part of the problem. And, more important, certain foods contain natural ingredients that can help protect against aging.

Since the 1950s a substantial body of evidence has shown how foods, properly selected, have a great deal of power to help us stay young. This evidence is now collectively known as the *free radical theory of aging*. While it was a heretical proposition in the 1950s, it is now widely accepted by scientists and nutritionists, who see free radicals as a contributor to skin aging, cataracts, arthritis, and, perhaps, to the most basic aspects of the aging process.

Certain foods slow the effects of time, while others speed them up. In addition, foods can change the amounts of hormones in the body. In turn, these hormones play a critical role in many bodily functions, from puberty to the onset of baldness.

In this chapter we look first at the signs of aging and how to guard against them: changes in our skin, our hairline, our eyesight, and our bones. Then we look at lifespan itself, and the factors that affect the speed with which we grow up and grow old.

Looking and Feeling Young

Can you keep your hair by eating right? Can your skin keep its youthful appearance? Are you doomed to wrinkles, osteoporosis, and cataracts? The fact is, there are fascinating new scientific findings in each of these areas. And enough specific information is available that you can put it to use right now.

Your skin is made of millions and millions of tiny cells, as is your heart, your brain, and every other organ in your body. Each cell has many jobs to do. Skin cells, for example, are not just bricks in a wall. They are very busy repairing injuries, neutralizing the effects of too much sun or various toxins, and taking in nutrients and modifying them for use as needed.

But cells are fragile things. They have only so much capacity to survive. If a small sample of your cells was put into a laboratory dish and given all the nutrients that the cells needed, at first they would grow. Each cell would divide into two, and their progeny would also grow and divide again. But sooner or later they would stop. Typical cells can go through the cycle of growth and division only about fifty times before becoming exhausted.[1] That is biologically predetermined, although the time between one division and the next can be hastened or slowed.

So what does this mean to you? It means that if your body is constantly exposed to the damage of sun, toxins, tobacco, or alcohol, not to mention the chemical wastes produced by normal body processes, you might rapidly use up your cells' capacity to replace themselves. If, on the other hand, you have a way to protect yourself, your cells would need to replace themselves less often and would therefore be able to retain their youth much longer.

The changes that most of us attribute to the aging process actually have very little to do with the passage of time. Compare the skin on your face to the skin on the inside of your upper arm. The skin on your upper arm is not exposed to sun, and it keeps its youthfulness much longer. These protected skin cells also retain more of their ability to grow and multiply. Sun-damaged skin is nearer the end of its lifespan.[2] Although the surface skin cells are constantly being replaced, the underlying skin becomes wrinkled and leathery and loses its resilience.

Skin samples taken during facelifts show the same thing: There are dramatic differences between areas as close together as the skin in front of your ear, which is sun-exposed, and the skin behind it, which is not: the sun-exposed areas age prematurely.[3]

There is, in fact, very little evidence of normal skin aging before age fifty. What passes for aging is mostly sun damage, or *photoaging*, which starts early in life. Photoaging gradually causes rough skin texture, wrinkles, distorted blood vessels, and spots of too much or too little pigment. If you were to examine sun-damaged skin under the microscope, you would see that the tiny elastic fibers that keep the skin supple are damaged, the outer skin cells have overgrown, and the blood vessels are dilated and damaged, too.[4] If you put a skin sample from a sun-protected area under the microscope, however, its baby's-bottom youthfulness is still there.

How can we protect ourselves from this destruction? We can avoid sunburn and even try to stay out of the sun, but there is no way to avoid it completely, nor would we want to. What is more important is a chemical reaction that occurs in the skin, and also in all other parts of the body. This chemical reaction is a chief suspect in the gradual destruction of the body we call the aging process.

Like all the cells of your body, your skin cells need oxygen. It is the very basis of animal life, including ours. But oxygen is biology's double-edged sword. As sunlight slowly bakes your skin,[5] oxygen molecules often become extremely unstable. They pick up too many electrons, or carry electrons in unstable orbits. These destabilized oxygen molecules are called *free radicals*. They are also produced, but to a lesser degree, in the course of the normal workings of the cells.

Free radicals are unstable, destructive molecules. They come in a variety of chemical forms, but all have one thing in common: They can attack and damage bystander molecules, rendering them unstable and ready, in turn, to attack yet other molecules, starting a chain reaction of cellular destruction. They attack the very tissues that make up your body.

If you were a tiny observer cruising through the blood vessels in a microscopic submarine, you would see free radicals attacking the cells of the body. They attack cell membranes and the tiny intracellular machinery. They can even damage DNA, the cell's central control machinery, causing normal cells to turn into cancer cells. These attacks occur in the skin, the heart, the brain, and other organs. If we did not have a means to neutralize these free radicals, we would self-destruct in short order.

The damaging effects of free radicals are not a recent discovery. Physician and researcher Dr. Denham Harman is a professor at the University of Nebraska School of Medicine and is head of the American Aging Association. In the 1950s, he was studying free radicals, which at that time were mainly of interest to chemists dealing with vats of industrial products. Harman suggested that free-radical damage might play a part in the aging of the human body.

What was to become one of the most important theories in human biology began with a bit of daydreaming. "After I had completed medical school and an internship in June 1954," Dr. Harman said, "I went to work as a research associate at the Donner Laboratory of Medical Physics in Berkeley. My time was my own except for one morning a week in the Hematology Clinic; I could have spent most of my time playing tennis if I had wanted to. But I used my free time to pursue my long-time interest in aging." Much was already known about the biology of aging, and about the chemistry of free radicals in our environment. But the two had never been put together.

"You know how sometimes you are struggling with a problem and cannot seem to find the answer to it, and then some time when you're thinking about something else, or maybe even dozing off to sleep, all of a sudden the solution hits you." One morning in November 1954, Dr. Harman was sitting in his office reading, and suddenly it struck him that free radicals were not just sitting in vats of chemicals in our factories and warehouses. They might actually be forming minute by minute in the blood coursing through our veins, attacking the insides of our arteries, aging our skin, sparking the cellular havoc of cancer. Could free radicals be the key to aging processes? Could they play a role in cancer or heart disease?

"I spoke with people on the Berkeley campus about this possibility," Dr. Harman said. "Most thought it was too simple an idea." But other researchers took an interest in the theory. There is now a huge body of research showing that free-radical damage occurs every minute of every day in the human body. "Evidence began to build up," Harman said, "and now, about forty years later, many scientists accept this, both for disease processes and for aging *per se.*"

NATURE'S "MEDICINE"

Plants are hit by direct sunlight hour after hour, day after day. They don't shrivel up and die; they thrive on it. Instead of being bleached or burned by the sun, they are able to use its energy to power the chlorophyll machinery of their leaves, turning water and minerals from the earth and carbon dioxide from the air into building materials.

The fact is, plants would rapidly be damaged by the sun if they did not have one vital chemical in their leaves: *beta-carotene*. As the sun beats down on plant leaves, free radicals form just as they do in your skin, but beta-carotene removes the free radicals before they can do their damage. Beta-carotene is a vital chemical all chlorophyll-containing plants use to neutralize free radicals as they are formed. In the 1950s, another researcher in Berkeley, California, developed a mutant single-celled plant that lacked beta-carotene. When he exposed this plant to light and air, it was wiped out in short order.[6]

The technical term for a protective chemical like beta-carotene is *antioxidant,* meaning that it neutralizes free radicals and blocks the tissue oxidation that they could cause. Antioxidants work by allowing themselves to be attacked and damaged by free radicals, sparing the cell itself.

As our ancestors plucked plants from the ground and fruits from trees, they took beta-carotene for themselves. It passed into their bloodstream and became part of their own defense against toxic molecules. Today, when you add a leaf of fresh spinach to a salad or bite into a carrot, this natural chemical enters the cells of your body. You cannot feel it, but it is busy knocking out free radicals that would age the skin or damage your heart or other organs.

Chemically, beta-carotene is made up of two molecules of vitamin A. In the body, some beta-carotene splits, yielding its two molecules of vitamin A, which also has some protective effect. But beta-carotene has antioxidant powers that vitamin A lacks. The skin cream Retin-A, which made headlines for its ability to reverse the signs of aging skin, is a relative of beta-carotene.

Beta-carotene helps protect the skin against the damaging rays of the sun, and makes it harder to sunburn and easier to tan. People who are extremely sensitive to the sun owing to genetic skin diseases can tolerate the sun much longer when they have beta-carotene-rich diets or supplements.[7,8] But beta-carotene's effect on the skin is not news to researchers. As long ago as 1926, a clinician named J. H. Bendes wrote in a Minnesota medical journal that,

in such patients as the high-typed blondes, the red-haired individuals who would not tan, various methods were used to aid in the tanning, such as a diet of green vegetables rich in vitamines. . . .[9]

In 1972, Boston researcher Micheline Matthews-Roth studied the effect of beta-carotene on the skin. In an unusual experiment, she fed beta-carotene to inmates at the Arizona State Prison for several weeks, then brought them out to the desert, where small areas of their backs were exposed to the sun for varying lengths of time. She found that beta-carotene made it harder to burn and easier to tan.[10]

This effect is relatively small, and it cannot protect you against prolonged sun exposure. On the other hand, sun damage to the skin is accumulated gradually. Day after day, the sun on our skin results in the effects we see later on. People who have the protection of a vegetable-rich diet every day may well have a long-term edge on the effects of the sun.[11] Almost certainly, the beta-carotene dose has to be subtantial. Vegetable-rich diets are effective, as are supplements, but a tiny pile of green beans on the corner of your plate will not help much.

Beta-carotene is easy to find. Yellow and orange vegetables such as carrots, sweet potatoes, and pumpkins contain enormous amounts. All other green and yellow vegetables and fruits also contain beta-carotene: broccoli, spinach, peaches, cantaloupes, kale, collards, mustard greens, and so on. People who consume extremely large amounts of carrots or other beta-carotene-rich vegetables can even develop a temporary orange coloring in their palms and soles.

I do not recommend that you rush out and buy a beta-carotene pill. It is no substitute for vegetables. First of all, plants do not contain just beta-carotene. There are dozens of other antioxidants in plants, each with a slightly different role in protecting the body. In fact, there are dozens of relatives of beta-carotene, called *carotenoids*, found naturally in plants, and there are other vitamins in vegetables that work as part of the body's antioxidant team. In addition, consuming a concentration of one antioxidant may reduce the body's absorption of others.[12] Vegetables, along with fruits, grains, and beans, provide nature's balanced mix of antioxidants.

Sun is not the only thing that attacks the skin. Tobacco is very harmful to the skin, and over time causes an aged appearance. Antioxidants do have a limited capacity to counteract tobacco's cancer-causing effect and possibly other tobacco effects, although this is not license to smoke. The effects of tobacco are so strong that vegetables cannot undo the risk to the lungs and other body parts.

The Body's Antioxidant System

Each cell in the body has an entire antioxidant system that it uses to neutralize free radicals. Beta-carotene is just the beginning. Vitamin C circulates in the bloodstream and is a very potent weapon against free radicals in the blood plasma.[13] Like beta-carotene, vitamin C even has a limited power to protect against the free radicals formed by cigarette smoking.[14]

Where does one get vitamin C? Of course, there is vitamin C in citrus fruits, but there is lots of vitamin C in green vegetables. People who build their menus with vegetables and fruits get vitamin C at every meal. Unfortunately, meals in Western countries are typically not based on vegetables; they are based on meat and dairy products. Beef, pork, poultry, and fish contain virtually no vitamin C. Likewise, milk, yogurt, cheese, and other dairy products are very low in vitamin C. As you will see shortly, these animal products are not just lacking in the protective nutrients; they can actually increase the production of free radicals and create hormone havoc.

If vitamin C is in short supply, free radicals in the blood plasma can approach the cells of the body. At the outer surface of the cell is a membrane that carefully regulates what will and will not enter the cell. Free radicals attack that cell membrane, and can severely damage the microscopic machinery inside your cells.

Cell defenses in the membrane include stored vitamin E. This vitamin does not prevent the formation of free radicals, but it does stop chain reactions of molecular damage. Molecules of vitamin E are chemically altered in the process of neutralizing free radicals, but they are restored to fighting form by vitamin C.[15]

So, as you can see, these vitamins make a good team. Vitamin C patrols the bloodstream for free radicals. When it finds them, it knocks them out. Free radicals that get through to the cell membrane have to face vitamin E, and when vitamin E is damaged, it is "repaired" by vitamin C. Beta-carotene, which works in areas with different oxygen concentrations from those in which vitamin C is effective, completes the team.

Vitamin E is found in many vegetables, beans, grains, and fruits, especially beans, corn, and sweet potatoes. Nuts, such as almonds, are loaded with vitamin E, although their fat content is high.

Unfortunately, no one yet knows just how much beta-carotene or vitamin C or vitamin E is the optimal amount. The Recommended Daily Allowances

(RDA) were developed with an eye toward meeting the body's basic needs, and generally do not take into account emerging information on the role of vitamins in immunity, cancer prevention, or slowing the aging process.

Researchers use doses of beta-carotene in the range of 15 to 30 mg per day, and in some cases as high as 180 mg per day. Beta-carotene is apparently safe even at considerably higher doses. The RDA for vitamin C is only 60 mg per day, but people interested in its antioxidant effects generally use larger amounts, ranging from about 500 mg to several grams per day. The RDA for vitamin E is 8 mg per day for women and 10 mg per day for men, but the optimal dose as an antioxidant is as yet not determined.

My own suggestion is to get these nutrients from foods rather than from supplements. Foods provide safe amounts of these nutrients, along with

Table 1 *Antioxidants in Foods*

	Vitamin C (mg)	Beta-carotene (mg)	Vitamin E (mg)
Apple (1 medium)	8	0.04	0.9
Broccoli (1 cup*)	98	1.3	1.0
Brussels sprouts (1 cup*)	96	0.67	1.3
Carrot (1 medium)	7	12	0.4
Cauliflower (1 cup*)	68	0.01	0.1
Chickpeas (1 cup*)	2	0.02	5.1
Corn kernels (1 cup*)	10	0.22	9.5
Grapefruit (1 medium)	94	0.38	0.6
Navy beans (1 cup*)	2	0	4.1
Orange (1 medium)	80	0.16	0.3
Orange juice (1 cup)	124	0.30	0.5
Pineapple chunks (1 cup)	24	0.02	0.2
Brown rice (1 cup*)	0	0	4.0
Soybeans (1 cup*)	3	0.01	35.0
Spinach, raw (1 cup)	16	2.3	1.7
Strawberries (1 cup)	85	0.02	0.4
Sweet potato (1 medium*)	28	15	5.9

* Figures refer to cooked servings.
Sources: J. A. T. Pennington, *Bowes and Church's Food Values of Portions Commonly Used* (New York: Harper and Row, 1989); and P. J. McLaughlin and J. L. Weihrauch, "Vitamin E Content of Foods," *Journal of the American Dietetic Association* 1979;75:647–65.

other helpful nutrients. Table 1 shows how much of each is in typical foods.

In addition to antioxidant vitamins, the cells of the body have built-in enzymes designed to break down free radicals. One of these, called *glutathione peroxidase,* is an enzyme whose name you do not need to remember. But it is worth knowing that, to work properly, this enzyme needs a certain mineral called *selenium.* Selenium is present in the soil, and plants take up selenium and bring it through grains to you in the form of bread, pasta, and so on. Unfortunately, the selenium content of the soil varies enormously from one area to another, so some doctors recommend taking small supplements of selenium—on the order of 50 to 100 micrograms (mcg) per day. If you choose to do this, do not exceed this amount, as selenium is toxic at high doses. If you also take a vitamin C supplement, take it at a different time, because vitamin C may interfere with absorbing selenium.

STOPPING FREE RADICALS AT THE SOURCE

So far, we have looked at ways to soak up free radicals. Most people do not spend their evenings in the medical library, and therefore have never heard of free radicals. Vegetables, for them, may be nothing more than a side dish as they eat chicken breasts and skim milk, not realizing that healthful eating is something quite different—as the remainder of this book describes in detail. Among the consequences of a vegetable-depleted diet is that it does not produce adequate defenses against free radicals. The resulting damage occurs in the cells of the skin and the internal organs.

And there is something else you should know. There are ways not just to neutralize free radicals that form but to actually reduce their production in the first place. The key is to avoid foods that cause free radicals to form. What kinds of foods are they? Vegetable oils, fish oils, and iron all stimulate the production of free radicals. While they have enjoyed an undeserved good reputation in the lay press, they can be a big part of the free-radical problem.

First, let's look at oils. All types of fats and oils promote the production of free radicals. Doctors correctly counsel patients to steer clear of saturated fat, such as that in beef or chicken, so many people thought there was no reason to be concerned about vegetable oils. The fact is, while animal fats are every bit as bad as you've heard, vegetable oils are not such health foods, either. Granted, they are not likely to elevate your cholesterol level, but they do contribute to free-radical production. The moral of the story is to keep *all* fats and oils to a minimum.

This is not to say that you should have no oil at all. A small amount of oil is intrinsic to foods—corn contains corn oil, for example, and all other vegetables (even broccoli) have small amounts of intrinsic oil. The key is to avoid the added oils that are used in frying or in salad oils.

Even worse are fish oils, which actively encourage the production of free radicals. As you may know, fish oils have been popularized as an aid against everything from heart problems to arthritis. While not all of these claims have held up, scientists have taken an interest in a certain type of fat in fish called *omega-3 fatty acids* because they can reduce the level of triglycerides in the blood, which play a role in heart disease. (The name "omega-3" is simply a chemist's term describing the structure of the fat molecule.) The bad news about fish and fish oils is that omega-3s in fish oils are highly unstable molecules. They tend to decompose and, in the process, unleash dangerous free radicals. Researchers from the University of Arizona[16] and Cornell University[17] addressed this problem in the *American Journal of Clinical Nutrition,* reporting that omega-3s are found in a more stable form in vegetables, fruits, and beans. And vegetables and fruits also provide antioxidants to help neutralize the free radicals that are produced. The body needs only a tiny amount of omega-3s, and vegetables, fruits, and beans provide the benefits of omega-3s while avoiding the more unstable forms. They concluded, "Significantly, the consumption of green leafy vegetables and fruits is consistent with these criteria."[17]

Later on we look at cooking tips that keep oil use to a minimum. Happily, foods rich in antioxidants also tend to be very low in fat; broccoli, spinach, carrots, and other vegetables are loaded with beta-carotene and vitamin C, but are extremely low in fat. Beans and grains contain vitamin E, and are also very low in fat.

IRON: THE DOUBLE-EDGED SWORD

Another way to reduce your body's production of free radicals is to watch your iron intake. Yes, after decades of popularity in the lay literature, iron's reputation has started to erode. While everyone knows that we need iron to carry oxygen in the blood, few people are aware that, in excess, iron is actually a catalyst for the damage caused by oxygen. Just as iron and oxygen work together in the form of oxidation we recognize as rust, something similar happens within the body. Iron encourages the formation of free radicals and their damaging effects. Other metals, including copper and aluminum, have also come under scrutiny for their complicity in free-radical damage.

Dr. Randall B. Lauffer is a biochemist at Harvard University. His book *Iron Balance* shows that iron can be like a detonator in a munitions warehouse.[18]

"Iron is a key component of the free radical theory of disease," Dr. Lauffer said. "This was discovered some time ago, and as we have learned more over the years, we have found that iron sort of sits right in the center of all that chemistry." Iron catalyzes the formation of free radicals, which then damage the tissue around them. Do we have lots of extra iron in our bodies? Unfortunately, the answer is yes. Men accumulate iron throughout adulthood. For most women, iron accumulation becomes a problem only after menstruation ceases.

"In general, as you age, you accumulate iron in your body," according to Dr. Lauffer. "Your body is really a sort of dead end for iron. There's no way to get rid of it in a regulated fashion. We can always get rid of extra sodium if you eat too many potato chips. But with iron, there's really no way to get rid of it. It stays in your body. Most men have 1,000 to 2,000 extra milligrams of iron in their bodies, and that's iron that they're not using. It's just waiting to cause trouble."

Trouble is an understatement. As you will see in later chapters, iron-catalyzed free-radical damage is now thought to be the spark that can set off both heart disease and cancer, in addition to aggravating aging processes.

So where are we getting all this troublesome iron? From meat, first of all. Meat contains a form of iron that is absorbed a bit more easily than iron from vegetables. This used to be thought of as an advantage, but it is now known that more people get into trouble because of iron overload than iron deficiency. The meat-based diets that are routine in Western countries contribute a huge load of a perfect catalyst for free-radical formation. Vegetables, beans, and grains do contain iron, but the body is better able to limit absorption from these sources.

"The dietary modifications that people are trying to make now to reduce their fat and cholesterol will tend to reduce iron levels, as well," Lauffer said. "So, the push toward a more vegetarian-style diet—less meat, and more fruits and vegetables and whole grains—this is totally consistent with all the iron information as well."

Does that mean that people who build their menus from grains, beans, vegetables, and fruits are going to become iron deficient? "Absolutely not,"

Dr. Lauffer said. "There are many studies in vegetarian populations where the iron levels are lower than they are in a meat-eating population, but they're certainly adequate—more than adequate, in many cases."

Some people aggravate the problem by taking iron pills, vitamins with iron, or fortified cereals when they are not actually iron deficient. Of course, children and pregnant and nursing women do have a higher need for iron, compared to people at other stages of life, and some women may become iron deficient during their reproductive years. But many people falsely conclude that they are iron deficient because of the popular myth linking fatigue and iron.

"Fatigue is, of course, very common," Dr. Lauffer said. But there are many causes of fatigue, and the old wives' tale that you need more iron, more red meat or liver to boost your iron-poor blood is largely false. Anemia is not the most likely cause. You can have a virus, you can have depression or other psychological disturbances, or there could be other dietary deficiencies or diseases."

To check your iron status, Dr. Lauffer suggests that you ask your doctor for the following specific tests, in addition to the more general hemoglobin and hematocrit that are usually run. Although general guidelines are given here, the tests should be interpreted by your doctor:

> Serum ferritin (normal values are 12–200 mcg/l of serum)
> Serum iron
> Total iron binding capacity (TIBC)

Doctors divide the serum iron value by the TIBC. The result should be 16 to 50 percent for women and 16 to 62 percent for men. Results below these norms indicate iron deficiency. Results above these norms indicate excess iron. A further test sometimes used to check for iron deficiency is the *red cell protoporphyrin* test. A result higher than 70 mcg/dl of red blood cells is considered abnormal. If two of these three values (serum ferritin, serum iron/TIBC and red cell protoporphyrin) are normal, iron-deficiency anemia is not likely. Serum iron and total iron binding capacity should be done after fasting overnight.

Unfortunately, the body has no way to rid itself of excess iron. Even if you are iron-overloaded, the body still jealously guards its iron stores. The only way to predictably reduce your iron stores is by donating blood. So this altruistic act can have health benefits for the donor as well.

CATARACTS

The eye is, by design, constantly exposed to light. As a result it is a place where free radicals tend to form, gradually causing sections of the lens to turn from transparent to opaque.[19] These opaque parts are cataracts, a common cause of loss of sight and a common reason for surgery.

Granted, ophthalmologic surgeons are happy to remove your lenses and put in brand-new synthetic ones. But scientific studies have shown that certain foods can help keep your original equipment in good working order.

Vitamins C and E and beta-carotene pass from the plasma into the eye. The eye contains very concentrated vitamin C in particular, and together these vitamins offer substantial protection against cataracts. If you are not getting your daily fruits and vegetables, you are not protecting your eyesight. Scientists have actually measured the risk: People who eat less than three and one-half servings of fruits and vegetables per day have nearly six times the risk of cataracts, compared to those who eat more.[20] Supplements of vitamins C and E also offer some protection.[21]

Iron and copper apparently increase the risk of cataracts[22] by encouraging the production of free radicals, and smoking adds to the problem by decreasing vitamin levels. And there are other contributing factors. People who spend long hours outdoors without protective glasses run an increased risk. The problem is the ultraviolet light, particularly for cataracts in the outer part of the lens.

Another interesting contributor is milk. Populations that consume large amounts of dairy products have a much higher incidence of cataracts than do those who avoid dairy products.[23] The problem is not the milk fat, which, like all saturated animal fats, has lost popularity in recent years. The problem appears to be the milk sugar, *lactose,* and nonfat dairy products are under just as much suspicion as is whole milk.

Chemically, lactose is a *disaccharide* molecule—that is, a double sugar. In the digestive tract, it breaks apart, yielding two simple sugar molecules, glucose and galactose. It is the galactose that is suspect in cataracts. When blood concentrations of galactose increase, it can pass into the lens of the eye. There, galactose degrades into various molecular waste products that can lead to opacities of the lens.[24]

Nursing children can generally handle galactose with no problems at all. They have active enzymes in their liver, kidney, and blood cells that break it down. But nature designed the body to be weaned from milk products after infancy, and, as we age, many of us lose much of the capacity to break down galactose. There are even some rare cases of genetic defects in which children cannot break down galactose. These children can form cataracts within the first year of life.

This problem is not the same as lactose intolerance. In fact, those who cannot digest milk, and who get all sorts of digestive problems when they drink it, are probably the lucky ones because they will avoid milk and all the problems it can cause. As we will see in Chapter 6, there is a great deal of evidence that milk contributes not just to cataracts but to diabetes, iron-deficiency anemia, and a surprising range of other health problems. Less fortunate are those people who can digest milk without any apparent symptoms. During digestion, their lactase enzymes break the lactose apart, releasing its load of galactose, which passes quietly into the bloodstream, contributing to problems that may not become evident until many years later. Ironically, commercial products are now sold for the purpose of aiding in the digestion of lactose. These do not reduce the galactose problem and, in fact, have the effect of increasing galactose exposure.

Investigators agree that milk sugar can contribute to cataracts—at the very least for those whose capacity to break down galactose is impaired. The problem is, we do not know who they are. We all lose some of this capacity as we leave our nursing years. Those who make dairy products a regular part of the diet are betting—or hoping—against the evidence.

Foods for Staying Young

So far, we have seen that foods can help protect us from free radicals. A menu of vegetables, fruits, grains, and beans provides beta-carotene, vitamins C and E, and selenium. Such a menu is very low in fat and contains no cholesterol at all. These foods not only help neutralize and eliminate free radicals as they form; they also actually reduce the production of free radicals by keeping fat and iron intake at appropriate levels and providing omega-3 fatty acids that are more stable than those in fish products. What were once thought of as modest foods are actually enormously powerful foods for health.

There is much more to this story than free radicals, however. Foods also affect hormones in both men and women, with very surprising effects.

FOODS AND HAIR RETENTION

Some men keep full heads of hair into their seventh and eighth decades. Others begin balding in their twenties. Until recently, men squinted at the slow recession of their hairlines, resigned to the idea that nothing could be done. Potions of all kinds, whether rubbed onto the scalp or swallowed, were all but useless. The march of time left a wide trail across the male scalp.

Several pieces of evidence might make men more optimistic. Studies have shown that while heredity is an important factor in baldness, it does not fully account for it. Within families, one male might have more aggressive loss of hair while others are spared somewhat. Also, certain drugs—most notably minoxidil—affect hair growth. Originally prescribed to reduce blood pressure, minoxidil has a limited ability to wake up dormant hair follicles, particularly at the crown. While most men get very little effect from it, some do see results and that, again, indicates that baldness is not only a matter of genetics.

If baldness is not just genetic, what else contributes to hair loss? It is caused by an interplay of heredity and hormones. Heredity, of course, is not within our control. But scientific evidence shows that the action of hormones on hair follicles may be affected by what we eat. There are hints that one's hairline may not be so easily eroded when dietary factors are on our side. First, let us look at how hormones affect hair loss. Then we will take a look at the role of foods in that process. Keep in mind that exploration in this area is far from finished, but a substantial amount is known right now.

In 1942, J. B. Hamilton published a series of observations that have been quoted by dermatologists ever since.[25] He had studied men who had had the misfortune to have their testes removed owing to medical problems. The reasons for the surgery varied, but Hamilton noted that, as the years went by, none of these men became bald. Even those whose family trees gleamed with bald heads never lost their hair. Later, many of these men received testosterone injections. The results were rapid: their hair fell out, and their baldness approached that of other male family members. If the testosterone injections were stopped, the baldness stopped advancing. And if the men came from families with little baldness, then the hormones did not cause much hair loss.

Hamilton's studies showed that testosterone is critical: without it, you won't go bald. Testosterone affects women, too. In families where baldness is common, women also carry the genetic capacity to become bald. They will usually not show it, because women have far less testosterone than men. But if enough male hormones find their way into a woman's bloodstream, either through medication, a hormone-producing tumor, or other abnormality, she can develop male-pattern baldness. (This is different from diffuse hair loss, which occasionally occurs in women and which should be evaluated by a dermatologist.)

In the hair follicle, testosterone is converted to a much more powerful hormone called dihydrotestosterone (DHT). Under the influence of DHT, normal hairs become thinner, then are replaced by tiny fine hairs, and eventually the follicles die off.[26,27] Those parts of the scalp affected in male-pattern baldness—the frontal hairline, the temples, and crown—are more sensitive to testosterone and are quicker to convert testosterone and its precursors into the more powerful DHT.[28,29]

DHT is a paradoxical hormone. It causes hair to grow on the face and chest. At the scalp, it makes hair fall out. Some speculate that baldness is nature's way of keeping the head cool, compensating for the beard's blanket effect on the face.[30] It is true that the area of skin denuded by baldness is about the same size as the beard area, but shaving off your beard will not slow your hairline's retreat.

While hormones are, in part, controlled by heredity,[31,32] they are also affected by the foods we eat. As is true in so many other health concerns, fingers are pointing to fatty diets. People on Western-style diets—that is, the pork chop and roast beef diets on which most of us in America were raised—have more testosterone in their blood than do people on lower-fat diets or vegetarian diets.[33–39]

Lest anyone think it is manly to eat foods that elevate testosterone levels, it has to be pointed out that the same foods also increase estrogen, the female sex hormone, in both men and women.[34,40] In addition, body fat actively converts testosterone into estrogen. As fatty diets add to one's girth, more and more estrogen is produced, which is why overweight men often have breast enlargement, as is evident on every beach in America. Obesity actually lowers the amount of testosterone in your body and increases estrogen. And foods affect hormones very quickly—within just a few weeks.[38,34]

None of this would matter much if testosterone were kept under control. But fatty diets do not just increase the amount of testosterone in the blood. They also reduce the amount of *sex hormone binding globulin,*[41] a protein whose job is to hold on to sex hormones and keep them inactive until needed. With less of this carrier protein in the bloodstream, more testosterone roams free, ready to enter the hair follicle.

Different people are affected by hormones differently. The amount of testosterone that will cause hair loss in one person may not have an effect in another. Can a boost in testosterone caused by foods lead to early or more aggressive baldness? Scientific studies so far give us only clues, but they do indicate that changes in hormone levels can affect how many hairs go down the bathtub drain.

For all of us, the amount of testosterone in the blood changes seasonally. It is lowest in the spring and peaks in the fall.[42-45] And during the springtime lull in testosterone levels, hair growth is maximal. As hormone levels rise toward fall, there is substantial hair loss, averaging about sixty hairs per day—more than double the rate at which hairs fall out in the spring. The annual cycle is apparently similar in men and women.[46]

This seasonal variation has had an interesting effect on hair research. Dutch researchers recently tested a Chinese herbal extract, dabao, for its ability to promote hair growth. The research subjects began using the herbal treatment in September and, as spring approached, they reported a significant increase in hair growth. The investigators also tested a placebo, and found that it, too, helped hair grow.[47] The problem was that hair always grows more as spring approaches. (Even so, dabao did show somewhat more effect than did the placebo.)

Nature's hormone peak every fall causes a transient thinning of the hair. But people on meaty Western diets have a sustained hormone elevation of about the same magnitude[34,39] as the autumn hormone peak, perhaps causing a year-round tendency toward hair loss.

What is important in baldness is not the amount of hormones in the blood,[48] but the amount in the hair follicle itself. In balding areas of the scalp, the oil glands in the hair follicle are larger.[29] These oil glands hold the enzyme machinery that converts testosterone into DHT.

In 1985, a Japanese researcher, Masumi Inaba, published a novel theory. He noted that, as diets in Japan become more like diets in the West, with rice being replaced by burgers and roast beef, the Japanese are experiencing an increasing incidence of baldness.[49] He hypothesized that the increased intake of animal fat causes the oil glands in the hair follicles to grow in size. The result, Inaba wrote, is accelerated production of DHT and more rapid damage to the follicle in genetically prone parts of the scalp. It is also known that higher amounts of circulating hormones, which occur in higher-fat diets, can increase the activity of these glands.

Blood tests have shown that American men have significantly more of the enzyme that converts testosterone to DHT, compared to Chinese men, and correspondingly more body hair and scalp baldness.[50] Although these differences are almost certainly influenced by genetics, dietary factors may play a part as to how soon and how aggressively the effects occur.

Researchers have also found that men who have high cholesterol levels or heart problems are more likely to be bald, compared to healthy men.[51] It could well be that the same diet that contributes to heart problems aggravates a tendency toward baldness.

If there is an effect of diet, a reasonable guess is that it might delay hair loss but not prevent it forever in genetically prone individuals. In other words, if nature calls you to start balding at twenty-five, you will eventually lose your hair no matter what you do, but with the proper diet you might not begin balding until years later.

It will take a long research study to test whether food choices can minimize the effect of testosterone and DHT on the follicle, and spare hair growth as young men pass into their thirties and forties. Such a study has not been done yet. But the diet that should be tested is one that eliminates animal fat, keeps vegetable fats to a minimum, and boosts antioxidant vitamins and fiber. This is the same dietary prescription to keep cholesterol levels and cancer risk at their lowest.

Coincidentally, my mother noted some time ago that, of her four sons, I was the only one who showed no perceptible thinning of hair. At the time, I was the only one who had abandoned the typical Western menu on which we all had grown up in Fargo, North Dakota. In fact, thinning of my hair did eventually begin but not until about a decade later than my brothers. Does diet get the credit? Only research will tell, but I suspect so.

Keeping Strong Bones

Part of youthfulness is straight posture and resilience in the limbs and spine. If, on the other hand, bone tissue wastes away, hips and wrists become fragile, and the spine bows into a stooped appearance. This bone loss is called *osteoporosis,* and is particularly common in women after menopause.

Some populations have less osteoporosis than others. Changes in diet and life-style may help prevent it, although the foods that are effective may not be the ones you would expect.

The dairy industry has used osteoporosis as a marketing tool, but milk does not seem to be the answer. In countries where dairy products are commonly consumed, there are actually *more* hip fractures than in other countries. When put to the test, most studies show that dairy products have little effect on osteoporosis.[52] As surprising as that may be, when researchers have measured bone loss in postmenopausal women, most have found that calcium intake has little effect on the bone density of the spine. There is also little or no effect on bone at the hip, where very serious breaks can occur. Some studies have found a small effect from calcium intake on bone density in the forearm.[53] The overall message seems to be that, as long as you are not grossly deficient in calcium, supplements and dairy products do not have much effect. *Science* magazine (August 1, 1986) noted "the large body of evidence indicating no relationship between calcium intake and bone density."[54]

Why not? For one thing, the amount of calcium in the bones is very carefully regulated by hormones. Increasing your calcium intake does not fool these hormones into building more bone, any more than delivering an extra load of bricks will make a construction crew build a larger building.

If milk, or calcium intake in general, is not a good hedge against bone loss after menopause, how about before menopause? That, too, seems to follow the pattern. Researchers in Madison, Wisconsin, compared the diets of 300 premenopausal women aged twenty to thirty-nine and measured their bone density. Calcium had no measurable effect on bone density. Very low calcium intakes would probably lead to deficient bone formation, but calcium intake spanning the normal dietary range made no difference: high-calcium diets led to no stronger bones than the lower calcium diets.[55]

Milk does contain calcium. But milk neither assures strong bones in childhood nor does it protect bones in adulthood. For the vast majority of people, the answer is not boosting calcium intake but, rather, limiting calcium loss. As surprising as it sounds, one major culprit in osteoporosis may be protein. Diets that are high in protein, especially animal protein, cause more calcium to be excreted.[55A, 55B] When volunteers eat high-protein meals, they lose calcium in their urine. If they consume more modest amounts of protein, they lose much less calcium in their urine. What is apparently happening is this: Amino acids, which are the building blocks of proteins, cause the blood to become slightly more acidic. To neutralize this acidic effect, bone material is dissolved, which is believed to lead to the loss of calcium in the urine.

The problem is not just the quantity of protein consumed but also the type of protein. Meats are high in a type of protein building block called *sulfur-containing amino acids.* These are particularly likely to aggravate calcium loss. Meats also contain large quantities of phosphorus, which can impair calcium balance.[56] Although the role of phosphorus in osteoporosis is far from clear, scientists believe that diets in which phosphorus and calcium intake are roughly equal help keep calcium in the body, while diets in which the two are unbalanced are thought to harm calcium balance. Beef has a high phosphorus-to-calcium ratio, about 15:1. Chicken breast is similar, about 14:1. For comparison, vegetables have calcium and phosphorus in much better balance. Carrots have a ratio of about 1.7:1, a peach is about 2:1. Boiled broccoli has a phosphorus-to-calcium ratio of about 0.4:1.

Green leafy vegetables provide generous amounts of calcium without the animal protein of meaty diets. In fact, green vegetables such as broccoli, collard greens, and kale are loaded with calcium. A recent report in the *American Journal of Clinical Nutrition* found that calcium absorbability was actually higher for kale than for milk and concluded, "greens such as kale can be considered to be at least as good as milk in terms of their calcium absorbability."[57] One cup (8 fluid ounces) of milk contains 291 mg of calcium. That is a substantial amount. But only about 30 percent of it is absorbed, and that glass of milk also contains 8 grams of animal protein to encourage the loss of calcium. Green vegetables, beans, and enriched flour are rich in calcium, and fortified orange juice supplies substantial amounts of calcium.[58] Table 2 shows the calcium content of many common foods.

Fruits and vegetables also provide boron, an element which appears to be important in preventing the loss of calcium, according to Dr. Forrest H. Nielsen, a research nutritionist with the U.S. Department of Agriculture. The best way to get boron, according to Dr. Nielsen, is through a balanced diet containing an abundance of fruits, vegetables, nuts, and legumes. Wines also contain appreciable amounts of the element. Animal products, including milk, have little or no boron. No one yet knows how much boron the body actually needs, but Table 3 on page 23 shows what foods are rich sources of boron.

Hormones play a major role in bone structure. After menopause, bone loss is often aggressive, and as a result, doctors often prescribe hormone replacements. Such treatments are effective in delaying osteoporosis, although their overall health risk remains controversial. Exercise is also important.[55,59] If bones are not being used, they have little reason to preserve their strength. In addition, alcohol and tobacco aggravate bone loss.[53,55]

Although the calcium craze has been founded largely on myth, this does not mean that the body does not need calcium. If you really are consuming very little calcium—say, below 500 mg per day—you may run into trouble.[60,55] However, it is very easy to meet your calcium needs. The sample menu below shows how easy it is to get a day's supply of calcium.

If you choose to supplement, calcium-fortified orange juice has an advantage over milk in that it contains no animal protein and is a form of calcium that is more easily absorbed than that in calcium carbonate supplements.[58] When replacement hormones are used, calcium supplements have been shown to be a helpful adjunct in slowing bone loss.

A Day's Supply of Calcium

Breakfast:

Pancakes (3 medium)	140 mg
1 orange (1 medium)	56 mg

Lunch:

Campbell's Lentil Soup (1⅓ cups)	54 mg
Salad of romaine lettuce (1 cup) and ½ tomato	24 mg
English muffin (1 muffin)	92 mg

Dinner:

Vegetarian baked beans (1 cup)	128 mg
Broccoli (1 cup, cooked)	178 mg
Cornbread (2-ounce piece)	133 mg
Total Calcium	805 mg

Table 2 *Calcium in Foods*

. . . .

	Calcium (mg)
Vegetables	
Broccoli (1 cup, boiled)	178
Brussels sprouts (8 sprouts)	56
Carrots (2 medium)	38
Cauliflower (1 cup, boiled)	34
Celery (1 cup, boiled)	54
Collards (1 cup, boiled)	148
Kale (1 cup, boiled)	94
Onions (1 cup, boiled)	58
Potato, baked (1 medium)	20
Romaine lettuce (1 cup)	20
Squash, butternut (1 cup, boiled)	84
Sweet potato (1 cup, boiled)	70
Legumes	
Chickpeas (1 cup, canned)	78
Great northern beans (1 cup, boiled)	121
Green beans (1 cup, boiled)	58
Kidney beans (1 cup, boiled)	50
Lentils (1 cup, boiled)	37
Lima beans (1 cup, boiled)	52
Navy beans (1 cup, boiled)	128
Peas, green (1 cup, boiled)	44
Pinto beans (1 cup, boiled)	82
Soybeans (1 cup, boiled)	175
Turtle beans, black (1 cup, boiled)	103
Tofu (½ cup)	258
Vegetarian baked beans (1 cup)	128
Wax beans (1 cup, canned)	174
White beans (1 cup, boiled)	161
Grains	
Brown rice (cooked, 1 cup)	23
Corn bread (1 2-ounce piece)	133
Corn tortilla (1 medium)	42
English muffin (1 medium)	92

	Calcium (mg)
Pancake mix (¼ cup, 3 pancakes)	140
Pita bread (1 piece)	31
Wheat bread (1 slice)	30
Wheat flour, all-purpose (1 cup)	22
Wheat flour, calcium-enriched* (1 cup)	238
Whole wheat flour (1 cup)	49

Fruits

Apple (1 medium)	10
Banana (1 medium)	7
Figs, dried (10 medium)	269
Orange, navel (1 medium)	56
Orange juice, calcium-fortified (1 cup)	300**
Pear (1 medium)	19
Raisins (⅔ cup)	53

. . . .

Source: J. A. T. Pennington, *Bowes and Church's Food Values of Portions Commonly Used* (New York: Harper and Row, 1989).
*Pillsbury's Best brand
**Package information

Table 3   *The Boron All-Stars*
. . . .
(mg per 100 ml fluid or 100 mg dry weight)

Applesauce	.279	Grape juice	.202
Broccoli stalks	.089	Green beans	.046
Broccoli tops	.185	Orange juice	.041
Carrots	.075	Peaches	.187
Cherries	.147	Pears	.122

. . . .

Source: J. McBride, "Banishing Brittle Bones With Boron?," *Agricultural Research* (Nov.–Dec.), 1987, 35(10), p. 13.

HEALTHY KIDNEY FUNCTION

High protein intakes have been found to contribute to progressive kidney damage. The kidneys are the bloodstream's filter, and high-protein diets push the kidneys to work extra hard. Protein breaks down in the body to amino acids and then to urea, both of which cause the kidneys to excrete more water. Thus, a high-protein diet raises the fluid pressure in the nephrons, which are the filter units of the kidney. The result is progressive destruction of kidney tissue.

Researchers have suggested that the human kidney may not be able to cope with frequent, large protein loads. Early humans ate meat rarely, if at all, and so they did not generally have to deal with large amounts of protein. With the current daily high intake of protein, though, the kidneys are called upon to constantly overwork in an effort to rid the body of the by-products from the breakdown of protein.[61]

This is of particular concern for people who have a history of kidney infections or other kidney problems. But evidence suggests that excessive protein also causes a gradual decline in kidney function for those who are otherwise healthy, while lower protein intake helps preserve kidney function.[61-64] Already, physicians recommend protein restrictions for people who have lost some kidney function, but that is good advice for everyone else as well.

The average American diet contains far more protein than anyone needs. The reason is that meats, poultry, and fish are simply combinations of protein and fat. They contain virtually no carbohydrates and no fiber. It is difficult to include these foods in the diet without the protein content climbing rapidly. And as problems of osteoporosis and kidney disease indicate, it is important not to overdo your intake of protein.

Food to Stretch Your Lifespan

Average years of life have not been dealt out fairly. A mouse gets only two years. A dog lives about a dozen years, or as long as eighteen in some exceptional cases. On the other hand, a turtle can easily outlive a human.

Human life expectancy in America is now about seventy-five years. This is an average, and includes not only those who live a full lifespan but also those who die in childhood or early adulthood. For people who have already cleared enough hurdles to make it to fifty, the average lifespan is longer— about seventy-nine.

Women live longer than men, and lifespan is not currently the same for all races. African-Americans have a shorter life expectancy than whites, in part owing to higher rates of cardiovascular disease, stroke, and cancer. And the gap in mortality figures between African-Americans and Caucasians is widening. Yet neither African-Americans nor Caucasians in America live as long as most Asians.

The good news is that our bodies do not carry an expiration date. Lifespan can be altered. The foods we chose for breakfast, lunch, and dinner can not only help keep us free from life-threatening illnesses but can affect a more basic part of our body's timetable. For instance, diet influences how fast children grow up and the age at which they reach puberty. Diet also influences the speed with which we race toward maturity, and may, in turn, influence how quickly the whole race ends.

Growing Up Slower

A puppy reaches maturity in a matter of months, much earlier than a human baby. But growing up quickly may not be such a blessing. The slowly maturing human child will far outlive his or her canine companion.

During my medical education I worked for a time at an inner-city clinic in Washington, D.C. There, girls of twelve and thirteen often came in asking for birth control pills. Many had already given birth to their first child. Some had been sent in by their mothers, who did not want them to become pregnant again. I wondered why nature was so cruel as to design the human body to become sexually mature at an age when a boy or girl is not old enough to care for a child or even to sustain a long-term relationship.

Well, perhaps nature was not to blame. Evidence suggests that the body is designed to reach puberty much later. The World Health Organization has for many years gathered statistics on the age of puberty worldwide. In 1840, the average age of puberty in girls in Western countries was not 12.5 years of age, as it is today; it was 17. The age of puberty has been measured in the United States, England, Norway, Denmark, Finland, and other Western countries, where it has slowly but surely been dropping in every instance.[65]

Researchers have gathered much more information on girls than boys because the onset of menstruation is much easier to pinpoint in time than is any biological change in boys. Nonetheless, there are suggestions that boys are maturing earlier, too. Researchers in England have observed that it is harder to fit children on bus seats than it was a generation ago, and, in fact, recent measurements showed that the average thirteen-year-old English boy is about two inches wider across the shoulders than in the 1950s.[66] It is believed that the difference is not the adult size they will reach, but the speed with which they will reach it. Other researchers have found that both boys and girls in Norway are reaching physical maturity earlier than they were in the 1920s.[67]

The most likely explanation has to do with diet. Puberty in girls depends on female sex hormones called estrogens, of which the principal one is *estradiol.* The level of estrogens in the blood is affected by the foods we eat. The customary Western diet of meat, poultry, dairy products, and fried foods increases the quantity of estrogens in the blood.[68,69,70] The results are seen in the accelerated pace of puberty and in the likelihood of cancer in organs that are sensitive to sex hormones, as we will see in Chapter 3.

What part of the diet is to blame? It may be the large amount of fat we tend to eat. About 37 percent of our calories come from fat. That is much higher than it was in the 1800s, when high-fat diets were limited to a small, wealthy portion of the population. But the low age of puberty may also be due to something that is missing. Grains, vegetables, fruits, and beans have lots of fiber, but when they are displaced by high-fat foods, the fiber content of the diet is reduced.

One way the body rids itself of estradiol is through digestion. The liver pulls estradiol from the blood, chemically alters it, and sends it down the bile ducts into the intestinal tract. There, the fiber from grains, vegetables, fruits, and beans escorts excess estrogens through the intestine and finally out the door as waste. At least that is how the system is supposed to work. But chicken breasts, beef, eggs, cheese, and all other animal products contain not even a scrap of fiber. As these products have assumed a larger and larger portion of the American plate, they have pushed off the grains, vegetables, beans, and fruits. Without adequate fiber to hold them in the digestive tract, estrogens are reabsorbed into the bloodstream, where they once again become biologically active. Recycling programs are a great thing for bottles and newspapers. But recycling hormones adds to human problems, apparently contributing to a lower age of puberty.

If a woman changes her diet to favor grains and vegetables, her estradiol level drops noticeably in short order. For instance, if you were to measure the amount of estradiol in the blood of vegetarians, it would be less than in meat-eaters. But this is just the beginning of the story, because what is important is not just the level of estradiol in the blood but also whether it can affect the reproductive organs. Estradiol, like testosterone, is carried around in the bloodstream on the special carrier protein, *sex hormone binding globulin*, whose job is to keep the hormone inactive until it is needed. Vegetarians have less estradiol to start with, and they also produce *more* of this carrier molecule. So more of their estradiol simply waits politely on its carrier protein rather than jumping in and directing the development of the breasts and other organs at inappropriate times.[71] Precisely the same thing happens with testosterone in males.

Certain foods have special effects. The soybean, for example, is a mainstay of Asian diets. It is sprouted, or steamed and eaten right out of the pod. It is turned into tofu and tempeh, and also into simulated hot dogs, burgers, and cold cuts, not only in Osaka and Tokyo, but also in Asian groceries and natural foods stores in America. Soybeans contain natural chemicals called *phytoestrogens*. These are very weak estrogens that can compete with and blunt the effect of normal estrogens. Estrogens attach to special receptors on the cells of the breasts and reproductive organs, like boats docking at a port. But if all the "docks" have been taken by phytoestrogens, there is nowhere for the estrogen to attach, and it will not affect its target organ. When the diet is rich in soybeans or soy products, phytoestrogens moderate the effect of estrogens.

If a change in diet is responsible for the drop in the age of puberty, then we would expect that, in countries that still follow a predominantly vegetable diet, puberty would occur at a later age. The Chinese diet, for example, is centered on rice and vegetables, with little meat and virtually no dairy products. I recently asked Dr. T. Colin Campbell, a biochemist at Cornell University who directs the massive China Health Study, about the age of puberty there. His findings confirm the theory. In China, puberty in girls occurs at an average age of about seventeen, ranging between fifteen and nineteen. And they not only have a higher age of puberty but also enjoy phenomenally low rates of heart disease, obesity, and cancer. In Japan, Westernization of the Japanese diet has been accompanied by a drop in the age of puberty in girls from 15.2 to 12.5 in the past four decades.[72]

Dr. Denis Burkitt, the surgeon whose research discoveries established the value of fiber in the diet, confirmed this in his years of research in Africa.

In rural African villages, the average age of puberty in girls is seventeen. In Johannesburg, it is thirteen, and the chief suspect is the Westernized diet in the urban setting.[73]

Further confirmation comes from the Netherlands, in a recent study involving sixty-three girls. Researchers recorded the amount of grains, vegetables, and other foods the girls ate. They took blood samples so that hormones could be measured, and they noted the age at which puberty began. Again, the results were unequivocal. The girls who ate more vegetables and grains had a later age of puberty. Those who ate less of these foods had more estradiol coursing through their veins, and, not surprisingly, an earlier onset of puberty.[74] The Dutch researchers also noted that, while they saw a definite effect of different vegetable intakes in the girls they studied, none ate nearly the amount of fiber that vegetarians do. The Dutch girls who ate the most vegetables still only got about 20 grams of fiber per day, while typical vegetarians average about 30.[70] So the rather subtle differences in diet between the girls in the Dutch study did affect the age of puberty, but not to the extent that a vegetarian diet would be expected to.

Not long ago, after a college lecture I gave on this subject, a woman from the audience told me that she had always wondered why she and her sister, who had grown up in Asia, had reached puberty in their mid-teens while their youngest sister, who had been raised in the United States, reached puberty at nine. In the third sister's case, the rice-based Asian diet had been abandoned for roast chicken and fried foods.

In addition to diet itself, there is also the questionable effect of ingesting hormones from other sources. Many people remember news stories about children in Puerto Rico reaching puberty at age four or five because of hormones fed to chickens to make them grow more quickly. Hormones are routinely used in the United States, too. If you were to look behind the ears of cattle raised on America's farms, you would find a small implant about the size of the end of a sharp pencil. The implant contains hormones that are used to make cattle grow faster. Ranchers actually use five different hormones. Three occur in the body normally: estradiol, testosterone, and progesterone. Two are synthetic: trenbolone acetate, which is a synthetic testosterone; and zeranol, which is a synthetic estrogen. In 1989, the European Economic Community banned imports of U.S. beef from cattle given hormones. But American farmers use these hormones routinely, contending that, while the hormones affect the animals, they are not concentrated enough in animal products to affect your health.

The effect of the hormone implants is probably minor compared to the effect of the beef itself in your body. Even the most chemical-free meats have enough fat in them to cause your hormone levels to rise measurably. Coupled with the fact that meats have no fiber, and actually displace fiber-rich foods from the plate, they give a predictable and unnatural boost to hormones.

It is sad to think of children of ten or eleven trying to make sense of breast development and the onset of periods, when nature almost certainly did not intend reproductive maturity so far in advance of psychological maturity. Think how different the adjustment to sexual maturity would be if children had four or five more years to anticipate it.

LONGER LIFE THROUGH BETTER EATING

The effects of diet do not start at puberty. Food choices exert noticeable effects much earlier, even in the toddler years. Vegetarian children may, in some cases, grow up a bit more gradually. At first, researchers worried that these children might be growing too slowly. But it turned out that they reach essentially the same height as other children do, but slightly later. A vegetarian diet in effect extends each phase of life. Children grow up more gradually, reach puberty later, are much less likely to die of heart disease or cancer in mid-life, and overall live years longer than people raised on typical Western diets. The standard American diet has an effect reminiscent of anabolic steroids. Athletes who inject steroids have overly rapid growth and an early onset of atherosclerotic heart disease ("hardening of the arteries").

But if we live years longer, what will we die of? Personally, I plan to die at age 120, while racing in the Monte Carlo Grand Prix. People who maintain healthful life-styles do not just add years to their lives. They also often avoid disease and the protracted decline of function that accompany cancer, stroke, diabetes, or obesity. Chances are, they aren't just trading their "golden years" for "Medicare years," or wasting their time shuttling between the doctor's office and the prescription counter.

If you thought living longer means a longer period of illness or disability in old age, think again. Dr. Robert Kohn, of Case Western Reserve University, examined the cause of death of people who died at a very old age, eighty-five and later. He found that many had no identifiable cause of death. So far as anyone could tell, they had no illness, no particular infirmity. They just eventually died "of old age."[75] So adding years to life need not mean years of infirmity. And when the end of life finally comes, it can be without the protracted misery that marks the last chapter of so many people's lives.

There is little doubt that the best diet is based on grains, vegetables, fruits, and beans. "Now some people scoff at vegetarians," says Dr. William Castelli, director of the Framingham Heart Study, "but they have a fraction of our heart attack rate and they have only 40 percent of our cancer rate. They outlive us. On the average they outlive other men by about six years now. And they outlive other women by about three years. The average age of death of a vegetarian woman is already up in the eighties, well ahead of where other women die."

Most people are not aware that they have any control over the effects of time on their bodies. But the best scientific evidence shows that you don't necessarily have to develop wrinkles at the corners of your eyes and across your forehead—or at least not so soon. You can keep strong bones and maybe keep your hairline a while longer, too. And as we will see in the next few chapters, you can also have a trim waistline, a teenager's cholesterol level, and much more control over your own health, once you know how to go about it. Time will play some of its dirty tricks on us no matter what we do. But the new way of eating you are about to begin has tremendous power to shield you from damage that would otherwise age your body prematurely.

2

Preventing and Reversing Heart Disease

Fort Mason is a group of buildings next to San Francisco's Golden Gate Bridge. I entered Building F at the appointed time, and was offered a seat in a circle of chairs. The other participants were heart patients, and they were palpably excited. The chest pain that had meted out increasing punishment to them over the years had given them a reprieve. Like prisoners freed from captivity, they were now doing all sorts of things they had thought they could never do again. These patients had all suffered from significant heart disease. And they got better, not with surgery but with an effective program of life-style changes.

In the not-so-distant past, doctors felt that little could be done to slow the progression of heart disease. That idea has been exploded by new scientific research. Not only do we have powerful new approaches to preventing heart disease, we also have ways to reverse it—to make even advanced disease go away without drugs or surgery, as Dr. Dean Ornish's patients made very clear.

Cholesterol is as important a factor as we ever thought, but we know that there is a cholesterol threshold below which heart disease is very rare, and it is not the 200 value that is frequently quoted. Emerging research also shows that iron, long thought to be a purely healthful nutrient, can act as a co-conspirator with cholesterol in the poisoning of the heart.

On the other hand, we have better defenses than ever. New heart protectors—natural constituents of vegetables and fruits—can add a layer of defense. And oat bran is not the only game in town; many foods provide soluble fiber that can drive cholesterol levels down.

This chapter covers all these areas, including the dramatically effective new program used for its reversal. And in terms of prevention, the prescrip-

31

tion in this book is much stronger than that offered by federal guidelines or most other cholesterol-lowering programs. The reason is simple: If you want to reduce your risk of a heart attack, and especially if your goal is to reverse existing heart disease, those programs are simply too weak. As we see in this chapter, there are stronger approaches with scientifically proven effectiveness.

But first, what exactly is heart disease?

The Assault on the Heart

Common heart disease, or *atherosclerosis,* is a disease of arteries. The coronary arteries are perhaps the most important arteries in the body because they carry blood to the heart muscle itself. The name *coronary* comes from the fact that they ring the heart like a crown.

When a person experiences the chest pain of heart disease, the heart muscle is not getting enough oxygen. Something in the coronary arteries is stopping the flow of blood to the heart. If you could look into the artery, you would see a raised bump, called a *plaque.* It impedes the flow through the artery, just as a wad of gum stuck on the inside of a pipe would slow the flow of water.

Plaques are composed of cholesterol, fat, debris, and accumulating cells growing from the muscle layer that sheathes the artery. As plaques gradually grow, the passageway for blood becomes more narrow. When the heart is taxed by exercise or excitement, chest pain *(angina)* occurs. When the blood supply is completely blocked, part of the heart muscle dies. This is called a heart attack or, in technical terms, a *myocardial infarction.* Doctors often must treat blocked arteries surgically, with plaque-crunching angioplasty or a coronary bypass, in which arteries or veins from another part of the body are transplanted onto the heart.

We do not have just one plaque forming in our arteries. Starting in childhood, this sequence of events takes place in major arteries throughout the body. This is not a normal part of life, however. Postmortem examinations of American soldiers in the Korean and Vietnam wars showed that, while atherosclerosis had already started in these young men, their Asian counterparts did not have atherosclerosis.

Researchers set about to learn how to prevent plaques from forming and, more recently, how to make them go away. Before long, it became clear that certain characteristics help doctors predict who is going to have a heart attack and who is not. High cholesterol levels, smoking, high blood pressure, and a sedentary life-style are the best-known risk factors. In addition, your risk of heart disease is increased by diabetes, obesity, a family history of heart disease, stress, and the "Type A" personality (a need to excel, bossiness, and impatience). In addition, if your body contains too much stored iron, or your diet is low in vitamin-rich vegetables and fruits, you run an increased risk because of the free-radical damage they encourage.

DIFFERENT TYPES OF CHOLESTEROL

If you had a bit of cholesterol on the end of your finger, it would look like wax. Cholesterol is not the same as fat. It is a specialized substance made in the livers of all animals, including the human animal, for use as a biological raw material. It is used to make cell membranes and hormones, among other functions.

Cholesterol is a dangerous substance. It contributes to the deaths of half the people in America and Europe. In a sense, cholesterol is like petroleum. Petroleum is a raw material that can be used for many purposes, but a tanker full of spilled petroleum, combined with a lit match, can be deadly. So petroleum must be very carefully contained and transported.

The body has its own oil industry, as it were. The liver manufactures cholesterol and sends it out to be used in the manufacture of hormones and cell membranes and other important parts of the body. When cholesterol is transported in the bloodstream, it is packed into special containers called *low-density lipoproteins* (LDL) and *very low density lipoproteins* (VLDL). LDL is sometimes called the "bad cholesterol" because, although it is necessary in limited quantities, a high LDL cholesterol level can dramatically increase your risk of a heart attack.

LDL delivers cholesterol to various parts of the body. When cholesterol is released from dead cells, it is picked up for disposal in another kind of package called *high-density lipoprotein* (HDL), the "good cholesterol." The more HDL you have, the lower your risk of a heart attack. Cholesterol levels are usually measured in milligrams of cholesterol per deciliter (mg/dl) of blood serum.

Cholesterol: The 150 Goal

If there were suddenly a huge influx of oil trucks coming from Canada or Mexico, statisticians could calculate how the risk of a deadly accident increases. The more oil trucks there are on the turnpike, the more likely a spill is to occur. The same is true of cholesterol. The more you have in your blood, the more likely you are to have a heart attack.

For four decades, the Framingham Heart Study has studied who gets heart attacks and who does not. Framingham is a small town outside Boston, which is like any other New England town except that it is a short drive from the Boston area universities. So its population has been studied by researchers for most of this century. If you had set up shop with these researchers, you would have seen something remarkable. For an entire year of the study, no one with a total cholesterol level below 150 mg/dl had a heart attack. The same thing happened the next year: not a single person whose cholesterol level was below 150 had a heart attack. And this continued the next year and the next. No one thought much about it at first. But after thirty-five years went by and no one whose cholesterol stayed below the 150 threshold ever had a heart attack, it began to seem pretty remarkable.

In many studies, researchers have found that higher levels of cholesterol are linked to higher risk. In fact, for every 1 percent increase in the amount of cholesterol in your blood, your risk of a heart attack rises by about 2 percent. That means that if your cholesterol were to go up 20 percent—say, from 200 mg/dl to 240 mg/dl—your risk of a heart attack would rise by 40 percent.[1]

Happily, it's a two-way street. If you lower your cholesterol, you get a two-for-one *improvement* in your risk. So if you lower your cholesterol level by 20 percent—say, from 200 down to 160—your risk goes down by 40 percent.

As your cholesterol level approaches 150, there is no statistical benefit to going lower. "We think there is a threshold in cholesterol, and that it's 150," says Dr. William Castelli, director of the Framingham Heart Study. "We've never had a heart attack in Framingham in thirty-five years in anyone who had a cholesterol under 150." The ideal level, then, is below 150 mg/dl. At that point, heart attack is not impossible, but is very unlikely.

You might be asking, if 150 is the threshold, why do we hear that 200 is a desirable cholesterol level? The National Cholesterol Education Program set 200 as an arbitrary goal: levels below 200 mg/dl are called "desirable." For higher levels, increasing degrees of medical scrutiny are indicated, and people with lower levels receive a measure of reassurance. Unfortunately, a lot of people whose cholesterol levels are 190 or 200 go on to have heart attacks. A level of 180 is better, and 170 better still, and so on until you reach about 150.

We know that 200 is not an ideal cholesterol level. In fact, it is quite close to the national average cholesterol level of 205. In a country where half the people die of heart disease, being near the average is not such a great thing. So why was 200 used as a goal? Because it was easy to reach. For most people, it is not difficult to lower the cholesterol level to 200. Unfortunately, setting the "desirable" level at 200 falsely suggested to people with cholesterol levels of 190 or 180 that there was nothing to worry about.

When doctors measure cholesterol levels, they first look at your *total* cholesterol level because it is a good, quick guide to your risk. Then, for a more exact guide, they divide your total cholesterol by your HDL level because they know that the lower your total cholesterol, the better and the higher your HDL ("good cholesterol") the better. The ratio of total cholesterol to HDL should, ideally, be about 3.0 to 1. Most Americans, unfortunately, are nowhere near that level. The average American male's ratio is 5.1 to 1. A recent study showed that Boston Marathon runners have an average ratio of 3.5 to 1. Vegetarians do the best, averaging about 2.9 to 1.[2] Smoking and obesity appear to lower HDL, but HDL can be raised somewhat by vigorous exercise and vitamin C-rich foods.[3]

TRIGLYCERIDES

Triglyceride is simply a technical term for the type of fat the body stores. From the various foods we eat, triglyceride molecules are assembled in the liver, packed into VLDL, and sent via the bloodstream to your thighs and hips and abdominal fat areas, where they wait until they are needed. Sometimes, of course, they wait a very long time.

Triglyceride levels above 200 mg/dl are generally considered to be elevated. But let your doctor interpret this level in light of your other cholesterol measurements. Some studies have linked high triglyceride levels to increased risk of heart disease, but some researchers believe that this only applies to those who also have high cholesterol levels.

People who follow low-fat, high-carbohydrate diets tend to have very low cholesterol levels and a low risk of heart disease. But their triglyceride levels rise somewhat, which has puzzled some doctors. What is happening is that some of the carbohydrate in the diet is simply being converted to triglycerides for transport and storage in the body. This is normal, and apparently not related to heart disease.[4]

On the other hand, levels that are extremely high (greater than 1,000 mg/dl) can spell real trouble, particularly inflammation of the pancreas, and medical treatment is necessary.

How to Lower Your Cholesterol

Most people can lower their cholesterol levels quite dramatically. Do not be discouraged if the American Heart Association diet or a similar chicken-and-fish diet did not do much for you. These are very weak programs. Many people falsely conclude that they cannot lower their cholesterol levels because the diet they tried had little effect. Let's try a more powerful program.

There are foods that are valuable allies, which you will want to include in your regular menu. There are others that you will want to avoid. First, the problem foods.

Animal Products: Cholesterol and Fat

Animal products contain two ingredients that drive your cholesterol level up: cholesterol itself and saturated fat. They have other serious problems, too, including too much iron and an absence of fiber and antioxidant vitamins. First, let's look at cholesterol.

Cholesterol is something animals produce in their bodies, and *all animal products contain cholesterol.* If you eat part of an animal or a glandular secretion like milk, you will get a dose of cholesterol. In turn, this will increase the amount of cholesterol in your blood. Every 100 mg of cholesterol you eat in your daily routine adds roughly five points to your cholesterol level. (Everyone is different, and this number is an average.) In practical terms, 100 mg of cholesterol is four ounces of beef, or four ounces of chicken, or half an egg, or three cups of milk.

It may surprise you to read that chicken has the same cholesterol content as beef. It does—about 25 mg per ounce.[5] Chicken is not a health food. It has received an undeservedly good reputation because it can be somewhat lower in fat than beef, depending on how it is prepared. But cholesterol is primarily in the *lean* portion of meats. There is a relationship between cholesterol and fat, as we shall see, but *cholesterol and fat are not the same thing.*

All fish products contain significant amounts of cholesterol, too. Shellfish, such as shrimp, lobster, or crayfish, are higher in cholesterol, ounce for ounce, than beef. But the point to remember is that all animal tissues contain cholesterol.

Eggs are packed with cholesterol. A single egg contains 213 mg, entirely in the yolk. That is a huge load, the most concentrated cholesterol in any common food.

Some people may believe that, since our bodies use cholesterol, we need it in our diet. Wrong. Our bodies make plenty of cholesterol for our needs, and we do not need to add any. And when we do, the cholesterol is left where it does not belong—in plaques in our arteries. There is no "good cholesterol" as far as foods are concerned. Simply put, cholesterol in food raises your cholesterol level. Animal products are the only source of cholesterol in the American diet.

But saturated fat is even worse. *Saturated* is a chemical term that means the fat molecule is completely covered with hydrogen atoms. If it is not, it is called *unsaturated*. If there is room for just one pair of hydrogen atoms to add on, it is called *monounsaturated*. And if there is room for more than one hydrogen atom, it is called *polyunsaturated*. Saturated fats stimulate your liver to make more cholesterol, while unsaturated fats do not.

Luckily, saturated fats are easy to spot because they are solid at room temperature, unlike unsaturated varieties, which are liquid. Beef, chicken, and most other animal products contain substantial amounts of saturated fat. Getting animal fat out of the diet has a dramatic effect on cholesterol levels. But do not get the idea that trimming the strip of fat off the outside of a cut of meat will eliminate the animal fat. Meats have fat not only on the outer edge but also marbled throughout the lean part. In the leanest cuts of beef, about 30 percent of the calories are from fat. In the leanest chicken, the figure is about 20 percent. Both of these are far higher than grains, beans, vegetables, and fruits, which are comfortably below 10 percent.

Unfortunately, the food industry has not been entirely honest in presenting its products, and consumers have not gotten much help in deciding what to buy. McDonald's, for example, trumpeted the arrival of the McLean

Deluxe Burger, claiming that it was 91 percent fat-free. McDonald's was reporting the fat content *by weight*. But when dietitians or scientists measure the fat content of foods, they are not interested in the percentage by weight because water content can throw off the measurements. For example, whole milk is only 3.3 percent fat by weight because most of it is water. But if you were to separate out the water, as the body does in the process of digestion, and see what you were left with, fully 49 percent of milk's calories come from fat. That is the number dietitians care about.

As a percentage of calories, regular ground beef is 60 percent fat. Extra-lean ground beef is 54 percent. If you were to analyze the fat content of the McLean Deluxe burger patty by percentage of calories, you would find that it is 49 percent fat. This is not surprising because the burger's main ingredient is—you guessed it—ground beef. The bun and toppings dilute it down to 29 percent fat, but the 9 percent figure is a McFib.

Likewise, when Empire Turkey Pastrami slices are marketed as 96 percent fat-free, it is an utterly meaningless statistic. Yes, it is 4 percent fat by weight. But when you pull out the water and measure fat as a percentage of calories, these turkey slices come out with a whopping 45 percent fat. And beware of words like *light* and *lean*. Oscar Mayer Light Beef Bologna calls itself 80 percent fat-free, but by percentage of calories it is actually 64 percent fat. The words *meat* and *low-fat* should never be used in the same sentence.

Saturated Vegetable Oils: As Bad as Lard

Animal products are not the only source of saturated fats. A few vegetable oils are naturally high in saturated fat. These are known as *tropical oils*: palm oil, palm kernel oil, and coconut oil. As far as your cholesterol level is concerned, they are as bad as lard. To remember which ones they are, picture a palm tree, with coconuts on the top. These are products to avoid.

Other vegetable oils can be chemically saturated by a process called *hydrogenation*. These solidified fats are then used in products such as margarine, and like animal fats, they will stimulate your liver to make cholesterol. Commercial bakers prefer hydrogenated vegetable oils because they last longer on the shelf. The shelf life of a Hostess Twinkee is lengthened by the partial hydrogenation of the vegetable oils with which it is impregnated. Your shelf life, however, will not be improved if you make such foods part of your routine. Look on the labels of foods you buy, especially baked goods, for the words *hydrogenated* or *partially hydrogenated*. This means that the vegetable oils were chemically solidified into saturated fats, which will turn on the body's cholesterol-production machinery.

Liquid vegetable oils are much better than animal fats and tropical oils, but all fats and oils are natural mixtures of saturated and unsaturated fats. Beef fat is about half saturated fat and the remainder is a mixture of monounsaturated and polyunsaturated fat. Corn oil is mostly polyunsaturated, but about 13 percent of it is saturated fat. That is a lot less saturated fat than is found in beef or chicken, but it still contributes to heart problems. The same is true of olive oil: about 13 percent of it is saturated fat. What about peanut or safflower oils? Seventeen percent and 9 percent, respectively. While vegetable oils do less harm than animal fats, none of them do your coronary arteries any good. This chart shows the percentages of saturated fat in different kinds of fat:

Animal Fats:		Vegetable Oils:		Tropical Oils:	
Beef tallow	50%	Canola oil	12%	Coconut oil	87%
Chicken fat	30%	Corn oil	13%	Palm oil	49%
Pork fat (lard)	39%	Cottonseed oil	26%	Palm kernel oil	82%
Turkey fat	30%	Olive oil	13%		
		Peanut oil	17%		
		Safflower oil	9%		
		Sesame oil	14%		
		Soybean oil	15%		
		Sunflower oil	10%		

Source: J. A. T. Pennington, *Bowes and Church's Food Values of Portions Commonly Used* (New York: Harper and Row, 1989).

The saturated fat is the part that increases your cholesterol level, although the unsaturated parts have health problems of their own, including a tendency to increase free-radical production and an impairment of the immune system.

At this point, you may be wondering which oil you should use in cooking. Unfortunately there is not sufficient evidence to call any of them health foods. Liquid oils are certainly better than animal fats, tropical oils, and hydrogenated oils, but the best advice is to learn to prepare foods with little or no added fats or oils. In Chapter 8, we show how to do just that, with cooking techniques and ways to modify recipes that minimize oils.

DON'T BUY THE FISH STORY

What about fish? All fish products contain both cholesterol and saturated fat. Although a substantial amount of fish fat is unsaturated, all fish fats are mixtures too, and they all include saturated fat. Of the fat in chinook salmon, for example, about 24 percent is saturated. And while fishes vary tremendously in their fat content, virtually all—haddock, halibut, cod, bass, catfish, and the rest—contain a similar mix of saturated and unsaturated fat. The saturated portion is usually about 15 to 30 percent of total fat content. This is lower than beef and chicken, but still a problem. See Table 4.

Also a serious problem, fish fats are unstable chemicals, encouraging the production of free radicals—the very sparks that start the process of plaque formation, as we will see shortly.

Table 4 *Percentage of Fat in Fish*

	Total Fat Content	% of Fat That Is Saturated
Anchovy	33%	29%
Catfish	33%	25%
Cod	8%	17%
Haddock	8%	13%
Halibut	19%	15%
Oysters	33%	24%
Ocean perch	16%	14%
Salmon, Chinook	52%	24%
Sea trout	32%	29%
Snapper	12%	18%
Striped bass	22%	20%
Swordfish	30%	26%
White tuna	16%	29%
Walleye	11%	20%

Source: J. A. T. Pennington, *Bowes and Church's Food Values of Portions Commonly Used* (New York: Harper and Row, 1989).

Although fish oils can lower your triglyceride levels somewhat, they do not lower cholesterol, as some people believe. They also make the blood less likely to clot in response to injuries. And many scientific studies have shown that supplements made of fish oils can impair the body's immune responses to bacteria and viruses.[6,7] While some older authorities recommended fish and chicken, I believe you are better off without them.

By now, you can see why we are hearing the *V* word so much these days. Vegetarian foods are the most powerful foods for a healthy heart. You may be wondering how one goes about making such a change in diet, and what will be left to eat. I made this change myself several years ago and I know many other doctors and patients who have done so as well. Chapters 6 through 8 will guide you through the transition step by step, and I think you will be impressed by the power of this change and may well wish you had made it earlier.

When you do make the switch, give it a chance to work. Do not include small amounts of chicken or fish in your diet and expect to get the same effect. For many people, eliminating those last few bits of animal products can make a big difference.

Free Radicals: The Spark that Starts the Damage

What we have discussed so far is only half the story. It is important not just to lower the amount of cholesterol in the blood, but also to keep it contained so that it does not cause any harm.

To extend our earlier oil truck analogy for a moment, imagine what would happen if a stone were to fly up from the roadway and poke a hole in a tank truck. The truck is flagged over to the side of the road. Ambulances, police cars, and teams of investigators arrive on the scene, evaluating the risk of explosion and other hazards. Several lanes are blocked off, and traffic on the road is cut down to a trickle.

Something similar happens to your cholesterol transport packages. LDL packages can be attacked by free radicals, the dangerous molecules we learned about in Chapter 1. This free-radical damage is thought to be what actually sparks the formation of a plaque. When the LDL package is damaged, the cells lining the artery pull it out of circulation. In turn, these cells are damaged by the LDL they have taken in.[8] Muscle cells in the area start to multiply and overgrow. These muscle cells are normally in the wall of the artery, giving it strength like the steel bands in a tire. But as they multiply they form a raised bump—a plaque—within the artery wall. And as the plaque grows in size, less and less blood can get past it.

Protecting Your LDL from Damage

Our bodies have a way of fending off free-radical damage to the LDL particles. Vitamin C is a powerful antioxidant in the bloodstream that is quick to neutralize free radicals. In addition, vitamin E molecules are packed onto the outside of the LDL, averaging six vitamin E molecules per LDL particle. Some free radicals will get past vitamin C, but vitamin E aims to limit the damage they do. As vitamin E stops free-radical damage, it is chemically altered. And vitamin C restores vitamin E again.[9,10,11]

Beta-carotene also defends the LDL, working in areas of the body with different oxygen concentrations from those in which vitamin C is effective. For many years, the Physicians' Health Study has been examining the effects of beta-carotene on 22,000 doctors. The study is run by Charles Hennekens of Harvard University. After six years, those consuming beta-carotene supplements had only about half the number of heart attacks, compared to those on a placebo. The subjects were using a supplement rather than vegetables. Their dose was 50 mg per day, the amount in four carrots or two sweet potatoes.[12] No one knows the exact amount for optimal protection, but it is clear that a vegetable-rich menu provides antioxidants that help the heart.

The antioxidants are not foolproof, however. To further protect LDL, we need to cut down on free-radical production. That means avoiding the omega-3 fatty acids in fish, which are unstable molecules that oxidize easily, causing the production of free radicals. Omega-3s are needed by the body for healthy skin, eyes, and nerves, and as raw materials for building other biological molecules; but vegetables such as broccoli, spinach, lettuce, and beans provide omega-3s in a form that is more stable and also more modest in quantity.[13,14,15]

The value of fruits, vegetables, and grains, then, is not just that they contain no cholesterol at all and very little fat. They also supply antioxidant vitamins that offer some protection and hold a more stable form of omega-3 oils.

As we saw in Chapter 1, iron is part of the problem, too. It acts as a catalyst for free-radical damage. When iron is plentiful in the body, free radicals have a field day. In a study of nearly 2,000 men published in 1992, researchers in Finland demonstrated that iron stored in the body is a major contributor to heart attacks. The more iron you have in your body, the higher is your risk of heart disease.[16]

Luckily, the same kind of diet that lowers cholesterol levels also lowers iron. Cutting out meat doesn't just cut out cholesterol and fat. It also cuts out some of the iron that can damage the heart. "Meat is a one-two punch," said Harvard University biochemist Randall Lauffer. "It contains a certain form of iron that is very rapidly and easily absorbed. And it contains saturated fat and cholesterol. So every bite of meat is contributing to two problems in the body—both of which lead to heart disease and possibly other chronic diseases that are common in Western meat-eating cultures."

Iron makes atherosclerosis more likely to start. It also makes atherosclerosis more deadly. The reason, apparently, is that as circulation is restored after a heart attack or after a surgical procedure such as angioplasty, the influx of blood causes more free radicals to form, a process which is greatly increased by iron.

It is not just people with extremely large amounts of stored iron who are at risk, as Dr. Lauffer points out. "We are also very concerned that even moderately elevated iron levels could increase the risk of atherosclerosis—the blocking of the coronary arteries that supply blood to the heart—as well as making a person's heart more susceptible to damage when they do suffer a heart attack."

Iron may help explain why men and women have very different risks of heart disease. Before menopause, women have a much lower risk, but after menopause their risk rises to match that of men. Scientists have assumed that the difference must be due to hormones, but have found no compelling explanation. But it may be that men's higher risk of heart problems is because they start accumulating iron in their bodies at an earlier age. For women, menstruation naturally removes iron on a monthly basis. After menopause, iron accumulation rapidly occurs and heart disease rates climb.

"The iron levels match exactly the mortality rates of heart disease in men and women," Dr. Lauffer said. "Men get very high iron levels early in life, say twenty years old, whereas women's iron levels are held down by the natural loss of iron through menstruation. As soon as that ceases, however, their iron levels bound up quickly to that of men and, at the same time, the incidence of heart disease increases." As we noted in Chapter 1, vegetarians are not headed for iron deficiency. Rather, they have lower, safer amounts of stored iron in their bodies.

Some people have used the free-radical theory as an excuse to return to burgers and fried chicken. Who cares about cholesterol, they say, if you have lots of antioxidants in your body? Well, there are several things wrong with that thinking. First, these animal products contribute a load of fat and iron that *encourages* free-radical damage. Second, the more cholesterol you have in your blood, the more likely it is that some of the LDL will be hit by a free-radical assault.

We do not want high cholesterol levels any more than we want convoys of oil trucks continually traveling up and down every highway and street, even if they try to drive safely. Accidents happen, both on the road and in your body.

POWER FOODS: BEYOND OAT BRAN

It is no surprise that grains, vegetables, fruits, and legumes are powerful foods for a healthy heart. They contain no cholesterol at all. They have very little saturated fat. The iron they contain is less likely to contribute to iron overload, owing to more modest absorption. And plants contain enormous amounts of natural antioxidants.

Certain foods seem to have a particular cholesterol-lowering effect, and it is not just oat bran anymore. Oat bran, of course, displaces high-fat, high-cholesterol foods. Every spoonful of oatmeal you have for breakfast displaces the eggs and bacon you might otherwise have ingested. And oat bran seems to have an additional effect owing to the *soluble fiber* it contains.[17,18] (Soluble fiber simply means fiber that dissolves in water, as opposed to wheat bran, which does not dissolve.)

If you want a technical explanation of oat bran's effectiveness, here it is. The liver converts cholesterol into bile and sends it down the bile ducts and into the intestine. There, fiber carries it away along with the digestive contents.[19] In order to replace these lost bile acids, the liver pulls cholesterol out of the blood and uses it to make new bile acids. The result is lower cholesterol levels. If there is not enough fiber in your diet, however, the bile acids moving along the intestinal tract can be broken back down into cholesterol, which can be reabsorbed into the blood. Fiber also seems to block some of the absorption of fat from the digestive tract and may actually reduce cholesterol synthesis in the liver.[20,21]

The good news is that there are plenty of other sources of soluble fiber. Fruits, particularly apples and citrus fruits, are very rich in *pectins,* a soluble fiber found in their cell walls and between the cells. Cooks are familiar with pectin as something that is in some fruits and that gels as it cools to make jams and jellies. In scientific studies, pectins have been shown to help lower cholesterol levels.[22,23]

Even the humblest of foods, the bean, contains substantial amounts of soluble fiber. As little as four ounces of cooked beans daily has been shown to lower cholesterol and triglyceride levels more than 10 percent in just three weeks.[21] Chickpeas,[24] canned beans,[21] and other whole beans[25-28] and bean extracts such as guar gum (a bean extract often used in commercial food products) are all effective.

Researchers at the University of Toronto used pinto beans, chickpeas, kidney beans, and lentils in a cholesterol-lowering study.[29] The subjects lowered their cholesterol levels and triglycerides, and they also liked the addition to their diet. They kept the beans on the family menu after the study was over.

Barley, which is commonly used in soups, also contains soluble fiber and effectively reduces cholesterol levels. My suggestion is not to focus on the variety (e.g., oat bran, soybeans, or barley) that is getting press attention for the moment, but simply to build your menu from a variety of grains, vegetables, fruits, and beans—the real power foods for a healthy heart. Among them you will get lots of beneficial soluble fiber.

Other Contributors to Heart Disease

Although this is a book about healthful foods, I do want to touch briefly on some other contributors to heart disease. It is not much use having a healthful meal if it is followed by a cigarette. Researchers have studied other risk factors and found that these factors can affect your heart, just as a bad diet can.

46

Tobacco and Alcohol

There is no doubt whatsoever that tobacco use is a risk factor for heart disease. People who smoke have a much higher risk than others do. Moderation in tobacco use is not what should be recommended. It is essential to quit.

I used to smoke cigarettes on my way to the hospital during my internship. I knew how risky tobacco was, but it was very hard to stop. The answer, I believe, is simply to keep trying. It took me many tries, and eventually it stuck.

Regarding alcohol, there has been more conflict. There is a long-standing debate as to whether alcohol boosts HDL and whether it might actually help the heart. Some studies have shown that teetotalers do not live as long as moderate drinkers. On the other hand, some teetotalers are people who have been forced to stop drinking after years of alcoholism or in the face of illness, and it would be a mistake to conclude that what these people need is a good drink.

However this debate ends, martinis before dinner will not protect you against the steak that follows. And while there is no apparent harm with occasional use, regular alcohol use clearly contributes to other health problems, including an increase in risk of breast cancer.

Lack of Exercise

Regular physical activity cuts death rates dramatically. The good news for nonathletes is that most of the benefits come from light physical activity such as daily walking. There is relatively little difference in the value of intense physical activity versus modest exercise, such as walking. But there is a big difference between getting any form of physical activity and never getting any at all.[30,31] If you are spending long hours in your recliner, you may as well be test-driving your coffin.

Having said that, do not buy into the myth that exercise can undo the effects of a bad diet. This is simply not true. Take soldiers, for example. They get a lot of exercise, and tend to stay physically fit. But when doctors examined the hearts of 300 American soldiers killed in Korea, 77 percent had some atherosclerosis. In many, the plaques were of substantial size, and in some cases they had blocked off entire coronary arteries.[32] These young men had grown up eating the typical American diet, and they had no hint of the powder keg waiting in their hearts. If you looked at the soldiers who had plaques that were big enough to block at least half of the artery opening, they seemed fit. They were not overweight; their average weight was 153 pounds. They did not have high blood pressure. And their average age was under 23.[33] But their "physical fitness" did not keep their arteries clear.

Physical activity cannot counteract the effects of a fat-filled diet, but it can *add* to the benefits of a healthful life-style. A simple program for getting your muscles moving again is found in Appendix I.

STRESS

During World War II, the prevalence of heart disease dropped in some populations. This suggested to some that stress has nothing to do with heart disease, since there is probably more stress during wartime than at any other. The truth is, heart disease was rarer during World War II because meats and other fatty foods were greatly restricted. If one looks carefully at the effects of stress alone, it is clear that stress contributes to heart problems.

Researchers in Lebanon[34] found a clear relationship between exposure to the ongoing battles in that country and the demonstration of plaques on angiograms (X-rays of the heart). But you don't have to be dodging bullets to be under stress. Daily life is full of events that cause our hearts to beat a bit faster and drive our blood pressure up. When we are emotionally stressed hormones are released in our bodies that prepare us for rapid action. Over the long run, they take a toll on the heart. Even such tasks as performing arithmetic problems or public speaking cause our hormones to respond. In patients with heart disease these effects show up in bouts of abnormal heart function, often without the patient being aware that the stress has had any effect on the heart at all.[35]

The same thing occurs at the workplace. Stress drives blood pressure up and, over the long run, causes measurable changes in the heart.[36] The problem, researchers found, is not just a demanding workplace. The problem is a combination of high demand and little worker control over the workload. Reducing stress means keeping your challenges within the range you can manage. In addition, you cope better when you have had adequate sleep. There are special techniques that can help melt tension out of the body; these are found on pages 301–303.

A Word about Heredity

Most people do not have a hereditary tendency toward heart disease. Even in families where heart disease occurs in many members over more than one generation, the problem is not usually due to genetics, but to eating or smoking habits that persist across generations.

A small fraction of the population, about 5 percent, does have a true genetic tendency toward heart disease. Your doctor can tell you if you are in this group. If so, proper diet is vital. Since you are at particular risk of heart problems, you will want to follow the most healthful strategy you possibly can.

It is a mistake to conclude that you have a hereditary cholesterol problem just because a cholesterol-lowering diet prescribed by your doctor did not work. If the diet included lean meats, poultry, fish, eggs, or dairy products, it was not a good test. Many people who try a low-fat, pure vegetarian diet see dramatic results in a rather short time.

Foods and Blood Pressure

High blood pressure is potentially dangerous. And it is not only a risk factor for heart disease. It can also lead to strokes and other serious problems. Happily, certain foods can have a beneficial effect on your blood pressure.

When your blood pressure is measured, two numbers are checked: *systolic* blood pressure is the surge of pressure during each heartbeat; *diastolic* is the pressure in the arteries between beats. A blood pressure of 120/80 means that each surge of blood causes as much pressure as 120 millimeters of mercury within the artery, and that a pressure of 80 millimeters of mercury remains between beats.

By now everyone is aware that salt has an effect on blood pressure. It is easy to reduce your salt intake. Salt is an acquired taste, and you will adapt to a lower intake very quickly. When I was a medical student, one of my professors told me that he was following a no-added-salt diet. At the time, this struck me as quite a deprivation. However, somehow I inadvertently did the same thing. I stopped adding salt at the table. Then I gradually reduced the amount used in cooking. Today I seldom add salt to anything, either in cooking or at the table. While this may sound ascetic, it was a gradual change and I never actually miss salt at all.

But salt is only the beginning of dietary changes that lower blood pressure. Numerous studies have shown that vegetarians have lower blood pressures than nonvegetarians. It is not just that vegetarians tend to have healthier life-styles overall. There is something about the vegetarian diet that lowers blood pressure. For example, researchers have compared Seventh-day Adventist vegetarians with Mormons. Both groups avoid coffee, alcohol, tea, and tobacco, but Mormons eat meat, while about 50 percent of Adventists are vegetarians. The vegetarians had blood pressures that were eight to nine points lower, systolic, and six to eight points lower, diastolic.[37]

Researchers in Australia began a series of experiments in which they put patients on a vegetarian diet for six weeks. The result was a definite lowering of both systolic and diastolic blood pressure. They then switched the subjects back to their previous diet and their blood pressure promptly went up again. The researchers concluded that a vegetarian diet clearly lowers blood pressure, but no one part of the diet is responsible for this benefit.[38] Even without restricting salt intake, a low-fat, high-fiber diet can lower blood pressure by as much as 10 percent.[39]

Why does it work? It is not because people who eat vegetarian meals tend to be slimmer than meat-eaters, although that is certainly true. The drop in blood pressure occurs before any substantial weight change. The change in blood pressure may be due to the fact that high-fat diets increase the tendency of blood cells to clump together, and make the blood thicker (more viscous).[40,41]

Another part of the explanation may relate to the reduced iron storage that vegetarians enjoy. The Finnish researchers who found a strong link between iron and heart disease also found that iron contributes to hypertension in their study of nearly 2,000 men.[16] Vegetarians do not just avoid the fat and cholesterol of animal products; they also skip much of the risk of iron overload.

The omega-3 oils that are common in soybeans, as well as several kinds of vegetables, also seem to contribute to the blood pressure lowering.[42] And vitamin C, which, of course, is packed into vegetables and fruits, can also lower blood pressure slightly. Mild hypertension can be reduced by as little as one gram of vitamin C daily.[3]

High blood pressure can be extremely dangerous and some people do need medication. If you are on medication currently, be sure to discuss any dietary changes with your physician, because your need for medication may change.

Stroke

Plaques do not form only in the heart. They also form in the arteries leading to the brain. When a part of the brain dies from the lack of blood supply, it is called a stroke. A person may suddenly lose the capacity to form words, or to move a part of the body. When I first worked in hospitals, I found strokes much more frightening than heart attacks. To see a patient struggling to remember simple words, or to have to learn to become left-handed as his right hand hung limply by his side, was truly heart-wrenching.

Strokes can occur for reasons aside from accumulating plaques. A blood clot may lodge in an artery to the brain, choking off the blood supply, or arteries can break open and bleed into the brain. In addition, some strokes are caused by inborn defects in the blood vessels.

A stroke can be a dramatic, and sometimes fatal, event. Or small, barely perceptible strokes can occur repeatedly over months or years, each one killing a small part of the brain. As parts of the brain are sequentially killed off, the net result is dementia, often indistinguishable from Alzheimer's disease.

Most strokes are preventable. Controlling your blood cholesterol level and blood pressure can dramatically reduce your likelihood of stroke. And avoiding tobacco is important, too. There is a strong relationship between smoking and strokes,[43] as there is between smoking and heart disease.

Claudication and Impotence

Plaques form in the arteries to the legs, causing leg pains, called *claudication,* which comes from the Latin word meaning "to limp." This pain comes on when a person walks or climbs the stairs, and is relieved by resting. It progresses so that less and less activity is possible, and eventually pain can even occur at rest.

Plaques also form in the arteries to the genitals. By age sixty, one out of four men is impotent. Researchers in France examined 440 impotent men and found that the risk factors for impotence are essentially the same as for heart disease.[44] In other words, just as high cholesterol levels, high blood pressure, and smoking cause plaques to form in the arteries of the heart, the same process occurs in arteries throughout the body.

There are other ways that diet can lead to impotence. Fatty diets contribute to diabetes, which in turn can lead to impotence by accelerating atherosclerosis. (As we will see in Chapter 5, the New Four Food Groups are dramatically effective for diabetics.) Meat-based diets also contribute to high blood pressure, which aggravates atherosclerosis and, in turn, impotence. And some drugs (e.g., methyldopa [Aldomet] and guanethidine) used to treat high blood pressure also interfere with sexual functioning.

The threat to sexual potency may be a greater motivator than the risk of a heart attack. People do have trouble picturing their coronary arteries, while other parts of the male anatomy have a tremendous psychic presence. It might have been easier to convince men of the need for dietary change if I were to have titled this book *The Male Sex Power Diet*. Evidence shows that claudication is reversible, just as coronary heart disease is. Is impotence reversible through life-style changes? No researchers have investigated that question, but there is no reason to believe these plaques are different from those in the conditions we know more about—in which case the answer will prove to be a resounding yes.

Reversing Heart Disease

On July 21, 1990, a revolution took place in medicine. That was the day the prominent medical journal *The Lancet* published the findings of a young, Harvard-educated doctor now on the faculty of the University of California at San Francisco. Dr. Dean Ornish demonstrated that heart disease can actually be *reversed* without medicines.[45] At the time he published his findings, heart disease was the commonest cause of death (and still is), but most doctors were not even attempting to reverse the disease. Most believed that the plaques of cholesterol and other substances that clog the arteries to the heart could not go away. The way to get rid of them was to wait until they were severe, and then send the patient to the hospital for a bypass or angioplasty. Many doctors would prescribe a diet of lean meat, chicken, and fish. With this dietary regimen, heart disease usually was not stopped. It went on, ever so gradually, to kill the patient.

At Fort Mason in San Francisco, Dr. Ornish tested a new theory. He believed that if a more potent diet was prescribed along with other life-style changes, plaques might stop growing. Even better, the plaques might actually begin to dissolve. To test this theory, he selected patients who had plaques that were clearly visible on angiograms. He split the patients into two groups. Half were referred to a control group in which they got the standard care that doctors prescribe. That would usually mean an American Heart Association–recommended diet, advice not to smoke, and often various medications.

The special intervention group, on the other hand, got a very different kind of treatment. The patients began a totally vegetarian diet. And vegetable oils were kept to a minimum as well; the prescribed diet was less than 10 percent fat (by calories). They were also asked to begin a program of modest exercise, walking about a half-hour a day, or one hour three times a week. They had to learn to handle stress through breathing exercises, visualization, meditation, yoga, or other techniques. And, of course, they were not allowed to smoke.

The patients met as a group twice a week in sessions that combined education and group support, and they brought their spouses or companions along. They talked together about their successes with the new program, but also about their problems and how to integrate the new program into their day-to-day lives. In cooking lessons, they learned to make healthful foods at home, and take-home meals were also provided.

Early on there were hints that something was changing. Dr. Ornish's patients started to feel better, and they continued to improve over the course of the year. Even though they had been struggling with the crushing chest pain of heart disease, that changed very dramatically. "Most of them became essentially pain-free," Dr. Ornish said, "even though they were doing more activities, going back to work, and doing things that they hadn't been able to do, in some cases, for years."

Their cholesterol levels dropped. And dropped. And dropped—lower than had ever been found in any previous diet experiment. "We found reductions in blood cholesterol levels that were comparable to what can be achieved with cholesterol-lowering drugs," Ornish said. With no side effects.

The people on the more traditional medical routine did not do so well. They followed the diet their doctors recommended, but their chest pain did not go away. It became more severe, and it struck more often. After a year, Dr. Ornish put the patients to the real test. They underwent another angiogram so the plaques in their coronary arteries could again be measured. Most of the patients on the standard treatment were not getting better.

"The majority of patients who made more conventional changes in their diet and life-style actually got worse overall," Ornish said. "Their arteries became more blocked rather than less blocked." The plaques in their coronary arteries were continuing to grow, cutting off blood flow to the heart a bit more with every passing day. These patients were still inching toward death.

But the special intervention group was getting better. "What we found after a year was quite dramatic," Ornish said. "Overall, 82 percent of the patients who followed this program showed some measurable reversal of their coronary artery blockages." Their coronary arteries were actually opening up. The plaques that had been growing in their hearts for decades were actually *starting to dissolve* within one year, with no medications and no surgery.

The work of Dr. Ornish and others has made previous recommendations obsolete, although not everyone has gotten the message. Many doctors still recommend "lean-meat" diets, even though such diets do not reverse heart disease for most patients and, in fact, are too weak even to stop the progression of the disease. "Our study and now four other studies have shown that, on average, people with heart disease who only make moderate changes—less red meat, more fish and chicken, taking the skin off the chicken, fewer eggs, and so on—overall they tend to get worse over time," Ornish said. "The arteries become more blocked." But for those who are willing to go further, the news is good indeed: "They begin to feel better, they have more energy, the chest pain tends to go away almost dramatically, and even the arteries become less blocked over time."

This does not mean that eating vegetarian meals a few times a week will reverse your heart disease. Dr. Ornish's program was meant to be followed seven days a week, and people who stuck to the program got the best results. And it was not just a diet. It was a life-style change. There is little point in a vegetarian diet if you continue to smoke, for example. A potent program frees your body from fat and cholesterol, from tobacco, from physical lethargy, and from stress to the extent possible. "We found, in fact, there was a direct correlation between the amount of change they made and the amount of improvement," Dr. Ornish said. "The more they did, the better they got."

Dr. Ornish's remarkable program is described in his book *Dr. Dean*

Ornish's Program for Reversing Heart Disease,[46] which includes excellent advice on handling stress, stopping smoking, increasing exercise, and modifying the diet. Of course, people who have heart disease should be under the care of a cardiologist. While life-style changes are very powerful for most people, they do not take the place of individualized medical care.

Dr. Ornish had weighed the question of whether it is realistic to ask patients to adopt such a diet. There was no doubt that a vegetarian diet is powerful. But would people who were raised on chicken and roast beef be willing to make the change?

The answer was yes. I had an opportunity to talk with Dr. Ornish's patients. I interviewed each patient in both the experimental group and the control group. I asked them how they liked the foods they ate, whether they found the new foods interesting, how their families felt about the diet, and how long it took to get used to the new menu. Dr. Ornish's patients did say that they had grumbled a bit. At the beginning, they didn't know what a lentil was. It took a little while to get used to a new way of eating—a month or two before they were totally adapted. But soon they found the new foods enjoyable and interesting, and began to lose their taste for foods that had damaged their hearts. And they loved what the program had done. For most, their cholesterol levels were dramatically lower, their chest pains had gone away, and they felt better than they had in years. They also lost weight. The average patient lost more than twenty pounds, without restricting calories!

The patients on the standard heart diet grumbled, too. They complained that their diet seemed to consist of nothing but chicken and fish, day after day after day. And they were not getting the benefits that would have made the change worthwhile. In talking to these patients, I found that people seem to grumble about any change in their dietary routine, and there does not seem to be any relationship between how much change is requested and how much they grumble. A more potent dietary regimen seems to get no more complaints than a weak one. And eventually tastes change. Within several weeks, people come to prefer their new routine. Moreover, the stronger program is so much more successful and rewarding that people want to stick with it.

"In some ways, it's easier to make big changes in diet than small ones," Ornish said. "You begin to notice the benefits so much more quickly when you make big changes that it becomes easier to stay on a diet like this. And the guidelines are very clear. We made recipes that were delicious and beautifully presented, as well as healthful."

Dr. Ornish's patients embraced their powerful new menu. One patient had an interesting reaction. He was angry—angry that no doctor had offered him this program before. Doctors were ready to crack open his chest, rearrange the plumbing in his heart, jump-start his heartbeat, sew him up, hope that he survived, and charge him tens of thousands of dollars. But not one doctor had even suggested that different foods and life-style changes might accomplish the same thing. I believe that before long there will be a substantial change in what doctors tell their patients. One day it may constitute malpractice for doctors not to inform patients of all their options, including the powerful new life-style steps that help reopen the heart.

Other scientists agree that heart disease can be reversed. "It will go away," says Dr. William Castelli, of the Framingham Heart Study. "Get your total cholesterol down to 150 and keep it there for five years. I don't care how you do it. Diet would be the best way, but if you have to use drugs you can still do it. You will reverse your lesions."

Dr. Ornish's research showed that doctors' recommendations have usually been too weak. If we want to die slowly, previous diets are fine. But if we want to reclaim health, we must adopt a truly healthful diet, along with other life-style changes. This is not to say that a vegetarian diet and a healthier life-style will make you live forever. They won't. But for most people they add years to life and help maintain a healthy body that can enjoy life, rather than surrender to an ever-increasing list of physical problems.

WHAT IS THE BEST DIET?

As we saw in the research of Dr. Ornish, people who are concerned about their hearts get little benefit from switching from regular meats to lean meats, or to chicken and fish. Some may have a reduced risk of heart attack compared to those who eat fattier cuts. But for most, atherosclerosis will still progress and they have little chance of reversing any existing heart disease.

Many doctors and even medical organizations still recommend diets that derive about 30 percent of their calories from fat, consisting of lean meats, fish, and poultry without the skin. Unfortunately, researchers have found that patients get worse on such diets.[45,47,48] It may be that plaques do not grow as rapidly on a lean-meat diet as they do on an unrestricted diet, but they still grow. In most patients, as they are busily pulling the skin off their chicken or trimming the fat off their meat, the blood supply to the heart is slowly and surely being choked off. The lean-meat, chicken, and fish diet just does not work very well for most people.

The power foods are foods from plants. Vegetarians have a much better menu for the heart. Lacto-ovo-vegetarians (those who shun meats, poultry, and fish but consume dairy products and eggs) do much better than those on lean-meat diets, while pure vegetarians who steer clear of all animal products do best of all.

If you were to switch from a standard American diet to a lean-meat diet in which you ate no more than two four-ounce servings of lean meat each day, and you kept your overall fat intake to 30 percent of calories, you would still only get about half the cholesterol-lowering effect that you would have gotten had you chosen a lacto-ovo-vegetarian diet, assuming your experiences were similar to those in research experiments.[49]

If you were to adopt a pure vegetarian diet, on the other hand, your cholesterol control would be better still. A pure vegetarian diet is sometimes called *vegan* (*VEE-gun*) and, of course, contains zero cholesterol, very little saturated fat, and lots of fiber. How powerful is the vegan diet? A research study in New England compared typical meat-eaters, lacto-ovo-vegetarians, and vegans. All the subjects were fairly young, ranging in age from twenty to forty-seven. The average meat-eater's cholesterol level was 173, which is lower than the average American's, but not unusual in a young population. The lacto-ovo-vegetarians' cholesterol levels were better, averaging 150. And the vegans' averaged—believe it or not—135.[50] A Harvard research study found about the same thing. Vegetarians who include eggs and dairy products in their diet ran cholesterol levels averaging 157. But vegans had an average cholesterol level of 124.[51] As you can see, both vegetarian groups had good cholesterol levels, on average. But remember, roughly half the subjects in the study will be above the average and half will be below it, assuming a normal statistical distribution. Since the lacto-ovo-vegetarians average cholesterol levels around 150, roughly half will be above this level. Many more of the vegans will be under that threshold.

As Dr. Castelli says, "Vegetarians have the best diet. They have the lowest rates of coronary disease of any group in the country." And those who pick from a purely vegetarian (vegan) menu are the best of these.

Yes, but how does it taste? That's the surprise. Although it does take a few weeks to adapt to any change in diet, people who switch to low-fat vegan diets come to prefer them. On your plate, this translates into linguine with tomato sauce, with broccoli and spinach on the side; or a bean burrito with Spanish rice and fresh vegetables; or miso soup and vegetarian sushi. In Chapter 8 you will find menus and recipes for any palate.

Imagine what would happen if the country were to establish such a diet as a new standard. One result, of course, would be a savings of phenomenal amounts of money. The cost of heart attacks is reflected in the billions of dollars for Medicare, Medicaid, private insurance, and out-of-pocket medical payments, not to mention the time lost from productive employment. And the dollars and cents mean nothing compared to the anguish of victims and their families as heart disease robs them of their ability to engage in daily activities or even walk without crushing pain, and ultimately leaves their spouses to grow old alone.

New research has given us more powerful tools than ever before. We now know that we can gain control over the health of our hearts.

3
Cancer and Immunity

When I was in medical school in the late 1970s, I was not taught that foods had the power to prevent cancer or improve cancer survival. Much of what we know today about the causes of cancer was, at that time, totally unknown. We did know that tobacco was carcinogenic. We had some inklings about fiber. But aside from that, we kept our scalpels sharp, our chemotherapy and radiation ready, and we waited.

No more. Eighty percent of cancers are due to factors that have been identified and can be controlled—if we choose to do so. Eighty percent is not my statistic. It is from the National Cancer Institute, and some estimates are even higher. And not only can we potentially prevent most cancers, we can also improve the survival of people who have cancer. Foods are extraordinary allies in our personal wars on cancer.

Cancer starts when one cell goes haywire. It could be one of the cells that make up your skin, or your lungs, or your digestive tract, or just about anywhere else in your body. In the center of the cell, in the nucleus, the DNA that directs its function becomes damaged. The saboteur may be a toxic chemical, radiation, or other cause. This kind of damage occurs commonly enough that our bodies have specialized white blood cells that patrol the bloodstream and body tissues, looking for damaged cells and removing them. But if one damaged cell is left to its own devices, it can begin to multiply. One cell splits into two. Two become four. Four become eight. And eventually this lump of cells is big enough to show up on a mammogram or a chest X-ray. This is cancer. It would not be so bad if this mass of cells would stay put. But it invades healthy tissues, and releases some of its cells to travel to other parts of the body, where new tumors form, eventually causing death.

What can we do about it? A lot. Thirty percent of cancers are caused by tobacco, according to the National Cancer Institute. Lung cancer is the most obvious example, but by no means the only one. Cancers of the mouth and throat are also caused by tobacco. And carcinogens in tobacco smoke are excreted in the urine, so along the way they cause cancer of the kidney and bladder. If you smoke, you would do well to stop. But it will take a while for your cancer risk to diminish, so you will want to pay close attention to the cancer-protection factors described later.

Foods are indicted in even more cancer cases than tobacco. The National Cancer Institute estimates that at least 35 percent of cancers are linked to foods, and some estimates are as high as 60 percent. Foods increase the amount of certain hormones in the body—hormones that can increase the risk of cancer. For example, several of the most common forms of cancer are linked to sex hormones. This is true of cancer of the breast, uterus, ovary, prostate, and perhaps other sites. The amount of hormones in our bodies and their actions are determined, in large part, by the foods we eat. Foods can help calm our hormonal storms and can also shore up our immunity.

Some foods also contain carcinogens, and others can increase the production of free radicals. On the other hand, some foods are protective. They help the body neutralize free radicals, eliminate carcinogens, and help the immune system knock out cancer cells.

Other factors, including radiation, pollution, genetics, and viruses, also play roles in certain forms of cancer. (See Table 5.) Sometimes factors work together to cause cancer. For example, tobacco and asbestos exposure can both contribute to lung cancer risk.

In this chapter, we learn about the dietary friends and enemies of cancer that we put on our plates every day.

Breast Cancer

Ask any doctor what women can do to prevent breast cancer, and the response will probably be to get an annual mammogram after age fifty, or perhaps after age forty. Mammograms help, but they do not prevent cancer. They *find* cancer. Biopsy, surgery, radiation, and chemotherapy then follow.

In the late 1970s, breast cancer attacked one in every eleven women. In

Table 5   *Estimated Percentages of Cancer Due to Selected Factors*

Diet	35–60%
Tobacco	30%
Alcohol	3%
Radiation	3%
Medications	2%
Air and water pollution	1–5%

Source: National Cancer Institute, *Cancer Rates and Risks* (Washington, D.C.: 1985); also R. Doll and R. Peto, "The Causes of Cancer: Quantitative Estimates of Avoidable Risks of Cancer in the United States Today," *Journal of the National Cancer Institute* 1981;66: 1191–1308.

the 1980s, the rate went up to one in ten. And in 1992, the rate was one in eight. In the sixteen years from 1973 to 1988, the annual number of new cases went from 73,000 to 135,000.[1]

Increasing scientific evidence shows that breast cancer is often preventable. In 1982, the National Research Council published a report called *Diet, Nutrition, and Cancer,*[2] showing the mountain of evidence already available at that time linking specific dietary factors to cancer of the breast and other organs. But brochures with watered-down recommendations have sat collecting dust at cancer research centers. There has never been an organized effort to give women the information they need to make decisions about cancer prevention.

As I mentioned earlier, when I was a medical student, the first room on the left on the hospital ward was occupied by a thirty-five-year-old woman whose breast cancer had spread to her bones. And in the very next room was another woman in her early forties with the same disease. This epidemic sent victims to every hospital in America. The only difference today is that the number of victims is higher than ever.

The link between diet and cancer is not new. An article in *Scientific American* in January 1892 printed an observation that "cancer is most frequent among those branches of the human race where carnivorous habits prevail." Asian countries, such as Japan, have low rates of breast cancer while Western countries have cancer rates that are many times higher. These differences are not due to genetics. Nor is it something in the air or water.

Many scientific studies have suggested that an important factor is the food we eat.[3,4]

When Japanese women Westernize their diets, as has been happening since the 1950s, particularly among the affluent populations of Tokyo, Osaka, and other major cities, the rate of breast cancer has increased dramatically. And when Japanese families move to the United States, the daughters have the same risk of cancer as the American women around them—many times higher than that in Japan.

Researchers have found that fat in the diet, especially animal fat, increases the risk of breast cancer. Although scientists continue to debate the role of fat in cancer, substantial evidence shows that the more fat there is in the diet, the greater the risk of breast cancer, as we will see. Alcohol also increases risk. And fiber, vitamins, and the mineral selenium help protect the body. As we look at these factors individually, it is important to remember that each one alone is just part of the puzzle. It is not fat alone that causes cancer, nor vegetables alone that prevent it, but rather the combined effect of the nutrients and poisons we put on our plate three times a day.

FAT: THE HORMONE BOOSTER

In Japan in the late 1940s, when breast cancer was particularly rare, only about 7 percent of the calories in the Japanese diet came from fat.[5] The American diet, of course, is quite different. Animal products are at the center of the menu, and there is no chicken or beef that is 7 percent fat as a percentage of calories. These products are all at least three times higher in fat, and the fat content on the average American plate is in the range of 37 to 40 percent of calories.

Countries with a higher intake of fat, especially animal fat, have a higher incidence of breast cancer.[3,6,7] This has been found not just once or twice but repeatedly in very carefully conducted studies. Even within Japan, affluent women who eat meat daily have 8.5 times higher risk of breast cancer compared to poorer women who rarely or never eat meat.[4] The Surgeon General's *Report on Nutrition and Health* stated: "Indeed, a comparison of populations indicates that death rates for cancers of the breast, colon, and prostate are directly proportional to estimated dietary fat intakes."[8]

When the link between fat and cancer was found, researchers did not have to look far to explain it. There are many ways that fatty foods affect the body.

First, as we saw in Chapter 1, high-fat diets increase the level of estrogens, the female sex hormones, in the blood. It is known that many breast tumors are fueled by estrogens. Estrogens are normal and essential hormones for both women and men. But the more estrogen there is, the greater the driving force behind some kinds of breast cancer. On high-fat diets, estrogen levels increase; on low-fat diets, they decrease.[9,10,11] When women begin low-fat diets, their estrogen levels drop noticeably in a very short time. Vegetarians have significantly lower estrogen levels than nonvegetarians, in part because of the lower fat content of their diet, and they have more of the carrier molecules, *sex hormone binding globulins,* which have the job of holding onto the hormone until it is needed. Fatty foods do the reverse. They increase estrogens and reduce the amount of the carrier molecule that is supposed to keep the estrogens in check. And every minute, the breast cells are exposed to a little more estrogen than is normal.

Animal fats are apparently a bigger problem than vegetable oils. Paulo Toniolo, of the New York University Center, compared the diets of 250 women with breast cancer to 499 women without cancer from the same province in northwestern Italy. The two groups ate about the same amount of olive oil and carbohydrates. But what made the cancer patients different was that they had habitually eaten more meat, cheese, butter, and milk. The women who consumed more animal products had as much as three times the cancer risk of other women.[12]

Vegetarian diets based on grains, vegetables, fruits, and legumes are the most powerful diets for health, but their power erodes if milk and cheese and other dairy products are added. Some studies of lacto-ovo-vegetarians have found that their cancer risk is almost as high as meat-eaters.[13,14] These vegetarians were avoiding meat but eating considerable amounts of dairy products that, like meat, contain animal fat and not a speck of fiber.

Even though cross-cultural comparisons have pointed a finger at animal fat as the principal problem, vegetable oil is also under some suspicion. Vegetable oils can probably affect estrogen levels and, as we will see below, increase the production of cancer-causing free radicals. So it is no good just replacing fried chicken with fried onion rings. The best diet not only eliminates animal products but keeps vegetable oils to a minimum as well.

Certain foods have special actions. As we saw in Chapter 1, soybeans contain natural compounds called *phytoestrogens.* These are very weak estrogens that can occupy the estrogen receptors on breast cells, displacing normal estrogens. The result is less estrogen stimulation of each cell. Soybeans are a mainstay of Asian diets, and may be an additional reason why these countries have low cancer rates.[15]

CHANGING HORMONE LEVELS

If a woman begins a low-fat vegetarian diet, can estrogen levels drop? The answer is yes, with measurable changes usually occurring within a few weeks of beginning a new diet.

The results are often dramatic. A patient once called me asking for Demerol, a narcotic painkiller. She was having intense menstrual cramps, and she had found that milder analgesics would not ease the pain. I agreed to prescribe pain medication, but asked her to modify her diet during the next month: no animal products of any kind, and no vegetable oil. This meant a vegan diet, and no potato chips, salad dressings, and the like. At the end of the next month, she called again. For the first time in years, her period had been essentially pain-free. The pain she had assumed to be simply part of "the curse" was actually gone.

If you or anyone you know has the same problem, try this dietary experiment. You may be surprised with the results.

HOW MUCH FAT IS TOO MUCH?

Will the 30 percent fat diet of lean meat, poultry, fish, and vegetables, long recommended by the National Cancer Institute, prevent cancer in the American population? I strongly doubt it. It is just too weak. In the 1950s, when Japan's cancer rates were very low, fat intake was about 7 percent of calories. In China, average fat intake is now about 15 percent of calories. The China Health Study looked at provinces with fat intakes ranging from 6 to 24 percent of calories, and found that breast cancer was more common in those provinces at the higher part of this range. Thirty percent is too high to be of any significant benefit.

A study at Harvard University suggested the same thing. Walter Willett and his colleagues followed a large group of nurses for an eight-year period, tracking their diets and their cancer rates. The nurses ate standard American diets; and those who had a bit less fat, about 27 percent of calories from fat, were not any better off against cancer than those consuming more fat.[16] Some have interpreted this to mean that diet has nothing to do with breast cancer. A more reasonable conclusion is that the diets these women followed were still high-risk diets. No groups with low fat intakes were tested in the study. A diet including regular consumption of animal products and drawing nearly 30 percent of calories from fat is much higher in fat than the Asian diets associated with low cancer risk. Just as reducing cigarette smoking from two packs a day to one pack a day will not lower your cancer risk much, minor changes in diet cannot be expected to, either.

The bottom line is that the National Cancer Institute's guideline—that fat be no more than 30 percent of calories—is far too high. Fat intake should probably be approximately 10 percent of calories.

But here is a key point: As important as it is to get the fat off your plate, that is only the beginning. Fat is not all there is to it. Other parts of the diet play important roles in your risk of cancer. Vegetables, fruits, grains, and beans are not just low in fat. They also provide fiber, vitamins, and minerals. Fiber, of course, is only found in plants and, as noted above, fiber is vital for helping the body to rid itself of estrogen. And the vitamin C and beta-carotene in vegetables and fruits are also linked to lower cancer risk. Numerous researchers have found that the more high-fiber, vitamin-packed foods women consume, the lower their risk of cancer.[17]

Selenium also has a protective effect. As we've seen, selenium is an essential element in the antioxidant system that works within the cells. It comes from grains, and women with higher amounts of selenium in the blood are less likely to develop breast cancer than women with lower amounts.[18]

Alcohol increases cancer risk. Although some have promoted modest alcohol consumption, hoping to lower risk of heart disease, even one drink a day can increase breast cancer risk by more than 50 percent, compared to nondrinkers.[19] That does not mean that your cancer risk is 50 percent. It means that it is half again higher than it was before. The effect of alcohol is mainly seen in younger women.

OTHER RISK FACTORS

Aside from diet, other factors have been identified that increase breast cancer risk.

• *Hormones.* Oral contraceptives appear to increase risk. Although newer birth control pills contain less estrogen and progesterone than older versions, evidence suggests some increase in risk from oral contraceptives.[20] The same may be true of supplemental hormones given to women after menopause.[21] In both cases, it makes sense for women to discuss the risks and benefits with their personal physicians.

• *Overweight.* Your weight affects your risk of developing breast cancer after menopause.[22] Before menopause, weight does not increase risk. For those who have cancer, overweight reduces survival, as we will see in more detail later in this chapter.

• *Radiation.* All the cells of the body are very sensitive to the damage of radiation, which can turn normal cells into cancer cells. This is why doctors try to avoid unnecessary X-rays and why your dentist gives you a lead apron during an X-ray. Of all the different parts of the body, the breast is probably the most sensitive to X-ray damage, and there is no doubt that X-rays to the breast can cause cancer.[23]

This poses an obvious dilemma. Since mammograms are X-rays, can they cause the very kind of cancer they are designed to find? Mammography does contribute to the radiation to which women are exposed. However, most concern arises from older X-ray equipment that emits more radiation. Mammography equipment manufactured in the past several years uses much smaller X-ray doses and is unlikely to contribute measurably to cancer risk. In fact, very compelling evidence shows that mammograms can be lifesaving for women over the age of fifty. Even though mammograms do not detect cancers until the tumor is eight to ten years old, they still can improve survival for women over fifty. Below that age, however, scientists are not so sure that there is any benefit to routine mammograms, although it is valuable to have one mammogram done before age forty for later comparison. The problem is that many cancers are missed on mammograms, and women have sometimes been falsely reassured by a negative mammogram, leading to delays in diagnosis and treatment. Women should discuss their own risks and benefits with their physicians, and should schedule mammograms only at modern facilities that do them regularly and maintain new equipment.

• *Genetics.* A genetic contribution to breast cancer exists, but is often overestimated. When cancer runs in families, it may well be due to dietary and other life-style factors that we learn from our parents, rather than from genetic inheritance. Even so, about 5 percent of cases are purely attributable to genetics.[24] In such cases, cancer is passed from parent to child as a dominant trait, and the family tree is riddled with the disease. And for a larger group of individuals, genetics probably makes a contribution in subtle ways. For example, it may well be that different genes influence one's susceptibility to carcinogens, the strength of the immune system to seek out and destroy cancer cells, the age of sexual maturation, body weight, and other factors that are relevant to cancer risk. Each of these is also influenced by diet.

• *Toxic chemicals.* "Better living through chemistry" was a corporate slogan, and Americans have certainly lived by those words. There are more than 25,000 chemicals in common use, and the long-term toxic effects of most of them are unknown. Some of the chemicals that we inhale or ingest tend to concentrate in our fatty tissues, and breast tissue is high on the list. Could these chemicals play a role in breast cancer? They may well.

Breast cancer is not evenly distributed geographically. Counties that house toxic waste sites tend to have higher than average rates of breast cancer.[25] That is true for other forms of cancer, too.

And you don't have to live near a Superfund chemical waste site to be concerned about toxic exposures. Toxic chemicals are available at any grocery store in the form of pesticides. Happily, organic produce is now more widely available. Chemical contaminants also end up in meats. Pesticides are sprayed on grains that are fed to cattle, chickens, and other livestock. In storage bins, feed grains are sprayed again. Animals concentrate these chemicals in their tissues and, if you eat the muscle tissue or mammary secretions of an animal, you are on the receiving end of their chemical concentration process.

Some evidence suggests that high-fat diets may encourage the absorption of carcinogens into the body. Researchers have observed, for example, that when the carcinogens in cigarette smoke are absorbed through the lung tissue, they tend to travel along with fats in the blood.[26] It may be that on a low-fat diet, the body is less likely to absorb and transport carcinogens.

Women who avoid eating animal products have much smaller concentrations of pesticides in their breast milk. In a 1981 study, vegetarians had only 1 to 2 percent of the national average levels of certain pesticides. And for all other chemicals tested except one, the breast milk of vegetarians was much freer of pesticides and industrial chemicals, compared to average Americans.[27] The exception was poly-chlorinated biphenyls (PCBs), for which vegetarians had levels comparable to meat-eaters. PCBs often come from fish consumption, and the chemical remains in the body for many, many years after exposure. Once PCBs are in the body tissues, avoiding contaminated fish will reduce PCB levels only very slowly.

Meat-eaters have far higher chemical concentrations in their breast milk, and their breast tissues bathe in these chemicals for years. There are obvious implications for a nursing baby, but what about the mother? Carcinogenic pesticides and industrial chemicals concentrate in the breast tissue, and the degree of their contribution to cancer remains unknown.

• *Time between puberty and first pregnancy.* The younger a girl is when puberty occurs, the higher her risk of breast cancer. Also, the later the age of her first pregnancy, the higher her risk. It may be that the early age of puberty has nothing to do with increased risk other than that it indicates an elevation of hormonal stimulation, as was described in Chapter 1. As high-fat, low-fiber diets have spread from the wealthy part of the population to, now, the entire population, the age of puberty has dropped dramatically, from age 17 in 1840 to 12.5 today. It may be that early puberty and cancer are both the result of a hormonal aberration.

On the other hand, it may be that the time period between puberty and the first pregnancy is one in which the body is particularly sensitive to carcinogens, and the longer this time period is, the greater the risk.

GETTING THE MESSAGE OUT

Occasionally people who have cancer report feeling that, if food plays a role in cancer, then they are somehow to blame for their disease. Guilt and blame often become concerns for people dealing with cancer. However, my belief is that these burdens are not useful. Besides, it makes no sense to blame anyone for things they had no way of knowing. Until major public education programs spread the word about the role of dietary factors and help people to change, cancer will remain an epidemic.

What we can do is not only boost our own strength against cancer but also break the cycle for the next generation. Of all the women born in America, one in eight will get breast cancer at some time in her life. If they do not have information on the disease, they are unable to decide for themselves what to do.

Although the National Cancer Institute takes the link between diet and breast cancer seriously and has issued guidelines (albeit weak ones) for cancer prevention, most American women have not gotten the message. In 1991, the Physicians Committee for Responsible Medicine commissioned a survey by Opinion Research Corporation of Princeton, New Jersey, asking how many women had not yet learned of the connection between diet and breast cancer. The results were dismal: 80 percent of women had no idea there was any link.

Why would the leading killer of young women not be the subject of prevention campaigns? Unfortunately, public attention is focused on *finding* breast cancer by mammography and self-examination, not on *preventing* it. Each October for the past several years has been designated National Breast Cancer Awareness Month. The president signs an annual proclamation, and television programs and magazines pick up the story. But every year since its inception, the materials disseminated to the press focus on mammography and self-examination. While that educational effort has merit, information on prevention is completely left out. What the press does not know is that National Breast Cancer Awareness

Month is sponsored by Imperial Chemical Industries (ICI), the makers of tamoxifen, an anti-estrogen drug used in the treatment of breast cancer. ICI provides the funds for promotional efforts for the October program, and retains approval rights over the materials that are used. And ICI has consistently decided not to include information that might prevent breast cancer. While tamoxifen is a very helpful drug for women with cancer, ICI's decision to focus only on *finding* cancer through mammograms and examinations has meant that lifesaving prevention information is effectively squeezed out of air play and out of press space.

The incidence of breast cancer cannot be reduced by early detection because mammograms and self-examination only find existing cancers and are intended to make treatment more successful. Finding cancer on a mammogram or examination will never be as helpful as avoiding cancer entirely.

Meanwhile, back in Japan a tragedy is unfolding. The U.S. government has been pushing Japan to accept American agricultural products, particularly tobacco and beef. As demand for these deadly products declines domestically, sagging sales are propped up overseas. And there is no shortage of patrons for McDonald's and Kentucky Fried Chicken in Tokyo and Osaka. Meat, poultry, and egg consumption has increased eightfold, and dairy consumption is fifteen times what it was in 1950. Fat intake in Japan climbed from less than 10 percent of calories in 1955 to 25 percent in 1987.[28] Meanwhile, consumption of rice and green and yellow vegetables has dropped dramatically.[29] Breast cancer death rates are increasing steadily, along with cancer of the colon, ovary, uterus, prostate, and pancreas.[28]

This is not to suggest that, without Western influence, Japan's diet would be perfect. The Japanese diet is too high in salt and too high in pickled foods. They pay a price in stomach cancer,[28] hypertension, stroke, and other health problems. But the Westernization of the Japanese diet is accompanied by Western diseases as well.

As the consumption of more meat, dairy products, and fried foods assaults women's bodies, and the protection of vitamin-rich vegetables and fruits is neglected, the effects are all too apparent: altered hormonal function, an unnatural age of puberty, and an impairment of the immune system that might otherwise knock out cancer cells. But a healthful diet can diminish the risk while building the body's defenses. To the extent that such a diet is put to work, we can hope to turn the tide on this epidemic.

Cancers of the Uterus and Ovary

The uterus and ovary, of course, are reproductive organs, and factors that affect hormone function can be expected to affect these organs as well. The risks of cancer of the uterus or ovary are higher in populations that have more breast cancer, suggesting that they may be caused by similar factors. Uterine cancer is linked to fatty diets and obesity,[3,30,31] although other factors, including hormone supplements, also play an important role. Ovarian cancer is also more common where people eat higher-fat diets.[3,32]

We now have some new clues to preventing cancer of the ovary from a study by Dr. Daniel Cramer of Harvard University.[33] Cramer studied hundreds of women with ovarian cancer, and had them record in detail what they normally ate. He compared them to a group of women who were similar in age and other demographic variables, but who had not developed cancer. There was one thing that the women with cancer had eaten much more frequently than women without cancer: dairy products, especially the supposedly "healthy" products such as yogurt.

The culprit may be a breakdown product of the milk sugar, lactose. As we saw in Chapter 1, lactose is broken down in the body to another sugar called galactose. In turn, galactose is broken down further by enzymes in the body. According to Dr. Cramer, when dairy product consumption exceeds the enzymes' capacity to break down galactose, there is a buildup of galactose in the blood, which may damage a woman's ovaries. Some women have particularly low levels of these enzymes, and when they consume dairy products on a regular basis, their risk of ovarian cancer can be triple that of other women. The problem is the milk sugar, not the milk fat, so it is not solved by using nonfat products. In fact, yogurt and cottage cheese seem to be of most concern because the bacteria used in their production increase the production of galactose from lactose. This is one of many reasons I recommend that dairy products be avoided, as we will see in more detail in Chapters 5 and 6.

Prostate Cancer: The Leading Cancer in Men

Just as women on high-fat Western diets have more estrogens circulating in their blood and a higher risk of cancer of the reproductive organs, a similar process occurs in men. High-fat diets alter the amounts of testosterone, estrogen, and other hormones in both men and women, as we saw in Chapter 1. One in ten men will develop prostate cancer at some point in his life.

The prostate gland is just below the bladder in men, where it produces semen, to be mixed with sperm cells. Cancer of the prostate is the most common form of cancer in American men,[34] occurring mainly in older men.

Cancer cells are found in the prostates of about 20 percent of men over the age of forty-five.[35] In most cases, these cancer cells do not develop into cancerous tumors that affect the overall health or lifespan of the individual. However, in many cases the cancer does grow, invades surrounding tissues, and spreads to other parts of the body. Although the disease varies greatly from one person to the next, the average patient loses nine years from a normal lifespan.[34]

Just as countries differ markedly in the prevalence of breast cancer, this hormone-related cancer varies in exactly the same way. Asian and Latin American countries have a much lower prevalence of prostate cancer, while it is very common in Europe and America. Ten men die of prostate cancer in Western Europe for every one who dies in Asia.[35]

Cancer of the prostate is strongly linked to what men eat. Again, animal products are consistently indicted. Milk, meat, eggs, cheese, cream, butter, and fats are found, in one research study after another, to be linked to prostate cancer.[36-45] And it is not just dairy products and meats. Some studies have also pointed a finger at vegetable oils.[3,37]

Who has a lower risk? Countries with more rice,[36] soybean products,[43] or green or yellow vegetables[46,47] in the diet have far fewer prostate cancer deaths. Vegetarians have less prostate cancer.[2] Scientists have long been interested in members of the Seventh-day Adventist church because of its vegetarian tradition. Adventist men have only one-third the prostate cancer risk of other men,[48] although Adventists also generally avoid tobacco, alcohol, and caffeine. Some evidence suggests that becoming a vegetarian in adulthood is helpful, but those who are raised as vegetarians have the lowest risk.[49]

How does a Western diet cause cancer? The prostate is very sensitive to hormones. As we saw in Chapter 1, men who consume diets based on animal products tend to have more testosterone and more estrogens, compared to men who eat healthier diets. This increase may be due to overproduction in the body or, because fiber in the diet is essential for the normal excretion of sex hormones, they are less able to get rid of them. The higher levels of these hormones make them the chief suspects in the epidemic of prostate cancer.

The protection that seems to come from including vegetables and fruits in the diet may be that every bite of broccoli is not a bite of beef. But, in addition, vegetables supply vitamins that are well-known cancer fighters, as we will see later.

Colon Cancer and Other Cancers
of the Digestive Tract

The colon is another name for the large intestine—that is, the second half of the digestive tract. The colon is assaulted day after day by our dietary indiscretions, and colon cancer can be the result.

The public already knows about the role of diet in colon cancer. Strong links have been found between the consumption of meats and other fatty foods and colon cancer.[2,50,51] When the past diets of cancer patients are studied, it is very clear that meat-based Western diets are linked to cancer. And comparisons of countries with different rates of colon cancer have supported this finding.

In order to absorb the fats that we eat, the liver makes bile that it stores in the gall bladder. After a meal, the gall bladder squirts bile acids into the intestine, where they chemically modify the fats we have eaten so they can be absorbed. Unfortunately, bacteria in the intestine turn these bile acids into cancer-promoting substances called *secondary bile acids*. The problem with meats is that they contain a substantial amount of fat, and foster the growth of bacteria that cause carcinogenic secondary bile acids to form. In addition, when meat is cooked, carcinogens form on its surface.

Happily, high-fiber diets offer a measure of protection.[2] Fiber-rich whole grains have a protective effect, as breakfast cereal commercials remind us. Fiber greatly speeds the passage of food through the colon, effectively removing carcinogens. And fiber has another interesting effect: it actually changes the type of bacteria present in the intestine, so there is reduced production of carcinogenic secondary bile acids. Fiber also absorbs and dilutes bile acids.

This humble part of the diet was largely ignored until a brilliant surgeon, Dr. Denis Burkitt, demonstrated the value of fiber, not only to protect against colon cancer but for dealing with a whole range of health problems. When the Physicians Committee for Responsible Medicine proposed the New Four Food Groups in 1991, Dr. Burkitt came to Washington to support the plan. Physicians have been very busy using surgery, chemotherapy, radiation, and other treatments to mop up the flood of disease, when the key, Dr. Burkitt said, is to stop the flood at its source: diet.

Even people who are at particular risk for cancer can be helped by a high-fiber diet. Jerome J. DeCosse, a surgeon at Cornell Medical Center, gave bran to patients with recurrent polyps of the colon. These are small growths that have a tendency to become cancerous. DeCosse found that within six months, the polyps became smaller and fewer in number. He believes that pentose fiber, which is plentiful in wheat, is the key to bran's power.[52]

Grains are not the only plant foods that help protect against colon cancer. Scientific studies have shown that populations consuming generous amounts of vegetables, particularly cruciferous vegetables such as broccoli, cauliflower, Brussels sprouts, and cabbage, also have a lower risk of colon cancer.[2] Precisely why this is so is not clear, but it seems to relate both to their fiber content and to specific cancer-fighting compounds they contain.

Other cancers of the digestive tract are also linked to dietary factors. In cancer of the esophagus, alcohol increases the risk, and alcohol and tobacco together exert a synergistic effect. Pickled foods and very hot beverages also increase risk, while fruits and vegetables reduce it. Stomach cancer is linked to smoked and salt-pickled foods, and again vegetables seem to have a protective effect. Liver cancer is linked to a carcinogenic chemical called aflatoxin, which is produced by a mold that grows on peanuts and corn. This disease is uncommon in most Western countries, but is very common in sub-Saharan Africa and Southeast Asia, where the mold is common. Pancreatic cancer has been linked to consumption of alcohol, coffee, and meat.[2]

Two themes consistently emerge from studies of cancer in many sites: vegetables and fruits help reduce risk, while animal products and other fatty foods are frequently found to increase risk.

Unfortunately, the terms *fiber* and *fat* tend to obscure the real dietary issues. People tend to think that fiber is something that one shakes out of a box when, in fact, fiber is found in whole grains, vegetables, fruits, and beans. (There is no fiber in any product from an animal.) So when you hear of the merits of fiber, think of whole-grain bread, rice, vegetables, fruits, and beans. And when you hear of the dangers of fats, think of meat-based diets aided and abetted by oily foods.

The Anticancer Defenses

VITAMINS

As we saw in Chapter 1, as oxygen is used in the body, some of the oxygen molecules become unstable and are called free radicals. These unstable oxygen molecules can attack cell membranes and can damage the DNA in the nucleus of the cell. It is this damage to DNA that is the beginning of cancer.

Natural chemicals called antioxidants, which neutralize free radicals, also help reduce cancer risk. Vitamin C, vitamin E, beta-carotene, selenium, and many other antioxidants are provided by a diet rich in vegetables, fruits, and grains.

People who include fruits and vegetables in their daily diets have lower rates of many forms of cancer, including lung, breast, colon, bladder, stomach, mouth, larynx, esophagus, pancreas, and cervix.[53] Effects have even been seen in childhood. When children with brain tumors were studied, it was found that their mothers consumed less vitamin C during pregnancy, compared to other women.[53] Again, there are many factors outside diet that contribute to cancer, from chemicals to radiation, but vegetables and fruits help counteract even these factors to an extent.

Even with vegetables and fruits in the diet, damage to the cellular DNA will occasionally occur. So the body has built-in repair machinery. Fixing DNA requires a B vitamin called *folic acid*, which is found in dark-green leafy vegetables, fruits, peas, and beans. The Recommended Daily Allowance of folic acid for adults is 400 mcg per day. As Table 6 below shows, beans and vegetables supply plenty of folic acid.

Table 6

Folic Acid in Foods

(mcg per 1-cup cooked serving)

Asparagus	176	Kidney beans	229
Baked beans, vegetarian	61	Lentils	358
Black beans	256	Lima beans	156
Black-eyed peas	356	Navy beans	255
Broccoli	108	Pinto beans	294
Brussels sprouts	94	Soybeans	93
Chickpeas	282	Spinach	262
Great northern beans	181		

Source: J. A. T. Pennington, *Bowes and Church's Food Values of Portions Commonly Used* (New York: Harper and Row, 1989).

Smokers have provided dramatic demonstrations of the power of vegetables and fruits. A fifty-five-year-old male smoker whose diet is low in vitamin C has a one-in-four risk of dying of lung cancer in the next twenty-five years. But if the smoker has a high intake of vitamin C, either through diet or supplements, his risk drops to 7 percent.[54]

People who quit smoking benefit from fruits and vegetables, too. Researchers at the University of Texas found that former smokers who do not eat many vegetables and fruits are five and a half times more likely to develop throat cancer compared to ex-smokers who eat more fruits and vegetables.[55] Even those who are at high risk for cancer—for example, asbestos workers who smoke cigarettes—are protected somewhat when their diet includes foods rich in beta-carotene.

The point is this: We are all exposed to cancer-causing chemicals, whether we like it or not. Some people are smokers, and, of course, quitting smoking is vital. But all of us are exposed to chemicals in the air, in the water, in our food, and in the household products we use, not to mention the carcinogens produced within our bodies as a part of our metabolic processes. While trying to minimize our exposure to carcinogens, we can also shore up our defenses against these assaults by including vegetables and fruits in our routine.

It is not just the vitamin C, beta-carotene, vitamin E, or fiber that makes these foods so powerful for health. It is these combined, and others besides. We are now at the point where it no longer makes sense to recommend just a beta-carotene–rich diet, or a vitamin C–rich diet, or a vitamin E–rich diet. What we need is a diet rich in vegetables, fruits, grains, and legumes, because every day we find more reasons why these foods are so powerful for health.

LIMITED IRON INTAKE

As we noted in Chapter 1, iron is a catalyst for the formation of cancer-causing free radicals. Gone are the days when nutritionists preached that the more iron there is in the diet, the better. Iron encourages damage to DNA, which can lead to cancer. "Iron is known to be a key catalyst for this process—one of the best catalysts you can imagine," said Harvard biochemist Dr. Randall Lauffer. "The body tries to safely sequester iron away in the cell and keep it away from the DNA." Of course, the body does need iron. But beyond the rather small amounts the body needs, iron becomes a dangerous substance, making DNA damage more likely.

In addition, cancer is a disease of uncontrolled cell division—cells dividing over and over, forming a tumor and sending cells to other parts of the body. Iron plays a role here. It is essential to cell division. "If the cell doesn't have iron around, it simply does not divide," Dr. Lauffer said. "So if you can restrict the amount of iron to a cancer cell, it actually slows down cancer growth."

Research has borne out that higher amounts of iron in the blood can mean higher cancer risk. "There are several studies in foreign countries and one very large study in this country with over 10,000 people examined," Dr. Lauffer said. "For men especially, it was clear that higher iron levels were associated with increased risk for certain forms of cancer. Iron-overload victims have an increased cancer risk. For example, a person with inherited iron-overload has 200 times the risk of liver cancer compared to a normal person."

A menu based on the New Four Food Groups keeps iron at a safe level.

On the other hand, meats encourage too much iron absorption. Chapter 1 gives details on how to determine your own iron status.

KILLER CELLS

There is one final piece to add to the cancer prevention puzzle: immunity. In spite of our best efforts, cancer cells will arise in the body from time to time. Left to their own devices, these cells will multiply and spread. Luckily, we have "soldiers" that roam our bloodstreams looking for these trouble-makers. These are the *white blood cells*. Some of them, called *natural killer cells*, are the foot patrols that seek out and destroy cancer cells and bacteria. They engulf and destroy aberrant cells before they can cause damage.

Like soldiers everywhere, they are not always given the very best rations. Some foods strengthen them, and others slow them down. It turns out that our natural killer cells work best when they are getting a healthy dose of beta-carotene–rich foods. The effect of beta-carotene on blood cells is dramatic. It significantly increases the percentage of cells in the body acting as natural killer cells and as T-helper cells,[56] which are a type of white blood cell that acts like an officer directing a battle plan. (Their name comes from the fact that they are conditioned by the thymus, a gland in the upper chest.) The effect of beta-carotene on these cells has been demonstrated both in

---

Steps to Cancer Prevention

Do not use tobacco in any form.

A varied menu of whole grains, vegetables, fruits, and beans supplies generous amounts of fiber, vitamins, and minerals, and less than 10 percent of its calories will be from fat.

Have more than one vegetable at a meal.

Avoid animal products and minimize added vegetable oils.

Minimize alcohol intake.

Maintain your weight at or near your ideal weight.

Avoid excessive sunlight and unnecessary X-rays.

human volunteers and in laboratory tests on blood cells.[57] Although vitamin A can be made from beta-carotene, the immune power comes from beta-carotene itself. The vitamin A packed into vitamins or contained in meats lacks much of the immune-boosting power of beta-carotene.

As we age, we lose much of our immune strength. Skin tests, such as the test that checks for exposure to tuberculosis, often act abnormally in older people, and the loss of immune function is considered normal. As the years go by, more and more of our white blood cells act as T-suppressor cells—that is, cells that turn off immune reactions.[57] New evidence shows that beta-carotene can counteract much of this age-related immune loss.[56] How much beta-carotene does it take to get these benefits? As little as 30 mg per day—the amount in two large carrots—causes the increase in natural killer cells and T-helper cells.

Although beta-carotene is safe, even in fairly substantial amounts, the best way to get beta-carotene is not in pills, but in the carrots, spinach, kale, and other packages in which nature supplies it. Why? Because we now know that beta-carotene is only one of perhaps two dozen related substances called *carotenoids* that occur naturally in vegetables and fruits, and which have varying degrees of biological activity.

Vitamins C[58] and E[59] and selenium[60] bolster immune function in addition to their antioxidant effects, but the importance of these effects against cancer is not yet clear.

Fats impair immunity, and cutting fat out of the diet helps strengthen the immune defenses against cells that turn cancerous. Researchers in New York tested the effect of a low-fat diet on immunity.[61] They put healthy volunteers on a diet that limited fat content to 20 percent, about half the national average. They cut down on all fats and oils, not just saturated or unsaturated fats. Three months later, the researchers took blood samples from the volunteers and examined their natural killer cells. The natural killer cell activity was greatly increased. These cells worked much better when the fat was out of the diet.

Although for heart patients vegetable oils are far superior to animal fats, when it comes to the immune system vegetable oils are no better than animal fats. In experiments, researchers have found that when they infuse soybean oil intravenously into volunteers, their white blood cells no longer work as well,[62] and test-tube experiments show similar results.[63]

Likewise, omega-3 fatty acids, which are found in fish oils, green vegetables, and soybean, flaxseed, and rapeseed oils, also compromise immune function.[64,65,66] The bottom line is to greatly reduce all fats and oils.

It will come as no surprise that vegetarians have the strongest immune systems. Since 1978, researchers at the German Cancer Research Center in Heidelberg have examined vegetarians. They weighed them (vegetarians weigh less than nonvegetarians); they measured them (their height is the same as nonvegetarians); they measured the vitamin content of their blood, finding more beta-carotene, compared to others. And recently, they tested the strength of their immune systems. They took white blood cells from vegetarians and tested their capacity to knock out cancer cells.[67] The vegetarians were compared against nonvegetarians working at the cancer center. Each day, blood samples were taken and their strength to kill cancer cells was checked.

The results were unequivocal. The vegetarians had more than double the ability of their nonvegetarian counterparts to destroy cancer cells. The researchers concluded that the immune muscle of vegetarians comes either from their having double the number of natural killer cells or from each cell having double the killing power. Whichever it is, vegetarians have a defense against cancer cells that is far beyond that of their meat-eating fellows.

The immune power of a vegetarian diet is partly due to its high vitamin content and partly due to its low fat content. There may be other contributors, too, such as reduced exposure to toxic chemicals and animal proteins. Thus, the wrong food choices can weaken our defenses against cancer, but a low-fat menu of grains, vegetables, fruits, and legumes allows the body's natural power to be brought to bear for greater health.

Surviving Cancer

BREAST CANCER

Not all cancers are the same. Some have a relatively good prognosis, and others have a very poor prognosis. For example, a tumor that is small and has not spread to the lymph nodes or other organs is less dangerous than a tumor that is larger and has spread. (Lymph nodes are pea-size collections of cells near the breast and other organs that are important to immune function.) Hospital laboratories also determine whether a breast tumor has receptors for estrogen or progesterone hormones. If it does, the tumor is slightly less aggressive than if it lacks receptors.

These prognostic factors are not due to chance alone. Thirty years ago Ernst Wynder of the American Health Foundation in New York observed that, aside from the fact that Japanese women are much less likely than American women to get breast cancer, when Japanese women do get the disease, they tend to survive longer.[68] Their improved survival is independent of age, tumor size, estrogen receptor status, extent of spread to lymph nodes, and microscopic appearance of the cancer cells.[69] It is not that Japanese women have better health care, because the same pattern has been observed in Hawaii[70] and California,[71] where Japanese women live nearby other ethnic groups and have essentially the same health-care system.

Researchers have begun to look at whether diet plays a role in survival. It does. Our old enemy—fat in foods—rears its ugly head once again. The more fat there is in the diet, the shorter a cancer patient survives. In a Canadian research study, women with cancer were more likely to have lymph node involvement if they had a high fat intake. This effect was found only for saturated fat and only for postmenopausal women.[72] Fat seems to have a measurable effect when cancer has spread to other parts of the body,[69] and little or no effect when the disease is localized.[73]

Researchers in Buffalo, New York, calculated what they believe to be the degree of risk posed by fat in the diet. For a woman who has breast cancer which has spread to other parts of the body, her risk of dying from the disease at any point in time increases 40 percent for every 1,000 grams of fat consumed monthly.[69] Of course, for any individual, there are many factors that play a role in survival. These figures were rough estimates drawn from groups of women both pre- and postmenopausal, in order to understand the magnitude of the effect of diet.

Let's compare three different diets, all of which contain 1,200 calories per day:

- On a low-fat vegetarian diet, about 10 percent of calories come from fat. This type of diet contributes about 13 grams of fat per day, or 400 grams per month.
- On a typical American diet, 37 percent of calories come from fat. This means about 49 grams of fat per day, or about 1,500 grams per month.

- On a diet with more fat than average—say, 50 percent of calories—fat intake would be 67 grams per day, or 2,000 grams per month.

If the researchers' finding holds, the typical American diet would lead to about a 40 percent higher risk of dying of breast cancer at any given point, compared to the low-fat vegetarian diet, while the high-fat diet would lead to a more than 60 percent increase in risk of dying. These figures do not mean that a woman's risk of dying in each instance is 40 percent or 60 percent. They mean that the risk is 40 percent or 60 percent higher than it would otherwise have been, assuming the individual is comparable to those studied. If, for example, a person's risk of dying, say, within five years were 35 percent on a low-fat diet, a typical American diet would boost the risk to 49 percent and the high-fat diet would boost it to 56 percent. This is not an enormous effect, but it is apparently a real one.

Other parts of the diet play important roles. Diets that are high in fiber, carbohydrate, and vitamin A seem to help the prognosis, while alcohol slightly worsens it.[74] Patients who have more estrogen receptors on their tumors (which indicates a better prognosis) tend to be those who had consumed more vitamin A.[74] For reasons that are not entirely clear, vegetables and fruits, and the vitamins they contain, help keep the cells of the body in better working order—one sign of which, for breast cells, is the presence of estrogen receptors. So vegetables and fruits are not only important in helping to prevent cancer but also in improving survival for those who have cancer.

Higher body weight increases the risk of dying of breast cancer.[73,75] Among postmenopausal women with breast cancer, slimmer women tend to have less lymph node involvement.[76] Heavier women have more lymph node involvement, higher rates of recurrence, and poorer survival.[72] It also makes a difference where the fat is on the body. One study found that, for reasons that are not clear, women who carry fat on the abdomen tend to have smaller tumors, less node involvement, and higher levels of estrogen receptors than women whose fat is proportionately more on their thighs,[76] although abdominal fat is linked to higher risk of other health problems, including heart disease, diabetes, and high blood pressure.

CANCERS OF THE UTERUS AND OVARY

The uterus and ovary, like the breast, are strongly influenced by sex hormones, and one might assume that the factors that improve survival in breast cancer might do the same for cancers of these organs. Unfortunately, aside from a smattering of research papers debating the benefits of assuring that patients get enough calories and the Recommended Daily Allowances of vitamins and minerals, researchers have essentially ignored this issue. Until more information is available, it seems most prudent for those with ovarian or uterine cancer to follow the same diet that helps prevent cancer in these organs and that keeps the immune system in good working order: a low-fat, pure vegetarian diet, with an abundance of vegetables and fruits.

PROSTATE CANCER

Diet may help improve survival in prostate cancer as well. When pathologists conduct autopsies of men over forty-five years of age who die from accidents or other causes, they find cancer cells in the prostates of about 20 percent of them.[35] These men did not know they had cancer and had no symptoms whatsoever. The prevalence of such latent cancers actually varies with location, the lowest rates being in Singapore (13 percent) and Hong Kong (16 percent), and the highest in Sweden (32 percent).[35] In most men, the cells never grow into a large tumor, never spread, and never affect life or health in any way. However, just as the prevalence of latent cancers varies from one country to the next, the likelihood that they will turn into symptomatic cancer varies in precisely the same way, suggesting that the same factors that cause cancer cells to form in the first place also encourage them to grow and spread. So while a Swede is twice as likely as a man from Hong Kong to have cancerous cells in his prostate, he is more than eight times more likely to die of prostate cancer.[35]

A low-fat, high-fiber diet can help eliminate the hormonal aberrations that are known to be linked with prostate cancer, and may help improve survival among those who have the disease. Unfortunately, there has not been enough research in this area to know just how successful dietary change might be.

Anthony J. Sattilaro was president of Methodist Hospital in Philadelphia, and became perhaps the most famous advocate of the use of diet against cancer. In his best-selling book *Recalled by Life*,[77] he raised the question as to whether diet can turn the tide on cancer, and the fact that there was simply not enough information yet available to speak with assurance.

Dr. Sattilaro was a young man when he was found to have prostate cancer. By the time it was diagnosed, it had spread throughout his body. Surgical removal was impossible; there was nothing for him to do but to get his affairs in order.

By chance, he happened to meet some young people who were advocates of macrobiotics, which is essentially a traditional Asian diet including generous amounts of rice and vegetables. There is a wealth of literature drawn from Asian traditional medicine on using diet in dealing with cancer and many other health problems. Although Sattilaro was skeptical, and initially taken aback by the idea of such a radical change in his diet, he felt he had nothing to lose. He began a macrobiotic program with the same rigidity that he had applied to his medical career. And as his book described, his symptoms began to fade. Before long, all trace of the cancer, including that on his X-rays, went away.

There were no double-blind studies, no control patients, or anything else that would suggest that what happened to Dr. Sattilaro will happen for anyone else, although there is a large cadre of people who report similar results.

I became interested in Sattilaro's story, so I went in search of him. He had resigned his job as head of Methodist Hospital and had moved to Florida. I met him in 1986. He was not only alive ten years after his anticipated death but youthful and vigorous. He had adhered to the macrobiotic diet and adopted a specific exercise program. He went swimming every day. His cancer seemed to be gone, and he kept X-ray films in a file for when he needed to remind himself of his remission. Sattilaro had been deluged with letters from other cancer patients, but always answered that he did not know if what had happened to him could also happen for them. He was not even sure that his dietary program should get the credit.

Eventually, he began to deviate from the diet, adding fish and chicken, as if to test whether he was cured or simply in remission. If it was a test, he failed. In July 1989, I called Dr. Sattilaro and found him to be gravely ill. His cancer had recurred—"viciously," he said. He was in good spirits, but harbored no illusions about the grim situation he was in. He knew that the end was very near. He had resumed the use of painkillers, which at times made him quite groggy.

Can the regimen he followed be given credit for his decade-long reprieve from cancer? Did his deviation from the diet compromise his defenses against cancer? These are questions that, while intriguing, are not answerable.

A group of patients with Kaposi's sarcoma, an AIDS-related cancer, tried the same macrobiotic diet, on the theory that a diet which boosts the immune system might help with AIDS. And it apparently helped.[78] Although AIDS patients generally lose certain types of immune cells (lymphocytes), these patients kept better lymphocyte counts. They were not cured, but their survival was improved.

Unfortunately, most AIDS patients get just the opposite. Their doctors prescribe a high-fat regimen sometimes called the "Häagen-Dazs diet" in order to counter the wasted appearance that comes with AIDS. Yet a high-fat diet would be expected to impair immunity. Obviously, no diet is a substitute for other intervention in a condition as severe as AIDS. On the other hand, it is a mistake to discount the benefits that a healthful diet might bring.

Colon Cancer and Other Cancers of the Digestive Tract

Researchers at the University of Arizona have found that people who have been treated for colon or rectal cancer have less risk of recurrence when their diets are rich in fiber. They found benefits from daily supplements of 13.5 g of wheat bran fiber (the amount in ½ cup of All Bran cereal) per day, but they speculate that other forms of fiber, such as oat bran, might have the same effect.[79] If you have bran cereal, I suggest topping it with soymilk rather than cow's milk to avoid animal fat, cholesterol, lactose, and animal proteins (see Chapter 6).

In addition, because colon cancer is encouraged by diets containing animal fat and discouraged by diets rich in vegetables, a low-fat, plant-based diet is important both for those seeking to prevent cancer and those who have already been treated for it. Vegetarian diets can easily boost fiber intake by 10 to 20 g per day.

Unfortunately, there is virtually no scientific information available on specific dietary steps to improve survival for those with other cancers of the digestive tract.

It is clear that much more needs to be learned about the power of foods to prevent cancer or to improve cancer survival. The good news is that the diet that helps protect against cancer is the same one that keeps cholesterol low and waistlines slim. Keeping animal products out of the diet, keeping oils to a minimum, and including generous amounts of vegetables, grains, beans, and fruits is a powerful prescription.

4

Real Weight Control

This chapter presents a new approach to losing weight. It is dramatically more effective than commercial diet plans. If the directions in this chapter are followed, weight control is usually permanent, without any calorie restriction.

Most diet plans are not very successful, and there are good reasons why. Many are simply too weak to get results. Others are geared only to the short term, with formulas that cause a temporary weight loss, often followed by a larger weight gain.

There is a much better way. Take Mark, for example. He was a successful businessman who traveled frequently and tended to circulate in upper-crust social circles. He was bright, well-dressed, and witty. But his weight had bothered him for years. He had been on every imaginable diet. He could lose some weight, and had many times, but could never maintain the weight loss. Like many other people, he was tempted to believe that his problem was a lack of willpower or that he had just been dealt a bad hand genetically. He had come to feel that diets were futile.

I first met Mark in July 1991. I was filming a series of medical instruction videotapes, and Mark had helped make the arrangements. At one point, we got to talking about the weight-control program in this chapter. He was skeptical at first, but decided to give it a try.

Mark's size 56 suit became a 54 suit. Then 52, 48, and on down. He called me a few months later. He had lost seventy pounds. By Christmas, he had lost more than a hundred. His suit size dropped to 44. In less than a year, his waist was sixteen inches slimmer. But what was most remarkable was that Mark was easily able to retain his progress. He bought a new set of clothes, and he can still wear them today.

Although I have changed his name, Mark is a real person. In this chapter, we first look at how old-fashioned diets failed him, and maybe let you down, too. And then we look at how to achieve permanent weight control.

The Failure of Most Diets

More than one-third of American women and one-quarter of American men are trying to lose weight. They spend $30 billion a year on diet programs and products. Often they do lose some weight. But if you check with the same people five years later, you will find that nearly all have regained most or all of whatever weight they lost. A National Institutes of Health panel sought data to show if any commercial diet program has long-term success. Not a single one could provide any. Meanwhile, frustration has spawned antidiet groups, carrying the message that people should accept being heavier than fashion might dictate.

While extreme thinness may be a twentieth-century fashion perversion, overweight is not just a cosmetic issue. It is clearly linked to cancer, diabetes, heart disease, and other health problems. It is not "natural" to be overweight. The fatty diet consumed in Western countries is not natural, the physical inactivity that is routine in America is not natural, and low-calorie dieting is neither natural nor a useful solution to the problem of overweight. The epidemic of obesity in America is the predictable result of these factors.

As we will see in detail, overweight is due primarily to the high fat content of our foods. People who consume grains, vegetables, fruits, and legumes tend to stay slim. Vegetarians are significantly slimmer than meat-eaters.[1,2,3] The typical meat-eating American gets nearly 40 percent of his or her calories from fat. Some federal programs call for a reduction to 30 percent. But both of these percentages are astronomical compared to the traditional diets of people in Asia or Latin America. A menu of grains, vegetables, fruits, and beans is easily under 10 percent fat. This is the key factor for the vast majority of overweight people. While there is gradually increasing recognition of this fact, most diet products and programs have still not quite put it to use. They still prescribe foods with a higher fat content than is advisable, and they get predictably poor results.

Diet Centers

Commercial diet centers have sprung up all across America. To their credit, most diet franchises offer more than just dietary information and food products. They also offer counseling, exercise, and other programs. Their dietary guidelines make a modest attempt at boosting complex carbohydrates by including pasta and vegetables in their meals. They also have come to appreciate the need to avoid overly restrictive calorie levels. But their food guidelines are extremely weak, and include about twice as much fat as they should.

I contacted representatives from Diet Center, Nutri/System, Jenny Craig, and Weight Watchers. For comparison, the plan I recommend, and which you will read in this book, derives about 10 percent of its calories from fat, but look at the fat content prescribed by these diet programs:

. . . .

	Fat Content
Diet Center	23%
Jenny Craig	20%
Nutri/System	30%
Weight Watchers	27%

. . . .

All have one serious flaw: they include substantial amounts of animal products and oil. The result is at least two times more fat than is optimal for weight control. The fat content of these meal plans is below that which is typical in America, but it is still too high to get good—and lasting—results.

If you patronize a franchise for its exercise or stress-reduction classes, be sure that it will allow you the flexibility to reduce the fat content of the diet and increase the carbohydrate content. The recipes in this book will help you do that. Unfortunately, some programs are extremely rigid because they are combating even worse diets in their customers.

Most frozen dietetic meals are high in fat too, but the manufacturers know that most consumers are not looking at the fat content. They are looking at the number of calories in each dinner. So they plan to put no more than 300 calories in the box, and make however small a serving is required to stay under that limit. This is a useless approach. As we shall see, it does not take advantage of what we now know about weight control.

Table 7 lists the average fat and calorie content of 25 Lean Cuisine and 23 Weight Watchers frozen entrees. Weight Watchers has a "regular" dinner line that is near 300 calories per dinner and an "Ultimate 200" line of smaller dinners that are 200 calories or less. As you can see, none of these product lines is low in fat.

Table 7   *Frozen Dinners: Small Portions, Lots of Fat*

	Fat	Calories
Lean Cuisine	25%	270
Weight Watchers	24%	275
Weight Watchers "Ultimate 200"	25%	179

SUPPLEMENTED FASTS AND HIGH-PROTEIN DIETS

Medifast, Optifast, and other high-protein formulas are designed for what their literature calls "supplemented starvation." They use a very low calorie, high-protein liquid formula instead of real food. The formulas are intended to remove all temptation to stray from the diet. Such diets can result in rapid and profound water loss, and can cause various metabolic disturbances. Older supplemented-starvation programs caused several deaths, so newer programs are designed to be used under a physician's supervision.

The maker of one program sends doctors a package of materials encouraging them to prescribe the program to patients. Prominently included is a detailed income prospectus stating that doctors could expect to pocket $15,700 *per month* in profits from selling the supplements, lab fees, and patient appointments. Also included is a newspaper article about a man who had lost ninety-two pounds on the program, with a picture in which he proudly displayed his old huge trousers. I telephoned the man. He said that while he had lost the weight at first, he had now gained about half of it back. Oprah Winfrey demonstrated the same Achilles' heel of the supplemented-starvation diets. She lost a phenomenal amount of weight, put it all back on, and became completely discouraged about any possibility of lasting weight control.

High-protein supplemented-starvation programs are impressive in the short run and disappointing in the long run. I do not recommend them. As you will see, there is a much more effective strategy. If, for whatever reason, you do begin a protein-supplemented fast, by all means do so only under a doctor's supervision.

Ultra Slim-Fast powders are made from various sugars and milk components, with added flavorings, vitamins, minerals, and fiber. They are to be mixed with low-fat milk, juice, or water, and consumed for breakfast, lunch, and as an afternoon snack, followed by a "sensible low-fat, well-balanced dinner." The three daily servings with milk supply fewer than 700 calories. The powders are fairly low in fat (16 percent), but their major nutrients are simple sugars, particularly sucrose (table sugar) and lactose. The overall program is basically an old-fashioned low-calorie diet, with supplements designed to avoid vitamin deficiencies. But as we will see, low-calorie diets don't take into account how the body works, and therefore cannot enjoy long-term success.

Some weight-loss plans, such as Dr. Atkins's *Diet Revolution,* have promoted diets that eliminate carbohydrates and push high-protein products like meat and eggs. There are several things wrong with that. First, they are not a formula for permanent weight loss. High-protein diets will cause a loss of water from the body, and fairly quickly too. But soon the weight returns because the body tissues require a certain amount of water in order to function normally. Water can be temporarily removed, but it quickly comes back. Besides, the weight that people carry in their abdomens, hips, and thighs is not mostly water, but fat.

There are also serious dangers in high-protein diets. The first is that high-protein products are usually high in fat. The "lean" beef, chicken, fish, dairy products, and eggs that are a big part of these diets are often accompanied by generous amounts of fat and cholesterol. Second, high-protein diets are strongly linked to osteoporosis and kidney disease. As we saw in Chapter 1, high-protein diets cause calcium to be lost in the urine, and may be a principal reason for osteoporosis in the United States. High-protein foods also release by-products that act as diuretics, forcing the kidneys to work much harder than they should, gradually wearing out the *nephrons,* which are the kidneys' filter units. Although we do need protein in the diet, scientists now know that the dangers of too much protein are very real indeed.

If you have a single eight-ounce serving of haddock, you eat the recommended daily allowance of protein for the whole day in that one serving. The same is true of any similar quantity of beef, pork, poultry, or other fish. Including such foods in your daily diet makes it very difficult to limit your protein intake to a safe level. The same problem applies to egg whites. Of the calories in an egg white, fully 85 percent are from protein. A person who has two eggs for breakfast gets 12 grams of protein with virtually no complex carbohydrate, no fiber, and no vitamin C.

Grains, beans, and vegetables contain more than enough protein, but not an excess. There is no need to combine these foods in any particular way. Any normal variety of plant foods provides the protein your body needs. Meats, chicken, fish, and high-protein drinks drive the protein content beyond what the body can handle safely.

Where Diets Go Wrong

If we discover that we are heavier than we want to be, there is a natural inclination to eat less food. We may skip lunch, eat only a tiny amount of our dinner, and hope that, if our body is not getting much in the way of food, it will burn off some of its fat. Many diets are based on the theory that overweight people got that way from overeating and the answer must be to cut back.

Nature will have none of this. Nature fights diets. The human body took shape millions of years ago, and at that time there were no diets. The only low-calorie event in people's lives was starvation. And those who could cope with a temporary lack of food were the ones who survived. So our bodies have built-in mechanisms to survive in the face of low food intake.

When you start a low-calorie diet, you know that you are trying to lose weight. But as far as your body is concerned, you must be starving. And biological mechanisms automatically kick into action to counter starvation. First, your metabolism slows down. Next, your body gets set to binge on the first available food. But let's take a closer look at what happens.

SLOWED METABOLISM

Our bodies are always active. Even when we are asleep, we are breathing, our blood is pumping through our veins, our body temperature is carefully monitored and regulated, and our minds are conjuring up dreams of our worries and desires. The body is expending a fair amount of effort every minute keeping its machinery in running order. When we awaken, the activities of the day demand much more of the body's energy.

To power all these activities, our bodies can use the energy of foods or the energy stored as fat. We use up these fuels the way an automobile burns gas. A car that is roaring up hills and zigzagging through traffic uses up a fair amount of gas, while a car that is idling or slowly moving along will leave a lot in the tank.

The speed at which our bodies consume energy is called the *metabolic rate*. In periods of food shortage the body slows down the metabolism to conserve energy. Just as a motorist who is running out of fuel tries to go easy on the accelerator and drive very smoothly to conserve gas, the body does the same sort of thing when food is in short supply. It turns down the metabolic flame to save as much of the fat on your body as possible until the starvation period is over, because fat is the body's fuel reserve. Body functions are turned down a bit, body temperature may fall, constipation will occur, and menstrual periods may stop.

If you go on a low-calorie diet, your body thinks you are starving. You can explain to your body that you are not trying to save your fat, you are trying to get rid of it. But your body is not listening. The more your food intake drops, the harder your body tries to keep from losing fat.[4] The effect is significant. On a 500-calorie diet, your metabolic rate can drop 15 to 20 percent below normal.[5]

This is very frustrating to dieters. They often find that, as the diet goes along, it becomes harder and harder to lose weight. Even worse, when the

Problems with Low-Calorie Diets

- Slowed metabolism
- Binges
- Unsatisfactory portions
- Persistent hunger

diet is over and they go back to eating normal portions, their slowed metabolism continues, so fat is rapidly accumulated again, often up to and beyond their starting weight. It takes weeks for the metabolism to speed up again. Researchers at the University of Pennsylvania found that five weeks after a group of individuals stopped a very low calorie diet, their metabolic rates had still not fully recovered.[5] This leads to the familiar yo-yo phenomenon, in which dieters lose some weight, then rebound to a higher weight than they started with.

The secret to keeping your metabolism from slowing is to make sure that your diet contains at least ten calories per pound of your ideal body weight. If you are aiming for a weight of 120 pounds, your daily menu should contain at least 1,200 calories. If you have less food than this, you run the risk of slowing your metabolism.

BINGES AND THE RESTRAINED-EATER PHENOMENON

The body's second defense against starvation is the binge. This is an automatic mechanism. Your body cannot differentiate a diet from a journey through the desert, where whatever food you come across could be the only food you will have for a long time. So it gets ready to take maximal advantage of any food source it finds. This is called the "restrained-eater" phenomenon.

Does this sound familiar? You have been dieting for several days. You had a tiny breakfast, skipped lunch, and then in the evening someone brings home a carton of ice cream. A little bit won't hurt, you decide as you take a taste, and before you know it you are scraping the bottom of the carton and digging around the cracks for every last bit. You then feel remorse for your "lack of willpower." The truth is that this has nothing whatsoever to do with willpower. Your body disconnected your brain, in effect, in order to accomplish a predictable biological phenomenon. Your body was operating on the assumption that the food in front of you might be the only food you would have for a while, so it demanded a binge.

Diets are not the only thing that leads to binging. Skipping meals also results in overeating later in the day. So if you have been a dieter whose self-esteem has been shot by binges, be kind to yourself. It is not a question of weak will or gluttony. The diet simply ran into something more powerful than itself—a built-in binge mechanism—and anyone would have had the same reaction.

But frequent binges can turn into bulimia: binge eating often followed by purging. Bulimia almost always begins with a diet and ends with a sense of shame and moral failing. Guilt leads to hiding food and secretiveness about eating habits, while the individual feels out of control and helpless. If this has happened to you, remember that binging is not a moral failing. It is a natural biological consequence of dieting. Many cases of bulimia would probably never occur if dieting were replaced with better food choices, which we will describe shortly.

Unfortunately, children in America are raised on a menu of fatty foods that makes many of them gain weight, especially in combination with an increasingly sedentary life-style. The predictable result is that many people become overweight. They mistakenly believe that the problem is the *quantity* of food they are eating, rather than the *type* of food, so many begin restrictive diets. The natural result is lowered metabolic rates, cravings, and binges.

Toward an Optimal Weight-Loss Menu

It is long past the time to set aside a popular misconception. This misconception is the role of the calorie. The myth is that heavy people got that way just by eating too many calories. Calories are a consideration, but overall they are not the cause of obesity in America. If you have been counting calories, it is time to throw the calorie chart away.

For the vast majority of people, overweight is caused not by *how much* they eat but by *what* they eat. Americans actually take in fewer calories each day than they did at the beginning of the century. If calories alone were the cause of overweight, we should all be thin. But we are not. Collectively, we are heavier than ever. Partly it is because we are more sedentary now. And the *content* of the American plate has changed dramatically. My grandparents ate beans, vegetables, fruits, bread, and rice; meat and butter were not everyday fare. But all that has changed. Today we eat meats—and all the fat they hold—two to three times a day, with cheese and fried foods adding even more fat. Indeed, there is 30 percent more fat in our diet today than in 1910.

You might say, so what? What difference does it make if we eat more greasy foods? It makes all the difference in the world. When researchers compare overweight people and thin people, they find that they eat roughly the same number of calories. What makes overweight people different is the amount of fat they eat.[6] Thin people generally eat less fat and more carbohydrate. As we will see shortly, fat in foods adds very easily to the fat on your body, while the carbohydrate in vegetables, grains, beans, and fruits helps your body burn up calories.

To follow are some simple but profound ideas for changing your diet that allow you to eat essentially unrestricted portions and maintain permanent control of your weight. The key is to base your menu on grains, vegetables, beans, and fruits. These foods are high in complex carbohydrate and fiber and very low in fat. But let's take a minute to see why these foods are so powerful for weight control.

Carbohydrates Boost Your Metabolism

Foods from plants are nature's only supply of complex carbohydrates. *Complex carbohydrate* is a chemists' term for molecules made up of many sugars linked together. When you eat the starchy white insides of a potato, or for that matter just about any other vegetable, the carbohydrate is gradually broken apart into simple sugars, which are absorbed and used by the body.

Not so long ago people believed that carbohydrates were fattening. Dieters would avoid starchy foods. They never went near bread, potatoes, or pasta. It turns out that carbohydrates were, in fact, innocent bystanders. People would take a piece of toast, which has only 64 calories, and slap on a pat of butter, which boosts the calorie content by more than 50 percent. Or they might take a baked potato, which has only 95 calories, and top it with a pat or two of butter, a spoonful of sour cream, some grated cheese, and some bacon bits. As they gained weight, they blamed the bread and potatoes. But the real culprits were the greasy toppings. In fact, carbohydrates are very important for permanent weight control.

For the calorie conscious, carbohydrates are naturally very low in calories. A gram (about 1/30 ounce) of carbohydrate has only 4 calories. Compare that to a gram of fat, which has 9 calories—more than twice the calorie content of carbohydrate. It is only when carbohydrate-rich foods are covered with fatty toppings that lots of calories are added.

Carbohydrate-rich meals are not just low in calories. They actually change your body. They readjust your hormones, which in turn boost your metabolism and speed the burning of calories. One of these hormones is thyroid hormone. Below your Adam's apple, your thyroid gland manufactures a hormone called *T4*, so named because it has four iodine atoms attached. This hormone has two possible fates: It can be converted into the active form of thyroid hormone called *T3*, which boosts your metabolism and keeps your body burning calories, or it can be converted to an inactive hormone, called *reverse T3*. When your diet is rich in carbohydrates, more of the T4 is converted to T3, and your metabolism gets a good boost. If your diet is low in carbohydrate, more of the T4 is turned into reverse T3, resulting in a slowed metabolism. The same thing occurs during periods of very low calorie dieting or starvation. Less of the T4 is converted to T3 and more to the useless reverse T3. This is presumably the body's way of guarding its reserves of fat; when not much food is coming in, the body conserves fat and turns down production of the fat-burning hormone, T3. But a diet generous in carbohydrates keeps T3 levels high and keeps the fat fires burning.[7,8,9]

Something similar happens with another hormone called *norepinephrine,* a relative of adrenaline. As carbohydrate-rich foods gradually release sugars into the body, more norepinephrine is produced, and it too encourages faster metabolism. Cigarettes do the same thing, which may be one reason why smokers are sometimes leaner. In an interesting experiment, researchers found that carbohydrate increases norepinephrine about the same amount as do cigarettes.[10] The moral of the story is not to have a cigarette, but rather to boost the carbohydrates in your diet. Vegetables, grains, fruits, and beans provide generous amounts of complex carbohydrates. In addition, fruits and vegetables are rich in potassium, which has been shown to boost the metabolism.[11]

Another important role of carbohydrates is that they are part of the cuing mechanism that tells the body when it has had enough food. Did you ever wonder why you stop eating? It is not just because your stomach is full. If it were, a few glasses of water would eliminate your appetite. It is also not the amount of fat in foods. If more fat were slipped into your foods, you would not find yourself responding by eating less; in fact, if you kept this up, the bathroom scale would register a bit more weight.[12] Carbohydrates are the cue the body needs to stop eating. The body adjusts the appetite based on the carbohydrate content of the meals

---

Calories in Nutrients

(per gram)

Carbohydrate	4
Protein	4
Fat	9

---

you eat. So you will eat more if there is little carbohydrate on your plate and less if there is a lot there.

Fruits contain a natural sugar called *fructose,* which may also play a role in the cuing process. Researchers found that when people consume a test dose of fructose, their appetites diminish.[13] In particular, they eat less fatty foods. It may well be that one way to cut your appetite for fatty foods is to bring home more fruit from the produce department. When you have a hankering for dessert, eat an apple, an orange, a pear, or a bowl of mixed fruit.

As we have noted, complex carbohydrates are found only in plants. Grains, vegetables, and beans are loaded with them, but there is virtually no complex carbohydrate in fish, chicken, beef, milk, or eggs. Along with carbohydrate, plants also supply fiber, which contains almost no calories, but adds texture to foods and makes them satisfying. Fiber is the part of plants that resists digestion in the small intestine—what people used to call roughage. The value of fiber was not appreciated until relatively recently, and so it was discarded in the process of refining whole-grain flour for white bread, and brown rice into white rice. Now we know that leaving the fiber in foods makes them more satisfying yet lower in calories.

To the extent that animal products or refined foods are included in the American diet, the fiber content of our foods is reduced. A healthful diet includes 30 to 40 grams of fiber each day. Yet Americans get only about half that because of their penchant for animal products and refined plant foods. When you build your menu from high-carbohydrate foods such as whole grains, beans, and vegetables, the fiber content of your diet will increase naturally.

Table 8   ## Plant Products vs. Animal Products

(Figures are percentages of calories)

Plant Products	Fat	Carbohydrate	Animal Products	Fat	Carbohydrate
Apple	5	94	Top loin	40	0
Banana	5	91	Top round	29	0
Peach	2	92	Halibut	19	0
Baked beans, vegetarian	4	89	Chicken, skinless (white)	23	0
Black beans	4	72	Roasted chicken	51	0
Broccoli	8	75	Short loin porterhouse	64	0
Peas	3	75	Atlantic cod	8	0
Potato, baked	1	93	Salmon, chinook	52	0
Spinach	7	76	"Extra lean" ground beef	54	0
Macaroni	4	85	Turkey, skinless (white)	18	0
Brown rice	5	86	Striped bass	22	0
White rice	1	89	Swordfish	30	0

Source: J. A. T. Pennington, *Bowes and Church's Food Values of Portions Commonly Used* (New York: Harper and Row, 1989).

High-Fat Plants

Nearly all foods from plants are low in fat. But the following are high in fat. Even though the fat is mostly unsaturated, it is more than you need. Figures are percentages of calories.

	Fat	Carbohydrate
Avocado	66	29
Cashews	73	23
Green olives	92	4
Sunflower seeds	77	13
Tofu	54	12

Fats: A Moment on the Lips,
Forever on the Hips

What are the most fattening foods? Meats, most dairy products, fried foods, vegetable oils, and salad dressings. What do these all have in common? They are loaded with fat, and fat is easily the most fattening part of the diet.

All fats and oils are extremely high in calories—9 calories in every gram. And fat in foods adds very easily to your fat stores. If you eat fat (animal fat or vegetable oil), it is added to your body fat with a loss of only about 3 percent of its calories in the process.[14] In contrast, if the body tries to store the energy of carbohydrates, it has to chemically convert it to fat, a process which consumes 23 percent of its calories. As an example, let's compare rice versus chicken. A ½-cup serving of rice holds 100 calories of carbohydrate. If the body tries to convert it into body fat, nearly a fourth of its calories are burned up and lost in the process. The rice contains almost no fat, only one-tenth of a gram. On the other hand, a chicken breast holds no carbohydrate at all. And nearly all the chicken fat can easily add to the fat on your body. If you were to eat two-thirds of a whole breast, you would have gotten 100 calories worth of chicken fat, only three of which are lost if it is converted to body fat. So not only are fats naturally high in calories; the calories from fat are more likely to increase body fat than are the same number of calories from carbohydrates.

To make matters worse, fatty foods have no metabolism-boosting effect. Researchers have put volunteers into experimental chambers that precisely measure how much oxygen they breathe in, how much carbon dioxide they breathe out, and how much heat their bodies generate. They have kept them in these chambers for days on end, feeding them different kinds of foods and measuring whether their metabolic rates increase or decrease. Although carbohydrates clearly boost the metabolism, fats do not.[15] A fatty meal causes no particular "burn." Part of the fat you eat is used up, and part is added to the fat stores you already have.

There are various kinds of fat. As mentioned in Chapter 2, the main categories of fat are saturated and unsaturated fat. Different kinds of fat have different effects on cholesterol levels. But for *weight control*, we need to be concerned about *all* forms of fat. As far as your waistline is concerned, animal fat is no better or worse than vegetable oil. Let's look at both.

ANIMAL FAT

Animal fat is an obvious problem. It was designed by nature specifically to store calories. The fat in beef, pork, chicken, or fish is the calorie-storage area of that animal. So if you eat animal fat, you are eating all those densely packed calories.

Many people have the misconception that if they trim the fat off the outside of a piece of meat, they have got rid of its fat. But because meats contain virtually no carbohydrate and no fiber, their main nutrients are protein and fat. Imagine that you took a sponge and poured oil into it, soaking the sponge with grease. Now, if you were to take one paper towel after another and wipe off the surface of the sponge, you would remove some grease, but the sponge would still be saturated with it. This is about what happens when people try to trim the fat from meats. You can remove some of the external fat, but it is impossible to remove the fat that permeates the cut of meat. If you are eating meat, you are eating another animal's fat and another animal's stored calories. Let's take some examples. For comparison, potatoes and rice are each about 1 percent fat; legumes such as peas or beans are only 3 to 4 percent fat; and most other vegetables tend to range between 5 and 10 percent fat (as a percentage of calories). In contrast, ground beef is about 60 percent fat. "Extra-lean" ground beef is not really so lean: 54 percent of its calories are from fat. Even the skinniest six beef specimens selected for the beef industry's "lean" advertisements could not find any cuts of meat that are anywhere near the fat content of beans, grains, or vegetables: round tip is 36 percent fat, top loin is 40 percent fat, top round is 29 percent fat. At its lowest, beef is still around 30 percent fat, which is several times the fat content of grains, vegetables, beans, and fruits. "Lean meat" is a contradiction in terms.

In the kitchen, the difference is even more obvious. Let's say we are making tacos using two different recipes for taco filling—one is made with ground beef and the other with beans. Three ounces of ground beef have about 225 calories. Beans, on the other hand, are very low in fat, and so three ounces of cooked beans have only about 110 calories. Which recipe do you follow to lose weight? And when you are eating out, any taco restaurant in the country will gladly substitute a bean filling for a meat one. It's cheaper for them, and it's better for you.

Let's say you are preparing a spaghetti dinner. A 1-cup serving of spaghetti topped with ½ cup of tomato sauce has about 200 calories. But if we add ground beef to the sauce, the dinner now has *365* calories. The ground beef has no carbohydrate at all and lots of fat, so it contributes a lot of calories.

The animal fat in dairy products is a big calorie booster, too. Look at what a little butter can do. A 1-cup serving of mashed potatoes made without butter or milk has 140 calories. Add a tablespoon of butter and what happens? Suddenly it holds nearly 250 calories.

Chicken producers have hoped that consumers would reject beef and choose their products instead. But chicken is no health food. The worst of the lot is the chicken frank, which weighs in at 68 percent fat. Roast chicken is 51 percent fat. Well, you may be asking, how about if I strip off the skin, throw away the dark meat, and use a nonfat cooking method? Even then, chicken is still 23 percent fat (plus 85 mg cholesterol in a 3.5 oz. serving), which is much higher than most grains, vegetables, fruits, and beans. The point is that chicken is much more like beef than it is like vegetables. It contains no carbohydrate or fiber, and it pushes these foods off your plate. As far as weight control is concerned, no matter how it is prepared, chicken lacks the power of a truly healthful food.

Fish has gotten more attention recently, particularly in discussions about cholesterol. But as far as your weight is concerned, fish fat is like any other fat: it contains 9 calories per gram. Of course, different types of fish differ greatly in fat content, ranging from high-fat varieties like salmon, to varieties like sole or haddock, which are similar to vegetables in fat content. That is their only similarity to vegetables, however. In all other respects, sole and haddock are typical animal muscles: no complex carbohydrates, no fiber, and a tendency to displace these foods from the diet. Plus, they contain significant amounts of cholesterol, far too much protein, and for many varieties serious contamination problems. So fish is not a health food, although certain types of fish are much lower in fat than are beef and poultry.

In summary, meats, poultry, and fish have two main problems for those concerned about their weight. First, they are muscles, and muscles are made up of protein and fat. Second, they contain no fiber at all and virtually no carbohydrate. So they not only give you a load of fat you don't want but also displace the fiber and carbohydrates that are essential to a satisfying and metabolism-boosting menu. Vegetarian foods—grains, vegetables, fruits, and legumes—are power foods for weight control.

VEGETABLE OILS ARE FATTENING TOO

In their defense, vegetable oils have no cholesterol and most are low in saturated fats compared to animal fats. But their calorie content is the same as any other kind of fat: 9 calories in every gram. All fats and oils are packed with calories, and it is no good becoming a vegetarian if meats are replaced with french fries.

Let's take an example. Only about 1 percent of the calories in a potato is from fat. And if it is baked or mashed, no extra oil is added. But let's say we cut a potato into french fries and drop it into some hot oil. Its fat content soars to 40 percent or more, while its calorie content doubles or even triples.

Here's another example. Doughnuts are fried and bagels are not. Which do you think have more fat? No contest. Half the calories in the doughnut are from fat, while the bagel's calories are only 8 percent from fat. Of course, if you add cream cheese or margarine to the bagel, the fat and calorie content quickly climbs.

Baked goods can be either very low or very high in fat. Bagels, pretzels, and many breads are quite low. On the other hand, croissants, cakes, pies, and cookies are usually loaded with fat. If you are baking, it is often easy to modify recipes, as we will see in Chapter 8. If you are buying commercial baked goods, check the label. Fat content is usually listed.

Tips for interpreting labels are given on page 102. If the fat content is not specifically listed, check the ingredients. These are listed in decreasing order of quantity, so if oil is one of the first ingredients, there is more of it than if it is one of the last items. The nutrition information label from a bag of potato chips is shown on page 102. What is important is the *percentage of calories* that comes from fat. This is easy to check. The top line of the label shows that there are 260 calories in one serving. Next to this, we see that 140 of these calories come from fat. To calculate the percentage, we simply divide the calories from fat by the total calories and then multiply by 100.

$$\frac{140}{260} \times 100 = 54\%$$

This means that a whopping 54 percent of the calories in these potato chips come from nothing but waist-padding fat. Potatoes themselves are nearly

Nutrition Facts

Serving Size 1 bag (50g/about 35 chips)
Servings per Container 1

Amount Per Serving

Claories 260	**Calories from Fat** 140

Total Fat 16g	
Saturated Fat 4g	
Cholesterol 0mg	
Sodium 170mg	
Potassium 650 mg	
Total Carbohydrates 24g	
Dietary Fiber 1g	
Sugars less than 1g	
Protein 3g	

fat-free, but when they are deep-fried they soak up an enormous amount of grease.

Salad dressings are another potential minefield—they can be packed with fat. Let's say we chop up a cup of romaine lettuce and half a tomato. So far, this has only 20 calories. But if we add a tablespoon of Catalina French dressing, the dressing is 76 percent fat and has more than three times the

What a Difference a Little Fat Makes!

(percentage of calories from fat)

Low-fat		High-fat	
Baked potato	1%	French fries	47%
Plain bagel	8%	Doughnut	50%
Plain popcorn	12%	Popcorn with butter	44%
Steamed cauliflower	6%	Cauliflower w/ cheese sauce	48%
Nonfat Catalina dressing	0%	Regular Catalina dressing	76%

calorie content of the salad it covered. Other dressings are as bad or worse: Good Seasons Zesty Italian is 95 percent fat: one tablespoon has 9 grams of fat and 85 calories. Even typical oil and vinegar has about 8 grams of fat and 72 calories per tablespoon.

For a better alternative, use a low-fat or no-fat dressing, now available at the grocery store, often sold in the dietetic foods section. Or sprinkle a little lemon or lime juice on your salad or vegetables. A tablespoon of lemon or lime juice has no fat and only 4 calories. Many people come to actually prefer the taste of fresh spinach, chickpeas, tomatoes, or other salad ingredients with no dressing at all.

One has to wonder why we are compelled to take perfectly innocent salads and vegetables and grease them all up. Why is it that a beautiful salad of deep green leaves with diced onion and tomato, green peppers, and chickpeas is not considered edible until spiced oil is poured on top? Why is

---

Best Bets for Nonfat Salad Dressings

Nonfat dressings are much better than regular varieties, which often have oil as their main ingredient. But read the label—some supposedly low-fat dressings have almost as much fat as the regular varieties. The following all have zero fat:

Lemon juice

Lime juice

Pritikin Italian

Pritikin French Style

Pritikin Garlic & Herb

Kraft Free French

Kraft Free Thousand Island

Kraft Free Catalina

Wish-Bone Healthy Sensation Thousand Island

Wish-Bone Healthy Sensation Italian

toast always topped with butter, a bagel with cream cheese, or a potato with butter and sour cream? We add flavored grease to many otherwise healthful foods.

Vegetarian Foods Are the Weight-Control Champs

So far we have looked at the different ways in which carbohydrates, fat, and fiber affect the body. If you like, you can forget about terms like carbohydrate and fiber. If your diet is made from grains, beans, vegetables, and fruits rather than from animal products, it will be naturally rich in both. Only a very few plant foods—avocados, nuts, seeds, olives, and some soy products—are high in fat. Other plants have a strikingly healthful profile: very low in fat and rich in complex carbohydrates. To the extent that animal products are added to your plate, complex carbohydrates and fiber are left off. Some supposedly dietetic commercial dinners include animal products, such as meat and cheese, but the most effective weight-control menus are vegetarian. For a comparison of plant and animal products, see Table 8.

Researchers have put vegetarians on the scale and found, not surprisingly, that the average pure vegetarian weighs substantially less than the average meat-eater.[1] If vegetarians also keep vegetable oil to an absolute minimum, their diet is even more powerful for weight control.

Some people who are still eating pork chops and beef instead of grains, vegetables, fruits, and legumes actually add concentrated fiber, such as Metamucil or oat bran, to their foods, trying to counteract the constipation, elevated cholesterol, and other effects of the fiber-depleted foods they are eating. They may also take vitamin supplements and try to mend their diets in other ways. But these repair measures are poor substitutes for truly healthful diets, as the rest of this book demonstrates.

Because Americans grow up eating meats, dairy products, and fried foods, fat contributes about 37 percent of the calories most of us get every day. For a typical 2,000-calorie menu, that is 740 calories each day just from fat.

A menu of grains, beans, vegetables, and fruits naturally contains only about 10 percent fat. That means that a huge number of calories have been eliminated from your diet. Let me give you a couple of figures. Over the course of a year, a standard American diet holds 270,000 calories of pure fat. A 10 percent fat diet based on grains, vegetables, fruits, and legumes cuts that figure to 73,000. Now, you can make up for some of that difference by eating other foods. But when the menu is naturally low in fat, a person can eat much larger portions without gaining weight.

When Dr. Dean Ornish puts patients on a low-fat vegetarian diet, along with an exercise program and other life-style modifications, his target is their heart problems. But these patients also lose a lot of weight. In fact, the average patient loses more than twenty pounds in the first year. "One patient lost almost a hundred pounds during the course of a year," Ornish said. They were not necessarily trying to lose weight. Dr. Ornish did not restrict the amount of food his patients ate. They could eat anytime they wanted and as much as they wanted, and they still lost weight.

"It's a different concept of dieting than most people are used to. In most diets, you still eat the same types of food, but you restrict the amount. So you're eating maybe a 30 percent fat or 40 percent fat diet, but you restrict the portion sizes, and people generally go around feeling pretty hungry. Sooner or later people get tired of feeling hungry. They go off the diet, they often gain most of the weight back, and then they feel even worse."

Dr. Ornish's program is just the opposite. "This is a diet based more on the type of food than on the amount of food. Within these guidelines, a person can eat whenever he or she is hungry. They often eat more frequently than before, and often even eat larger portion sizes than they did before. And yet, because the diet is so low in fat, they often lose weight."

An average weight loss of more than twenty pounds, with no calorie restriction, may be surprising to many people, but it is not unusual with low-fat vegetarian menus.

"They don't just keep losing," Dr. Ornish said. "They come down to something approaching their ideal body weight, and then they stabilize."

Similarly, international comparisons have shown that people who eat very low fat foods can eat more while staying slimmer. In detailed studies of sixty-five Chinese provinces, Dr. T. Colin Campbell of Cornell University found that the Chinese diet helps people stay slim. Is that because they are starving? Hardly. They actually eat more than Americans do.

"The quantity is actually greater than what we tend to consume in this country," Dr. Campbell said. "They consume a lot of rice, of course, enormous amounts of rice and some other grains. The total amount of food they consume is actually greater than what it is here."

Again, it's not *how much* you eat, it's *what* you eat. The grains and vegetables that make up the Chinese diet give it little fat and generous amounts of complex carbohydrates.

"On average, the fat intake as we measured it is 15 percent of calories, which is quite substantially below what we have in this country," Campbell said. Typical fat consumption in China ranges between 6 and 24 percent of calories.

When I was growing up, American parents tried to cajole their children into eating their dinner with images of "all the starving people in China." Well, the Chinese actually eat more than we do. And because their diets are so high in plant foods and low in fat, they stay slim while we go to Weight Watchers. The Chinese are also more physically active, which we will discuss shortly.

Once people are used to fatty foods, they tend to crave them, unfortunately. It seems that we have a "set-point" for fat. We get used to having a certain amount of fat in foods. If we get too much, we do not like it, and if we have less, we feel deprived. If we are used to butter on our potato, it seems bland without it. If we are used to having toast that drips with butter, we miss it when it's gone.

What I have found, however, is that these set-points are easy to change. For example, if you were to have a salad with no dressing at all, it would seem a little strange at first, but within just a few times of trying it this way, you would come to prefer it. Having set this new habit, you will find it strange to have salad oil added.

You can try the same sort of test with popcorn. If you are used to having butter on your popcorn, the first time you have it without butter it will taste bland. But if you have it several times without butter, you will become accustomed to the lighter taste, and buttered popcorn will then taste greasy.

For most people, the process of adjustment takes a few weeks. At the beginning, you may wake up in the night screaming for lard-covered doughnuts and chocolate fish sticks. But before long you'll reset your taste for fat to a new lower level. You will wonder how Americans can stand all the grease they consume and why they resign themselves to the health problems that are its predictable result. But don't tease yourself. I find that it is easier to cut out meats, chicken, fish, and fried foods *entirely*, and to set a new habit that leaves them out, than to tease yourself with occasional greasy foods. Many people experience such extraordinary health benefits from this dietary change that they never want to go back to greasy foods, even if they were not fattening.

Of course, we do need some fat in the diet. A healthful menu of grains, legumes, vegetables, and fruits, with only rare use of additional oils, will derive about 10 percent of its calories from fat. Even this is more than the body needs. Some doctors hold that children can (and perhaps should) have a bit more fat in their diet than is recommended for adults. It is risky to go too far with this, however. By the age of four or five, children get hooked on chicken nuggets and all the other greasy foods that spell obesity, cancer, and heart disease a few decades later. Ten to 15 percent of calories from fat is more than enough at any age, and at higher levels health problems are more likely.

There is no doubt which menu is the most powerful for cutting the fat: vegetarian foods are free of the animal fat that permeates meats, poultry, and fish. Staying away from fried foods and added oils is the other half of the food prescription. Although this sounds like a big change (and it is), there is a world of healthful foods waiting to fill the bill. Pasta dishes like linguine with a light basil sauce or spaghetti with tomato sauce, vegetable curries, bean burritos, and other vegetable entrees are ready to help you burn off the pounds.

Artificial Fats

Manufacturers are starting to push products that gratify the taste for fat without adding calories. The NutraSweet Company has launched Simplesse, which actually is a protein that simulates the texture of fat on the tongue. Simplesse cannot be used in baked or fried foods, however, because its consistency changes when heated. Procter and Gamble has developed Olestra, an indigestible and unabsorbable sucrose polyester designed to taste like fat. Is it safer than other chemical additives? This is still a matter of vigorous dispute, as some contend that Olestra may cause cancer and liver problems.

Fake fats may be a shot in the arm for manufacturers, but they are no answer to America's weight problems. Not only is their safety in doubt, but these additives reinforce the taste for fatty foods rather than help you break the habit.

Extra Calories in Alcohol

Alcohol's reputation continues to decline in health circles. The findings that alcohol increases the risk of breast cancer and birth defects, and contributes to many other very serious health problems, has cast a long shadow over the idea that a glass or two of wine might be good for your heart.

For some people, at least, alcohol adds to the padding on the waistline. Six ounces of wine adds about 130 calories to your dinner. One beer contains about 150 calories, light brands about 100. A 1½-ounce jigger of typical 100-proof liquor has 124 calories. In addition, alcohol temporarily alters body chemistry to impair the body's ability to burn off fat.[15] And for some people alcohol does not displace other calories. If you were to have a typical soda before dinner, the 155 calories it contains would cause you to eat slightly less at dinner, so that your overall calorie intake remains fairly constant. Some people use this same sort of compensatory mechanism with alcohol, but others do not. If they have a beer before dinner, the 150 calories it supplies are not compensated for by eating less later. Instead, the calories in alcohol *add* to their total.[16]

For alcoholics, things are very different. Alcoholism often causes people to consume less food, because in this disease alcohol disrupts the normal cues that regulate eating patterns. Alcoholics tend to be deficient in a host of nutrients.

Sweets: A Trojan Horse for Grease

Jelly beans, gum drops, and hard candies are just chunks of simple sugars, with no fiber. They are the most concentrated form of calories that can be found in a carbohydrate food. If you have a sweet tooth, you may well get more calories than the body needs. Even so, sugars are not nearly as calorie-dense as fats, and many people mistakenly attribute their weight problems to sugar, when in fact the problem stems from fat.

Sugars often act as a Trojan Horse for fat. Coconut cream pie may be sweet, but most of the calories are not from sugar, they are from fat—57 percent, to be exact. Häagen-Dazs ice cream runs between 50 and 70 percent fat. A Mr. Goodbar is a Mr. Fatbar: 59 percent of its calories come from fat. And a Hershey's Whatchamacallit bar is 50 percent you-know-what.

On the other hand, if your sweet food were a peach, it would be just 2 percent fat. An apple is 6 percent.

ARTIFICIAL SWEETENERS

What about artificial sweeteners? NutraSweet and saccharin have been huge commercial successes. But chemical sweeteners are no substitute for genuine dietary change. Many people consume beef, chicken, and french fries, and then use a diet soda to try to compensate. But they cannot undo the damage of a fatty diet. Replacing a teaspoon of sugar with a chemical sweetener saves you 16 calories. But just 2 grams of fat hold more calories than that teaspoon of sugar. This is not to say that sugar is a health food. The point is that artificial sweeteners are no substitute for what has to be done if permanent weight control is your goal, and that is to throw out the fatty foods and bring in the grains, vegetables, fruits, and legumes.

Normally, the body knows to stop eating when its nutrient needs are met. However, artificial sweeteners do not cue the body that it is time to stop eating. So an artificially sweetened food or beverage is likely to be followed with something else. Some scientific studies have shown that aspartame (the sweetener sold under the name NutraSweet) actually increases the appetite, although others have contradicted this finding.[17-22]

Chemical sweeteners also pose potential health risks. Cyclamates and saccharin have both been under suspicion for their cancer-causing potential. Some have suggested that NutraSweet may cause headaches and grand-mal seizures. There are also case reports of children whose behavior has become extraordinarily disturbed after drinking aspartame-flavored beverages. Others have concluded that, for most people, aspartame is safe. But while the toxicologists fight it out, there is little reason to be part of the experiment. This is particularly true for children and for pregnant women.

It is hard to find anything good to say about synthetic sweeteners. Their main benefit is to their stockholders, not to the consumer. People struggling with weight problems get no miracle cure from artificial sweeteners.

Overeating

Most people with weight problems do not overeat. They are the victims of a high-fat diet coupled with a sedentary life-style. In fact, they may well eat less than do thin people. Nevertheless some people do overeat.

We already looked at one kind of overeating, the restrained-eater phenomenon. If you have been trying to stick to a very low calorie diet, you are set up for the restrained-eater phenomenon. It is your body's attempt, in the midst of what it perceives as starvation, to take advantage of whatever food source becomes available. The result is a binge, often followed by enormous guilt. The answer is to avoid skimpy diets. There is no reason for such diets, anyway. The diet recommended in this book promotes natural and permanent weight control without calorie restriction.

A second form of overeating is carbohydrate craving, which has received a great deal of publicity from Judith Wurtman, who, along with her husband, Richard Wurtman, and other researchers at Massachusetts Institute of Technology in Cambridge, Massachusetts, broke new ground in showing how foods affect the brain.

Carbohydrate cravers can put away enormous amounts of carbohydrate-rich snacks. The foods can be sweet or starchy—taste is not the issue. The reason they consume these snacks is because, without them, they slump into depression. Carbohydrate cravers tend to become depressed in the winter months when the days are short, and foods may help normalize their brain chemistry.

Carbohydrates can increase a brain chemical called *serotonin,* which helps regulate moods, sleep, and other brain functions. The biological process involves several steps. During digestion, carbohydrates break down into simple sugars, which in turn stimulate the body to release insulin, which helps sugar pass from the bloodstream into the cells of the body. Insulin has the same effect on amino acids, which are the building blocks of protein, escorting them out of the bloodstream and into the cells. So after a carbohydrate-rich meal, insulin moves the sugar and the amino acids out of the blood and into the cells. As all this is happening, one particular amino acid is left behind in the bloodstream. It is called *tryptophan.* Without all the other amino acids around, tryptophan has less competition in getting into the brain, which is exactly what it then does. In the brain, tryptophan is converted into serotonin, a brain chemical which plays a very important role in your moods. One way many antidepressants work is to increase the amount of serotonin in the brain. Serotonin is also important in sleep, which is why you may have heard of people taking tryptophan supplements as a sleeping pill before they were withdrawn from the market, owing to what seems to have been a poisonous manufacturing contaminant. (The tryptophan found naturally in foods is safe.)

It turns out that carbohydrate-rich foods affect different people differently. Some people feel sleepy after they eat sugary foods. Others get grumpy. For particularly sensitive people, modest amounts of any sugar (even fruit sugars) can set off a depressed mood. Carbohydrate cravers, on the other hand, feel better when they have sugar or complex carbohydrates.

There is nothing wrong with eating carbohydrate-rich foods. Just the opposite, carbohydrates are essential for good health. But there are two keys for carbohydrate cravers: first, select foods rich in complex carbohydrates—such as rice and other grains, beans, and vegetables—rather than sugar candies. Second, steer clear of high-fat foods—pies, cakes, and cookies. These sugar-fat mixtures can add to weight problems.

Compulsive Eating

Compulsive eating is as painful as any other addiction. While most people with weight problems are not compulsive eaters, some are, and there are ways they can help themselves. Author Victoria Moran knew this problem intimately. She was on the binge-diet merry-go-round for years before she found her way off. She wrote a book called *The Love-Powered Diet*.[23] Of the various approaches to the problem, hers actually works. There are three key elements:

1. *Recognize the problem.* Look at how you handle eating. "Do you hide food?" Moran asks. "Do you sneak food? Do you eat one way when you're by yourself, another way when you're with other people?" Do you eat when you are not at all hungry? Do you eat in response to stress, anxiety, sadness, or anger? The biggest problem in recognizing compulsive eating is denial. Like any addiction, the victim can engage in nearly endless self-deception. However, once the problem is recognized, the solution is not so far away.

2. *Stick to the New Four Food Groups.* The New Four Food Groups allow people with weight problems to do something that they may never have been able to do before. "You can throw out the food scale, and throw out the calculator," Moran said. "You don't need to count anything anymore, because the food is low in fat and high in fiber." That's right. And throw out the calorie chart, too, because grains, vegetables, fruits, and legumes are naturally modest in calories. Animal products and oils, on the other hand, tend to be fattening and lead to the stingy-portion diets that are now customary in weight-loss programs.

3. *Try Overeaters Anonymous.* Treat compulsive eating as you would any other addiction. Doctors learned long ago that there was no program for addictions that had anywhere near the power of Alcoholics Anonymous and the analogous programs that address other habits. For compulsive eaters, there is no program better than Overeaters Anonymous. O.A. does not spell out a particular diet. It helps its participants break their food addictions through a twelve-step program.

"I recommend Overeaters Anonymous very strongly," Moran said. "Changing any habit is difficult, and it's always good to have support, but when you're dealing with an addiction, support is absolutely essential. You can call someone at any time of the day or night. There's also no charge for O.A., so if a person goes for six or eight meetings and says, 'This is not for me,' there's nothing to lose.

"The first step of the twelve steps that were originated by Alcoholics Anonymous is to admit powerlessness—over alcohol, food, unhealthy relationships, or whatever the problem is. That's a very interesting step to take, because when I say that I am powerless over food, or the way that I deal with food, then I am at a fork in the road. I have to take one path or the other. One is to allow the addiction to kill me, physically or emotionally: I'm going to die early, or at least have a miserable life for as long as I do live.

"But there's another road, and that is this: If I can't help myself, then there has to be some other power that can come in and take over where my weary will power no longer works. If you are a food addict of long standing, or someone who doesn't think it's terribly serious but who just can't change on his or her own, then you need a power that's stronger than your will. So that's the beginning: admit there's a problem, and just toy with the idea that perhaps there is some help that doesn't come from your own will power."

Overeaters Anonymous is listed in the phone book. Or write to P.O. Box 92870, Los Angeles, California 90009, for information on a meeting near you.

The secret to beating compulsive eating is, first, to recognize the problem. Then, use the combination of dietary change, including the New Four Food Groups, plus inner change through the support of Overeaters Anonymous. For the compulsive eater, dietary change alone is not sufficient, and psychological growth without better dietary habits is not enough either, as Moran notes: "I've had someone come up to me after a talk I'd given and say, 'I'm a registered dietitian, but I binge and throw up every night.' And I thought, this person needs to know about inner change. But I have also known people who were in Overeaters Anonymous who were no longer eating for a fix, whose lives had really turned around, yet who would carry little food scales to restaurants."

The combination of inner transformation and better food choices is the winning combination. "You can have freedom when it comes to food. You also get a happier, healthier life overall. It's a real gift. The beauty of this is that, even recovering compulsive eaters who may think, 'I'll never be able to enjoy food again' find out, 'Maybe I never enjoyed food before.' "

Use Your Body

A key to staying slim is physical activity. Unfortunately, our bodies are neglected. Many of us spend all day at a desk, all evening in front of the television, and we drive back and forth between the two. Does your body complain, "You never take me anywhere. When we were young, you used to take me out to tear up the town, but now we never do anything"? If you and your body have become a tired old couple, it is time to get to know each other again.

The physical activities that got our blood moving when we were younger tend to fall by the wayside as we grow older. And those who recognize a need to "burn off some calories" often feel daunted by the images it brings to mind: huffing and puffing down the road with other joggers, most of whom look totally miserable. I am not recommending jogging or weight-lifting or aerobic exercises to rock-and-roll music, unless you particularly enjoy these activities. I am recommending something quite different from exercise. But first, let's review what physical activity does that makes it so powerful for weight control.

First, all physical activity burns calories. Every movement of your body uses up some energy, and the more you move, the more calories you burn.

Second, when you are physically active, your body readjusts your metabolism to burn calories more quickly. This effect persists for a time even beyond the period of activity.

Third, when you stay active, your muscles keep their strength. If you do not, your muscles waste away from inactivity. This is important because your muscles are real calorie burners. Muscle tissue has a rapid metabolism and is much better than fat tissue at burning off the calories we ingest.

Fourth, physical activity helps keep the appetite under control. After a tennis game or an hour on the dance floor, people are actually less likely to overeat, even though they have just burned off a lot of calories. This mechanism helps you stay slim after you have shed unwanted pounds, but unfortunately will not help as you are losing weight. While you are overweight, your appetite is not likely to be affected by your physical activity.[24]

Fifth, people who use their bodies are better able to relax, and more likely to get a good night's sleep. This is important, because when you are chronically tired or stressed, you are much more likely to use unhealthful foods or other indulgences to prop yourself up.

Just as there are foods that naturally work to keep you slim, there are physical activities that do the same. The most important ingredient in any physical activity is enjoyment. If it is not fun, you won't stick with it. Physical activities do not need to be particularly strenuous, and they certainly do not have to be unpleasant. Remember, you can burn up all the gas in your tank in either a high-speed chase or a leisurely drive. The same is true of the fat your body has been storing. The simple program in Appendix I will help you get going. It is very easy, and it really works.

If a low-calorie diet has slowed your metabolism, change your dietary habits before you dramatically increase your physical activity. Even though physical activity increases the metabolic rate for most people, it can actually have the opposite effect on people who have been on severe diets.

It's Not All Genetic

For better or for worse, genetics does play a role in our size and shape. If your parents were tall, you are likely to be tall. If they were heavy-set, particularly early in life, you may well have the same tendency. The role of genetics has been clearly demonstrated in studies of identical twins who were raised apart. Their ultimate weights tend to be rather similar, in spite of differences in the diets of the families who raised them.[25] Genetics is not everything—they don't have identical weights—but there is clearly a tendency toward a similar body size.

We tend to inherit not just our size but our shape, too. If your parents and grandparents were apple-shaped, carrying their weight in their chests and abdomens, you are likely to be apple-shaped. If they were pears, carrying their weight in their hips and thighs, you are likely to have the same tendency.

Apples are more likely to have health problems, including heart problems, high blood pressure, and diabetes, as a result of their weight. To check whether weight problems will affect your health, take a tape measure and measure your waist and then the widest point of your hips. For women, if your waist is more than 80 percent of your hip measurement, your weight will add to your risk of heart disease, cancer, diabetes, and other problems. For men, health risks begin when your waist is bigger than your hips. Hip fat is less likely to contribute to health problems compared to abdominal fat, but unfortunately it is harder to get rid of.

As you lose weight, your size will change, but your basic shape may not; you may become a skinny pear, but you'll still be a pear.

Although genetics does affect size and shape, it is certainly not the last word. We give our children a lot more than just DNA. We give them recipes. We give them preferences for food that take hold at a very young age. We pass along our attitudes about the importance of food and its meaning. In my family, food was not a particularly important part of our family life, and was never used as a cure for depression or a reward for accomplishment. But for other families, food plays a central role in family matters, and love, nurturance, and rebellion can all take place between the spoon and the mouth. So when something "runs in the family," that does not necessarily mean it is coded on your chromosomes.

The Keys to Permanent Weight Control

What makes us grow heavy are diets centered on meats, dairy products, fried foods, and oils. Fat in foods adds all too easily to our own fat stores, and does not boost our calorie-burning mechanisms. Refined sugars and alcohol conspire against us, too. These foods give us lots of calories, without the complex carbohydrates and fiber that can help us stay slim.

Low-calorie dieting is no solution because it slows your metabolism and makes binges more likely. The answer for permanent weight control is, first, to build your diet from grains, vegetables, fruits, and beans. These foods are more powerful than any weight-loss diet. Most people can eat all they want, any time they want, and stay slim. If you really are overeating, you can help yourself overcome this, as many others have.

And don't forget to take your body for a walk, a game of tennis, or a night on the dance floor. You'll love the new you.

A Weight-Control Plan that Works

1. Build your menu from grains, vegetables, fruits, and legumes, as detailed in Chapters 6 through 8.

2. Use generous amounts of rice, using the recipe on page 252.

3. Include generous amounts of vegetables, including raw vegetables, such as carrots, fresh greens, and cucumbers.

4. Eliminate all animal products.

5. Keep vegetable oils to a minimum.

6. Add regular physical activity to your routine. Start with a half-hour walk every day or one-hour walk three times a week, or substitute any equivalent activity. See page 299.

5

Surprising New Leads with the New Four Food Groups

So far we have seen a powerful menu for lowering cholesterol, staying slim, preventing cancer, and maybe even slowing the effects of aging. But that is really only the beginning. Many other conditions never well addressed by previous diets are improved, prevented, or reversed by the low-fat New Four Food Groups program. Adult-onset diabetes can often go away, appendicitis and varicose veins can usually be prevented, and the course of multiple sclerosis can be changed substantially. Arthritis can, in many cases, be improved. And if you have been consuming milk and antacids for an ulcer, here's a new two-week treatment that cures ulcers in most patients. In this chapter we look at these and other surprising facts.

Arthritis

Arthritis means painful and swollen joints for millions of people. Arthritis is actually a group of very different diseases. Osteoarthritis is a gradual loss of cartilage and overgrowth of bone in the joints, especially the knees, hips, spine, and fingertips, apparently caused by accumulated wear and tear. At least 85 percent of the population above the age of seventy has osteoarthritis. Unlike rheumatoid arthritis, osteoarthritis causes only transient stiffness and usually does not cause major interference with the use of the hands, although it can cause painful episodes.

Rheumatoid arthritis is a more aggressive form of the disease, affecting over 2 million people. It causes painful, inflamed joints, and sometimes leads to severe joint damage. Rheumatoid arthritis is one of medicine's mysteries.

117

For one thing, the disease seems to be relatively new. There were no medical reports of the disease until the early 1800s; skeletons unearthed from medieval cemeteries have shown no signs of it. Some have suspected that a virus or bacterium may play a role, perhaps by setting off an autoimmune reaction. There may also be a role for genetics, perhaps in causing a susceptibility to the disease.

For years, people have suspected that foods play a role in causing rheumatoid arthritis. Many have noticed that their joints feel better when they steer clear of dairy products, citrus fruits, tomatoes, eggplant, or certain other foods.

Not long ago, I was giving a series of lectures and interviews in the Midwest. A woman who was driving me from one appearance to another told me that she had had painful arthritis. Now she was a picture of health, thin and athletic looking, and her arthritis was totally gone. What had made the difference? Dairy products were the culprit. When she left them out of her diet, her arthritis went away completely.

Shortly thereafter, my schedule brought me through Wisconsin. There I met another woman who also told me that her arthritis was clearly linked to dairy products. It pained her to say so, because she had been raised on a Wisconsin dairy farm. But she learned that staying away from dairy products was the key to getting rid of her symptoms.

Other foods have been blamed as well. A 1989 survey of over a thousand arthritis patients revealed foods they felt were most associated with their symptoms: red meat, sugar, fats, salt, caffeine, and nightshade plants (e.g., tomatoes, eggplant).[1]

At first, scientific studies did not find that eliminating such foods helped substantial numbers of people. So doctors stuck to using anti-inflammatory medications and painkillers in what is usually a losing battle against joint damage. However, an increasing number of research reports show that certain dietary changes are, in fact, helpful.

For instance, diets that boost polyunsaturated oils and add omega-3 supplements have a mild beneficial effect, and researchers have found benefits from vegan diets.[2] Diets that include dairy products are not helpful,[3] and diets that boost saturated animal fat cause arthritis to get worse.[4] Several studies have shown that supervised fasting can be helpful.[5]

A team of Scandinavian researchers hit upon a regimen that produced significant improvements in rheumatoid arthritis. The number of tender or swollen joints diminished, morning stiffness decreased, grip strength improved, and blood tests used in the assessment of arthritis also improved, although X-rays of the joints did not. The program was carefully tested in a comparison with standard medical treatment. *The Lancet,* a prominent British medical journal, published the report as its lead article on October 12, 1991.[5] Here is the treatment program the research team used.

The patients first began a modified fast for seven to ten days. During this period, they consumed herbal teas, garlic, vegetable broths, and juice extracts from carrots, beets, and celery. No fruit juices were allowed.

After the fast, the patients reintroduced a "new" food item to their diet every other day. If they had any worsening of symptoms during the following two days, this item was eliminated for at least seven days. If the item was introduced again, and again caused worsening of symptoms, it was omitted permanently.

For the first three to five months, they eliminated meat, fish, eggs, dairy products, gluten (a wheat product), refined sugar, and citrus fruits. In addition, salt, strong spices, preservatives, alcoholic beverages, tea, and coffee were to be avoided. After this period, gluten and dairy products could be reintroduced, but would be again eliminated if they produced symptoms.

Why does such a regimen work? The researchers felt that food allergy or intolerance may be a more frequent contributor to arthritis than is commonly recognized. Their dietary regimen excluded common problematic foods. It had other advantages, too: vegan diets dramatically change the amount and type of fats in the diet, which, in turn, can affect the immune processes that play a part in arthritis. The omega-3 fatty acids in vegetables may be a key factor, along with the near absence of saturated fat. And patients lose weight on a vegan diet, which contributes to the improvement.

In addition, vegetables are loaded with antioxidants which can neutralize free radicals. As we saw in Chapter 1, oxygen-free radicals attack many parts of the body and contribute to heart disease and cancer, and intensify the aging processes generally. Joints are not spared. Imagine that a runner's knee is injured slightly, perhaps owing to strain or exercising a bit too hard. A little fluid accumulates in the joint. If the exercise is continued, the joint movement causes the pressure in the joint to increase momentarily, which in turn causes the blood supply to the joint to be cut off for an instant. With every pounding step, the blood supply stops, then returns, over and over again.

The joint is set up for free-radical injury. As blood rushes back in and oxygen is restored to the joint tissues, free radicals are produced. Iron acts as a catalyst, encouraging the production of these dangerous molecules, which in turn attack the cells lining the joint, inflaming and damaging the tissues.[6]

The cells in the joint try to defend themselves. Vitamin C and vitamin E, which are plentiful in a menu drawn from vegetables and grains, help neutralize these free radicals. The body also tries to keep iron sequestered from the tissues. Iron is transported and stored in special protein packages, rather like the way explosives—and cholesterol—are packaged and transported with great care. Meat-based diets supply an overload of iron. And meat has no vitamin C and very little vitamin E. On the other hand, vegetables supply more controlled amounts of iron, with generous quantities of antioxidant vitamins. Antioxidants may have a role, not just in prevention but also in reducing symptoms of arthritis. Some treatments of arthritis, including nonsteroidal anti-inflammatory drugs, work at least in part by neutralizing free radicals. For the most part, however, vitamins and other antioxidants will prevent damage before it occurs, rather than treat an inflamed joint.[6]

Many doctors tell arthritis patients that dietary changes will not help them. Unfortunately, this conclusion is based on older research with diets that included dairy products, oil, poultry or meat.[7,8] It is clear that, at least for some people, a healthier menu is the answer to arthritis.

Gout

Gout is a form of arthritis that usually starts in the big toe. Severe pain ensues, often requiring hospital treatment. Tests show abnormally large amounts of a chemical called *uric acid* in the blood, and if the doctor draws a sample of fluid from the inflamed joint, uric acid will be found there as well. For some reason, men develop gout much more commonly than do women.

Some patients have attacks in joints other than the big toe, and as time goes on, more joints may become involved. Uric acid can also lead to kidney damage and kidney stones, and deposits in the skin, particularly in the ear, forearm, elbow, or Achilles' tendon. If these deposits break open, as they sometimes do, out comes a chalky or pasty material made largely of uric acid crystals.

The word *gout* comes from the Latin word *gutta*, which means a "drop," because in ancient times the disease had been thought to be caused by drops of mythological "morbid humors."

Patients improve with medication in the hospital. But the key to prevention of gout lies in changing the diet. Although some cases are due to inborn deficiencies of certain enzymes, the cause most often is the Western diet. Uric acid is a breakdown product released from diets loaded with animal products.

The New Four Food Groups are an ideal prescription for preventing gout. It takes time for uric acid levels to change, so if you are currently being treated for gout or high uric acid levels, do not stop your medication during the dietary transition, and do so only under the guidance of your physician. Dietary transitions are times of particular vulnerability for people with a tendency toward gout.

Multiple Sclerosis

Multiple sclerosis is a disease of the nervous system in which episodes of weakness or sensory symptoms come and go. The disease strikes young adults, usually between the ages of twenty and thirty-five. Early symptoms may be quite vague: fatigue, difficulty sleeping, or nervousness. Later on, visual blurring and other sensory symptoms occur, and the extremities become weak. At first, these symptoms usually resolve on their own. As time goes on, however, the symptoms become chronic, and eventually the individual may become incapacitated and ultimately die. A hot bath or any other source of heat can make the symptoms much worse. The disease was unknown until the early 1800s, and, like rheumatoid arthritis, may well be an affliction of modern times.

Until recently, there was little hope for MS patients. Medical treatments were not much help, and diet was the last thing anyone thought about. But one doctor has changed that. Dr. Roy Laver Swank's studies of MS began in 1948 in Montreal. The young doctor noticed that MS follows a pattern like that of typical diet-related diseases. It is rare in Asia, but relatively common in North America and Western Europe. In Montreal, the disease was considerably rarer among poorer residents, whether French- or English-speaking, than among wealthier citizens. He looked within other countries and found that MS rates were high where saturated fat intake was high and rare where fat intake was low. On the other hand, polyunsaturated oils seemed not to increase the risk.

Swank hypothesized that, in the presence of a genetic predisposition, fat may cause the clumping of platelets and blood cells, leading to sludging of blood in the capillaries to the brain. These microscopic clumps damage the capillary's capacity to be selective in what goes into the brain and what does not. Toxic products enter the brain, leading to damage and scarring of the brain cells and nerves. He spent a considerable amount of time proving various aspects of his theory and published over two dozen research articles in major journals.

Swank developed a diet that cut down on saturated fat. The dietary changes he recommended were modest compared to those necessary to reverse heart disease or prevent cancer. He limited saturated fat intake to no more than 15 grams (three teaspoons) per day. This meant no red meat at all for the first year, and only small amounts thereafter. Fatty dairy products and other sources of saturated fats were to be eliminated as well. He felt that, unlike saturated fats, polyunsaturated oils might actually be helpful, so he recommended from 20 to 50 grams of oil per day. He published his recommendations in *The Multiple Sclerosis Diet Book.*[9]

Dr. Swank tested his findings in Montreal and later in Portland in more than 2,000 patients, and followed these patients for anywhere from one to four decades. The results are impressive. The dietary treatment was most effective when begun early. For those who started the dietary treatment in the early stages of the disease, 95 percent either remained unchanged or actually improved during the next twenty years. Those who started the dietary changes later in the course of their disease did less well. After thirty-six years, only 30 percent of patients who did not go on the diet were still alive, compared to 79 percent of those who followed the diet.

Later, the suggestion to boost polyunsaturated oil was relaxed, as many patients did very well when they reduced both saturated and unsaturated fats.

Although Dr. Swank's research was published in major journals,[10] it still tends to be ignored by most physicians, perhaps because of their general discomfort with dietary treatments. Research, however, has been very supportive.

About a year ago, after I finished a lecture in Portland, a man in the audience came up to introduce himself. "I thought you might like to see

what one of Dr. Swank's patients looks like," he said. He had been diagnosed with multiple sclerosis three decades earlier and, unlike the patients
I had seen decline during my medical training, this man did not seem to have
lost any ground at all. He did not claim to know why the diet worked, but
he was not about to stop what might have saved his life.

Diablotes

My father specialized in the treatment of diabetes. He told me how, during
his training at Boston's Joslin Clinic, a competing institution received a
research grant for $25,000, an enormous amount of money at the time. Dr.
Joslin, who was then a prestigious diabetologist, responded: "Gentlemen,
we don't need a $25,000 grant. What we need is a good idea." Dr. Joslin
would have been delighted with the extraordinarily good ideas that have
helped diabetics in recent years.

Diabetes is, in essence, starvation. The cells of the body are starving for
their normal food, which is a simple sugar called glucose. Normally, the cells
use this sugar to run their microscopic machinery. The problem in diabetes
is that sugar has trouble passing from the bloodstream into the cells where
it can be used. It must be escorted into the muscle, liver, and fat cells by
a hormone called insulin, which can be thought of as a key that opens a door
in the cell membrane for glucose to enter. When insulin is absent or not
working properly, glucose simply waits in the bloodstream, unable to enter
the cells.

From this disarmingly simple beginning, diabetes leads to many problems. Sugar builds up in the blood and ends up being excreted in the urine.
Excessive urination leads to thirst and dehydration, along with weight loss
and weakness. In serious and untreated cases, the disease progresses to
labored breathing and coma.

Over the long run, the results of diabetes can be deadly. Diabetics can
develop aggressive atherosclerosis, leading to heart attacks and strokes. The
poor circulation to the legs, combined with trouble combating infections,
means that a simple foot sore can progress to gangrene and amputation.
There can even be damage to the tiny blood vessels in the retina, leading to
blindness, and in the blood vessels of the kidney, leading to kidney failure.

The technical name for the disease is diabetes mellitus. (*Mellitus* is a Latin word meaning "honey-sweet," referring to the sugar content of the urine.) There are two different types of the disease. In childhood, if the pancreas is somehow damaged so that insulin cannot be produced, the result is insulin-dependent diabetes, which means that the affected individual will need insulin injections for the rest of his or her life. This form of diabetes is sometimes called childhood-onset diabetes or Type I diabetes. It usually starts before the age of forty.

In the second, and much more common, form of diabetes, the problem is not a lack of insulin but simply that the insulin does not work effectively. This form of the disease is called non-insulin-dependent diabetes (or adult-onset or Type II). It typically occurs in overweight adults over the age of forty, and is usually treated with dietary changes and oral medications, although insulin injections are sometimes used.

Diabetes is not rare. About 7 million Americans have it, and the prevalence is higher in African-Americans, Hispanics, and Native Americans. Because diabetics frequently need medical treatment and lose time from work, the costs of medical care and lost productivity are enormous—over $20 billion annually.[11]

The New Approach to Diabetes

The combination of the New Four Food Group menu and regular physical activity has a powerful effect on diabetes. In a study of a low-fat, starch-based diet and regular exercise in patients with non-insulin-dependent diabetes, researchers found that twenty-one of twenty-three patients on oral medications and thirteen of seventeen patients on insulin were able to get off their medication in less than four weeks. At two- and three-year follow-up, most diabetics treated with this regimen retained their gains.[12,13]

Although non-insulin-dependent diabetics often find that the disease disappears with diet and exercise, people with insulin-dependent diabetes will need insulin injections regardless of the diet they follow. However, dietary changes are usually helpful in managing the disease and in minimizing complications. Diabetic treatments should always be individualized. The information in this book should be coordinated with the treatment prescribed by a physician for your own needs.

The cornerstone of the diet is, first, to keep fats and oils to a minimum because they interfere with insulin. When I was a medical student, we did not appreciate the importance of this. We thought sugar was all there was to it. It is true that diabetics tend to develop high blood sugar levels in response to sugary foods. We used to chase our patients around the hospital to make sure they never bought candy in the gift shop, because we did not want their blood sugar to rise. But all the while, the high-fat foods on the hospital trays were a much bigger problem because fats interfere with the action of insulin. Researchers have taken samples of cells from individuals on various diets and found that when patients are on low-fat, starch-based diets, insulin is able to bind to the cells more effectively.[14,15] This can also be seen in the reduced amounts of insulin that such patients require.

Although doctors used to believe that diabetics should steer clear of carbohydrates, we now know that just the opposite is true. Complex carbohydrates and fiber should be increased to allow a more gradual release of sugars into the blood. Many scientific studies[12–20] have shown that blood sugar levels are under better control on diets that are high in fiber and carbohydrate and low in fat.

The specific type of carbohydrate may make a difference. For example, beans seem to cause little rise in blood sugar levels, while the soluble fiber in fruits, vegetables, and legumes helps reduce blood sugar.[21,22,23]

A very low fat, high complex-carbohydrate diet also encourages weight loss, which improves insulin's action. Weight loss alone can make non-insulin-dependent diabetes disappear. A healthier diet may also reduce the complications of the disease. Researchers at the National Institutes of Health compared diabetic patients with eye damage to patients without it, and found that those who had not developed the characteristic retinal damage had consumed more carbohydrate and fiber, and less protein.[24]

A no-cholesterol, low-fat diet gives the diabetic the best defense against the risks of arterial damage. This diet is also modest in protein, so it helps preserve kidney function, as we saw in Chapter 1.

The diet currently recommended by the American Diabetes Association could stand considerable improvement. The cornerstone of the ADA diet is a set of exchange lists, which divide foods into six categories: milk, fruit, vegetables, starch and bread, meat, and fat. The foods within each group have a similar nutritional makeup, and the lists help the patient maintain fairly constant levels of fat, protein, and carbohydrate intake day after day. The main problem with the diet is that it is much too high in fat, cholesterol, and protein, and too low in complex carbohydrates. Up to 30 percent of the calories in the ADA diet come from fat.[25] This is too high, with the result being more insulin resistance than would occur on a lower-fat diet. And given diabetics' tendency toward aggressive damage to the heart, blood vessels, and kidneys, high-fat, high-protein foods are the last thing they need. The difference between the New Four Food Groups and the exchange lists is that the New Four Food Groups delete the milk, meat, and fat categories; encourage more generous amounts of grains, vegetables, and fruits; and add the legume group, yielding a much more powerful regimen.

Physical activity is also very important. Exercising muscles have a voracious appetite for sugar. They pull it out of the blood, even with very little insulin present. For this reason diabetics do well to maintain a regular program of aerobic physical activity. Caution is advised, however; a sudden increase in exercise can lower blood sugar too rapidly, and insulin doses will need to be adjusted by your doctor.

DIETARY LINKS TO THE CAUSE OF INSULIN-DEPENDENT DIABETES

Insulin is produced in specialized cells in the pancreas. Damage to these cells causes insulin-dependent diabetes in children and young adults. Mounting evidence shows that insulin-dependent diabetes is linked to dairy-product exposure in infancy. Epidemiologic studies of various countries show a strong correlation between the use of dairy products and the incidence of diabetes.[26] Cow's milk proteins can enter the infant's bloodstream and stimulate the formation of antibodies.[27] In turn, antibodies that can attack and destroy the insulin-producing pancreatic beta cells have been found in insulin-dependent diabetics.[28]

A recent report in the *New England Journal of Medicine* adds substantial support to the suggestion that cow's milk proteins stimulate the production of the antibodies, which in turn destroy the insulin-producing pancreatic cells.[29] Researchers from Canada and Finland found high levels of antibodies to a specific portion of a cow's milk protein, called *bovine serum albumin,* in every one of the 142 diabetic children they studied at the time the disease was diagnosed. Evidence suggests that the combination of a genetic predisposition and cow's milk exposure causes the childhood form of diabetes, although the genetic predisposition is fairly common, and there is no way of identifying with certainty all children who are predisposed. Antibodies can apparently form in response to even small quantities of cow's milk proteins, and it seems to make no difference whether the proteins come from regular cow's milk or cow's milk formula. Cow's milk proteins can even reach a breast-feeding baby if the mother drinks milk. These proteins pass into her bloodstream and into her breast milk.

The destruction of insulin-producing cells occurs gradually, especially after infections which cause the cellular proteins to be exposed to the damage of antibodies. Diabetes becomes evident when 80 to 90 percent of the insulin-producing beta cells are destroyed.

While the *New England Journal of Medicine* report was the first to bring the dairy-diabetes link to the lay public, researchers and clinicians have long suspected this possibility. It may well be that avoiding cow's milk would prevent the vast majority of cases of insulin-dependent diabetes.

Hypoglycemia

Hypoglycemia is a frustrating problem. The symptoms are often vague and may elude diagnosis. Doctors are frustrated with it, too, because they often find that people who believe they are hypoglycemic clearly are not, yet the true cause of their symptoms may remain unknown.

Hypoglycemia means low blood sugar. Symptoms include headache, poor concentration, fatigue, confusion, palpitations, anxiety, sweating, and tremulousness. These are caused by the brain not getting the glucose it needs, and also by adrenaline and related hormones becoming more active when blood sugar falls.

Hypoglycemic episodes are brief, lasting from minutes to hours. If the affected individual does not have some food or the episode does not correct on its own, the blood sugar will continue to drop and fainting, seizure, or coma will result in a matter of hours. A person who feels out of sorts for days on end should look for another cause of the problem.

The best-known type of hypoglycemia occurs after eating. It is rarely life-threatening, but it can be very annoying because of the weakness, faintness, or palpitations it causes. After a meal, blood sugar rises, and then begins to fall. If it falls too quickly, the symptoms of hypoglycemia can begin. The exact cause is unknown, but it is generally assumed to be due to the body's insulin, whose job it is to remove sugar from the blood, doing its job too well and reducing blood sugar too far. About 5 percent of people run low blood sugars (below 50 mg/dl) after meals, although it causes most of them no problem and they are usually not aware of it. What seems to be important in causing symptoms is *how fast* the blood sugar drops.

If hypoglycemia occurs after an overnight fast rather than after eating, it may be due to one of any number of medical conditions from hormone deficiencies to tumors, and is more serious than that which occurs after meals. Pregnancy can also disrupt normal sugar metabolism and lead to hypoglycemia.

Diabetics can become hypoglycemic. If they have used too much insulin, or have eaten less or exercised more than usual, they may begin to feel shaky and tired. They soon learn that sugar or other food will make these feelings go away.

Alcohol can reduce blood sugar, particularly in poorly nourished people who go on a drinking binge. When the liver is preoccupied with trying to break down and remove alcohol from the body, it loses much of its ability to maintain blood sugar adequately.

To test for hypoglycemia, doctors can check your blood sugar after fasting and after a test dose of glucose. They will look for blood sugar dropping below 50 mg/dl after a glucose test, or 60 mg/dl after an overnight fast.

The treatment for after-meal hypoglycemia used to be a low-carbohydrate diet. Doctors reasoned that since carbohydrate is what stimulates the release of insulin, a low-carbohydrate diet would keep insulin in check. Some people do feel better on such a diet, but unfortunately, when carbohydrate is taken out of the diet, there are only two things that can go in its place: protein and fat. So the low-carbohydrate approach can lead to far worse problems than it attempts to solve: heart disease, cancer, diabetes, and overweight, to name a few. In addition, some research suggests that when people begin low-carbohydrate diets, their ability to handle sugar gets even worse. In other words, a dietary indiscretion leads to worse hypoglycemic episodes than they had before they began the diet.

A better approach is to eliminate simple sugars such as candies and sodas, and to *increase* complex carbohydrates such as rice, vegetables, and beans. These foods tend to allow a more gradual absorption of glucose and a blunted insulin response. For some, it helps to select intact grain products such as brown rice, and avoid ground grains such as in pasta or bread. Some people also need to avoid fruit. Try frequent small meals instead of three large meals each day.

If you feel tired after meals, your problem may not be hypoglycemia. It may be due to one of two factors. First, fat in foods causes people to feel sleepy. After a greasy meal, the viscosity ("thickness") of the blood measurably increases. This may be a contributor to the after-meal slowdown that many people feel.

A second contributor is sugar, but by a mechanism totally unrelated to hypoglycemia. Sugar causes an increase in a brain chemical called serotonin, as described on page 110. In turn, serotonin makes us feel sleepy or irritable. The solution to this problem is a balanced menu from the New Four Food Groups.

The Fiber of Life

It is impossible to turn on the television these days without a commercial for the fiber in breakfast cereals; fiber in whole-grain crackers or bread; fiber in popcorn, oatmeal, and seemingly everything else. The explosion of awareness of the need for fiber began with a dedicated missionary surgeon in Africa, Dr. Denis Burkitt, whom we met briefly in Chapter 3.

Fiber was actually his second medical breakthrough. Dr. Burkitt first became famous for identifying, and later curing, the first human cancer found to be caused by a virus, and Burkitt's lymphoma and the Epstein-Barr virus are now studied by every first-year medical student. But on the heels of this discovery, Burkitt set about to find out why certain diseases were epidemic in England and Western Europe, yet were extremely rare in Africa. Appendicitis was very rare in Africa. Diverticular disease (small pouches in the wall of the large intestine) occurs in most older Western adults, but was quite rare in Africa. The same was true of hemorrhoids, varicose veins, hiatal hernia (part of the stomach rising into the chest cavity), and colorectal cancer.

He surveyed hospitals in Africa, India, and elsewhere and was able to track where diseases occurred. And he made a striking observation: in cultures that Westernize their diets, these conditions emerge gradually and in a particular order. Appendicitis is one of the first. Hemorrhoids occur soon thereafter, followed by varicose veins, colon polyps and colon cancer, hiatal hernia, and diverticular disease. This was exactly the same order as these diseases tend to appear in individuals. Appendicitis can occur in children, varicose veins and colon cancer in mid-life, and diverticular disease in later life. He reasoned that the same factors that cause these diseases in individuals must cause their emergence in cultures undergoing a transformation of diet.[30]

To make a long story short, the answer was fiber, although Burkitt soon added considerations about fat and other factors. Fiber is found only in plants, so traditional diets of grains, vegetables, beans, and fruits are loaded with fiber. Meats, dairy products, and eggs contain no fiber at all, so diets centered on animal products tend to be low in fiber. In addition, modern refining processes extract the fiber from grains as whole-grain flour is turned into white flour, and brown rice into white rice. The result of the modern fiber-depleted diet is a whole string of ills, from constipation to colon cancer, and even such unlikely problems as varicose veins and hemorrhoids. In the following sections these surprising links are detailed.

Constipation

Fiber is part of the body's waste removal system. In the digestive tract, fiber holds water, keeps stools soft, and moves wastes along quickly. A good way to become constipated is to build your diet on poultry, fish, yogurt, beef, cheese, or any other animal product. They contain no fiber at all, and the more of these you send down your digestive tract, the less fiber your body has to work with.

Advertisers would have us believe that fiber comes from breakfast cereals. Actually there is fiber in all grains, vegetables, fruits, and legumes, and the New Four Food Groups bring you plenty of fiber whether you eat breakfast cereal or not.

The diet of most Westerners supplies only about 10 to 20 grams of fiber per day. A menu from the New Four Food Groups can easily double that.

At the risk of evoking graphic recollections of Freud's theories about toilet training, it should be pointed out that the American habit of one bowel movement per day or even every other day is not the norm in countries where a high-fiber diet is prevalent; there it is typical to have two or more bowel movements per day. More frequent bowel movements and softer stools are easier on the intestinal tract than fewer, smaller, harder stools.

APPENDICITIS

The appendix is a small fingerlike tube that projects from the intestine in the right lower part of your abdomen. When the appendix becomes inflamed, there is little choice but to remove it surgically. What the surgeon finds is a swollen, red, and sometimes ruptured organ.

Appendicitis is still rare in societies on traditional high-fiber diets. But countries undergoing economic transformation and rapid dietary change soon need surgeons ready to excise the cause of the right lower abdominal pain.

Dr. Burkitt found that the first step in the cause of appendicitis is a blockage of the opening of the appendix by a small firm bit of stool. Infection, inflammation, and pain then follow. High-fiber diets keep the stools soft, so blockage of the appendix tends not to occur.[31]

It may well be helpful for people to keep their appendixes. There is some evidence that the appendix was not put in the body simply to give surgeons practice in a fairly simple operation. Like the tonsils, the appendix may have an immune function. Indeed, certain cancers, particularly Hodgkin's disease (a form of cancer arising in the lymph nodes), are more common among people who have had these organs removed.

VARICOSE VEINS AND HEMORRHOIDS

The cause of varicose veins is not exactly dinnertime conversation. But Dr. Burkitt's findings have explained what had previously been a medical enigma. So even though these facts are not very pretty, I will describe them in some detail.

The swollen tortuous veins we call varicose veins are common in North America and Western Europe, but rare in Asia and Africa. Medical texts have attributed the condition to pregnancy, the upright posture, and prolonged standing, but none of these explanations has held up. After all, there is no shortage of pregnancy, upright posture, or standing in Africa and Asia, where varicose veins are rarely found.

The heart pumps blood out to all parts of the body through a system of arteries. Veins return the blood back to the heart. The veins in the legs have quite a job to do. They not only have to send blood a long way back up to the heart, they also have to work against gravity. The leg veins have a system of valves that are designed to keep blood from falling backward toward the feet, not unlike locks in a canal.

People on constipating, fiber-depleted diets often strain to pass stools. One or two such episodes can be innocuous enough, but people who strain to pass stools on a daily basis are putting a considerable amount of force on their abdomens. This force pushes blood backward out of the abdomen and down the veins of the legs. Daily straining destroys the valves in the veins. One after another, from the top of the leg on down, the damaged valves lose their ability to keep blood from slipping back down. The result is swollen and distorted veins. Ordinary physical exertion, by the way, such as sit-ups or lifting heavy objects, tightens the abdominal muscles but does not greatly increase the pressure within the abdominal cavity, and is not likely to increase your risk of varicose veins.

The destruction of the valves has also been implicated in the formation of blood clots in the veins. These blood clots are of particular concern not only because of the damage they cause in the involved leg (phlebitis), but because pieces of the clot can dislodge and travel up to the heart, where they are pumped out again to lodge in the lungs. If you were to take X-rays of the pelvic area of a group of Americans or Europeans, you would see tiny shadows on the X-rays of most of them, right where the veins that come up from the leg are located. These are old clots that have become calcified. If you were to X-ray a group of Africans who consumed a traditional diet, you would find these old clots in fewer than one person in five.[32]

Surgeons in England reasoned that perhaps they could cut down on the risk of blood clots forming in their surgical patients by feeding them bran. That is exactly what happened.[31] There are other contributors to blood clotting besides disruption of blood flow, and other causes of disrupted blood flow besides fiber-depleted diets. Nonetheless, putting the grains, vegetables, fruits, and beans back in the diet is an easy and important step to take.

Just as abdominal straining can damage the veins of the legs, the same thing happens to the veins surrounding the anus. A British surgeon, Hamish Thomson, provided an explanation for hemorrhoids, which is as follows: Hemorrhoidal blood vessels are normal structures used to provide an effective closure for the end of the digestive tract just as the lips do for its beginning. Repeated abdominal straining engorges these vessels. Then the passage of hard stools pushes the enlarged vessels downward and out through the anal opening. The result is the engorged, painful masses we call hemorrhoids.

While some people may need surgery for hemorrhoids, trading a meat-based diet for a high-fiber, plant-based diet is an important step in preventing them in the first place and in preventing a recurrence of swelling.

HIATAL HERNIA

The stomach is located just below the diaphragm, and a passageway through the diaphragm allows the esophagus to reach the stomach. In a person with hiatal hernia, part of the stomach actually slips through the diaphragm into the chest cavity.

About one in every five people has a hiatal hernia, and most have no symptoms whatsoever. The rest are buying antacids for heartburn.

Dr. Burkitt hypothesized that the condition is another result of daily straining to pass stools.[31] This creates enormous abdominal pressures, pushing the stomach upward toward the esophagus. The prevalence of hiatal hernia seems to follow the same pattern as other diet-related conditions: wherever low-fiber diets abound, hiatal hernia occurs.

DIVERTICULAR DISEASE

Diverticula are small pouches that form in the wall of the large intestine, like a bicycle inner tube pushing outward through a hole in the outer tire. Diverticulitis is the medical term used when these small pouches become inflamed, sometimes causing a great deal of pain.

Doctors used to suggest low-fiber diets for patients with diverticular disease on the theory that they should keep the intestinal tract relatively empty. That treatment did not work very well. In fact, it turned out that hard, compact stools disrupt the normal movements of the intestinal tract, increase pressures in the intestine, and lead to the formation of diverticula.[33] A better solution is a high-fiber diet. Fiber holds water and keeps intestinal contents soft, allowing them to move along smoothly without damaging the intestinal wall.

Gallstones

The gallbladder is about the size of an uninflated balloon, and is used to store bile, a digestive juice manufactured in the liver. After a meal, the gallbladder squirts bile into the intestinal tract to assist in the process of digestion. Bile can crystallize to form small stones. If a stone sits in the gallbladder minding its own business, it will cause no symptoms at all. But if it lodges in the tube system between the gallbladder and the intestine, it can cause intense pain or jaundice. Women have a greater risk of gallbladder problems than men for reasons that are unclear, as do overweight and older individuals.

Every day, surgeons remove gallbladders from patients. They send the stones off to the laboratory, which reports to the surgeon what they were made of. The number one ingredient is cholesterol. The problem was that there was too much cholesterol in the bile for it to stay dissolved. Imagine that you were to stir salt into a glass of water. Some of it would dissolve. But if you were to put in more and more, eventually it would be unable to dissolve and would remain in crystal form. The same happens with cholesterol. If there is too much of it in the bile, it forms solid stones.

Plant foods are cholesterol-free and low in the saturated fats that cause the body to make cholesterol. The natural fiber in plant foods also helps by discouraging the reabsorption of the cholesterol back into the blood. It is not surprising that vegetarians are only half as likely as meat-eaters to develop gallstones.[34]

But be sure not just to eliminate animal products. Keep vegetable oil to a minimum as well, because it too is a stimulus for bile production. The high polyunsaturated-fat diet that is still used by some to promote cholesterol reduction is the wrong way to go, because vegetable fats can also cause gallbladder problems. The New Four Food Groups fit the bill perfectly, with a low-fat, no-cholesterol menu that also helps keep you trim.

Food Poisoning

What's live, infectious, invisible, and present on one out of every three chickens you buy at the grocery store?

When we think of food poisoning, we think of an unsanitary restaurant kitchen, or maybe home canning gone awry. But food poisoning is an everyday occurrence. If you had the flu recently, it might not have been caused by a virus. It might actually have been a bacterial illness you brought in the door with your groceries. Because one out of every three chickens has live salmonella bacteria growing right inside the plastic packaging. Or maybe salmonella got you when you decided, damn the cholesterol, full speed ahead, and you ate an egg. Eggs are increasingly a source of salmonella.

Animal products are surprise packages, with a seemingly endless array of contaminants. Salmonella causes an intestinal illness with vomiting, diarrhea, abdominal pain, and low-grade fever beginning anywhere from six hours to two days after infection. Usually, it passes in several days without any treatment. But sometimes it becomes very serious, spreading into the blood and to various organs. Most cases are never reported. The Centers for Disease Control estimates the true incidence to be anywhere from 400,000 to 4 million cases per year. The death toll has been as high as 9,000 per year.

To see why salmonella is so common, you have to take a look at modern farms. Chicken farms are now essentially factories. Many thousands of tiny chicks are put into a large steel building. Eight weeks later, they are boxed and trucked to an assembly-line slaughterhouse. During their two months of life in a crowded steel building, they are living in the accumulating excrement of thousands of birds. That excrement contains salmonella and other bacteria.

In the slaughterhouse, the feathers are beaten from their skin. In the process, feces containing salmonella are beaten into the skin. The chickens are eviscerated by machine. From time to time, the intestines are punctured, and feces are spread around even more. The carcass is then run through a water bath to cool. This water starts out clean, but rapidly accumulates feces and debris.

When you bring home a chicken from the store and cut the package open, a little bit of water dribbles out onto the counter. You might think it is "chicken juice." Well, chickens are not fruit; they do not have juice. What dribbled out onto your counter was a combination of cooling water, blood, lymph, and feces, which CBS News once called "fecal soup."

Under federal regulations, it is perfectly legal to sell salmonella-tainted products. And illness is inevitable. The federal government uses inspectors who actually look at every chicken carcass. The irony is that salmonella are not visible to the human eye. Thousands of inspectors and hundreds of millions of dollars go to inspect the 6 billion chickens slaughtered every year in the United States. They throw out birds with broken bones, but allow carcasses covered with salmonella to be wrapped up and sold. When researchers have gone to grocery stores and taken samples, they have found that one in three chicken packages has salmonella bacteria still alive in the package. This is true of all major brands.

Sickness is not usually the result of eating the chicken because salmonella are easily killed by cooking. Illness results from contamination of kitchen surfaces and cooking implements. For example, chicken is cut on a cutting board that is then used to slice lettuce and tomatoes for a salad, which then becomes thoroughly contaminated with the chicken's unseen bacteria. Or a sponge used to clean up "chicken juice" on the counter is then used to wipe off other surfaces.

In infants, the elderly, and people with immune disorders, salmonella can be especially serious and is often fatal. The highest incidence is in three-month-old babies, who may be victims of cross-contamination or from infection from others in the household. Infants are protected somewhat if they breast-feed. Within the breast milk are cells that can help the child knock out salmonella.[35] And they are protected much more when their parents don't bring animal products into the home.

Salmonella is not only found in chicken meat. Outbreaks have frequently occurred from beef and many other animal products and rarely from produce such as melons or tomatoes, apparently due to contaminated soil. (Washing produce removes bacteria.) And increasingly, eggs are bringing salmonella into households across America. Egg operations are intensely crowded, typically putting three to five hens into a single cage with a floor about the size of a folded newspaper. The salmonella that is spread from one bird to another can end up inside the eggs, even when the shells are intact.[36]

In October 1989, in an Atlantic City casino, a man was eating a chocolate mousse with his wife and their friends. He and more than 100 other people became ill. He got worse and worse, and finally died three months later. What was in the mousse? Salmonella, according to the New Jersey Health Department, apparently from a shipment of eggs.

In 1987, in a New York City hospital, 404 patients suddenly came down with salmonella, and 9 died. The source was the low-sodium tuna-macaroni salad, which was made with salmonella-laden eggs. The egg farm sent the chickens to slaughter and the ovaries were removed for inspection. More than two-thirds tested positive for salmonella, suggesting that chickens pass salmonella, not only in their feces but also directly from the ovaries into the eggs.[37]

Cooking eggs "sunny-side up" cannot kill salmonella, no matter how long the cooking continues.[38] The *Journal of the American Medical Association* observed that eggs should be boiled for seven minutes, poached for five minutes, or fried for three minutes on each side.[36] More prudent is to avoid eggs altogether, because of their load of cholesterol, fat, animal protein, and, of course, salmonella. Look out for hidden eggs, especially foods made with raw eggs: Caesar salad dressing, hollandaise sauce, eggnog, and homemade ice cream.

People can sometimes be infected with salmonella and carry the bacteria in their own intestinal tracts without being aware of it. Normal intestinal bacteria keep the salmonella from overgrowing, but if a person happens to take antibiotics for some unrelated condition, normal bacteria will be killed off. Salmonella, however, are often resistant to commonly used antibiotics because they came from farms where antibiotics are routinely fed to livestock as growth promoters. With the other bacteria killed off, the salmonella overgrow and can cause a very serious illness.

All doctors now recognize the problem of antibiotic-resistant bacteria, which is why they will not use antibiotics without clear evidence of a bacterial infection. But farmers are fostering bacterial resistance as they feed antibiotics willy-nilly to animals, not to stop infections but to promote more rapid growth.

Salmonella is not the only disease-causing bacteria that resides in the poultry department. As many as 65 to 80 percent of chickens are contaminated with a bacteria called *campylobacter*,[39, 40] and many strains are resistant to antibiotics. The result is at least 2 million cases annually of vomiting, diarrhea, fever, and abdominal pain, particularly in small children,[41] when it sometimes is mistaken for appendicitis.

There are other uninvited dinner guests, including yersinia, *E. coli*, and others, which cause a whopping intestinal illness and which all have one thing in common: they are transmitted primarily in animal products such as poultry and other meats, eggs and milk. Plant products tend to be free of these pathogens unless contaminated by contact with animal products.

One particularly worrisome bug is *Toxoplasma*, a protozoan (one-celled animal) present in 25 percent of pork products, 10 percent of lamb, and many other animal products. Millions of people are infected with *Toxoplasma* with no problem at all, but if a woman acquires toxoplasmosis during pregnancy, her baby is at risk for birth defects such as blindness or brain damage.[42] Miscarriage or stillbirth can also occur. People with impaired immune systems, including cancer patients receiving chemotherapy, AIDS patients, and transplant recipients who are on rejection-suppressing medications, can also have serious problems with toxoplasmosis.

Although cats have often been blamed for *Toxoplasma*, only about 1 percent of cats actually pass it in their feces, and this is a result of ingesting another *Toxoplasma*-infected animal. Cleaning the litter box within two to three days removes *Toxoplasma* before they can become infectious. The most common source of *Toxoplasma* is undercooked or raw meat. Thorough cooking destroys the organism but, like salmonella, the problem is cross-contamination. When raw meat touches the kitchen counter or the carving knife, *Toxoplasma* can be transferred to the new surface, where they can survive, waiting to contaminate other foods. *Toxoplasma* can also be transmitted from soil.

What about raw bars or sushi? Don't even think about them. Bacterial contamination is rampant, particularly in oysters. The Food and Drug Administration estimates that the bacteria *Vibrio vulnificus* are present in 5 to 10 percent of raw shellfish, and there is no way to tell an infected oyster from a clean one.[43] Shellfish live in waters that are often polluted with human and animal waste. The result is hepatitis, salmonella, or cholera. Any sushi bar in the world would be perfectly happy to make you vegetarian sushi using cucumber, carrot, or radish instead of raw fish. Take them up on the offer.

The fish you might buy at the store is a surprise package, too. Unlike cows and chickens, fish are cold-blooded. So the bacteria that live in them are quite comfortable—and even grow—at the temperatures in your refrigerator. *Consumer Reports* found that bacterial contamination is so common in fish that at least 40 percent have begun to spoil before they leave the grocery case.[44] And a slightly higher percentage contain fecal bacteria from human or animal waste. Fish pick up these bacteria in polluted waters and in the ironically named process of "cleaning" and handling. And you can smell it. The "fishy" smell that is so familiar in the nether regions of the grocery store comes from trimethylamine, a chemical produced as fish begins to spoil.

One final culinary nightmare is provided by poison-producing bacteria. The story begins with the innocent-looking bacteria that live on human skin, in the nose, or in the digestive tract. These were the critters your mother was thinking of when she said, "Wash your hands before you eat—you're covered with *Staphylococci* and *Clostridium perfringens*."

These bacteria generally do no harm. But what happens when, for example, a picnic guest who did not wash his hands happens to stick his finger in lunch to take a little taste. Bacteria incubate in warm foods. They are particularly fond of high-protein foods like chicken salad or chili.

When *Staphylococci* are allowed to sit in foods for several hours at room temperature, they produce a chemical poison that accumulates in the food. Then after the volleyball game, you root through the picnic leftovers. It takes about two to four hours for the symptoms to hit: nausea, vomiting, and diarrhea. The illness will be memorable, but it will usually go away on its own.

Let's say you were concerned that the chili has sat out too long, so you put it back on the stove before eating it. Unfortunately, a second heating will not always help. Although the bacteria are usually killed by heating, some bacterial toxins are heat-resistant. Bacterial contamination is discouraged by the more modest protein content of the recipes in this book. Even so, it is essential to maintain good hygiene and not to leave foods out at temperatures that encourage bacterial growth.

Ulcers

Ulcers occur in the first part of the intestine, called the duodenum, or, less commonly, in the stomach or the esophagus. They cause a burning pain, particularly after meals. The old method of dealing with ulcers was with antacids and, more recently, drugs to reduce acid production. And people often eliminated coffee, tea, and spicy foods from their diet.

All that is now changing. There is substantial evidence showing that ulcers can be caused by a particular type of bacteria called *Helicobacter pylori*. It is believed that we acquire the bacteria through human contact. *Helicobacter pylori* bacteria can actually survive in the acid conditions of the stomach. They cause gastritis and apparently lower resistance to the effects of acid.

About 95 percent of people with duodenal ulcers and 70 percent of people with stomach ulcers are infected with the bacteria, and treating the infection eliminates peptic ulcer disease in most. Researchers at Baylor College of Medicine have tested medicines to destroy the *Helicobacter* in their ulcer patients. One experiment showed that when ulcer patients are treated with acid-reducing medications alone, 80 percent relapse within six months. However, when anti-*Helicobacter* medications are added to the regimen, the relapse rate was cut to 6 percent. This treatment is new and still somewhat controversial among gastroenterologists, some of whom prefer to stick to the acid-reducing medications.

The other major cause of ulcer-related problems is aspirin. Not only can aspirin irritate the stomach, but it also interferes with blood clotting, making bleeding more likely. So steer clear even of coated aspirin if you have any tendency toward ulcers, gastritis, or other cause of bleeding.

Enthusiasts of Latin American cuisine can take heart. In spite of their reputation as an ulcer-causing food, jalapeño peppers got a not-guilty verdict from researchers who fed them to volunteers and then—believe it or not—passed endoscopes into the volunteers' stomachs and looked around for any sign of damage. Aspirin caused damage, but jalapeños did not.[45]

If you still take antacids, be careful: many contain aluminum. The name Maalox, for example, is a shortening of magnesium and aluminum hydroxide. Some evidence has linked aluminum to Alzheimer's disease, and while it is uncertain whether or not it actually causes the disease, you may not wish to be in the experimental group! Milk is used by some as an antacid. However, although milk reduces acidity in the short run, it can actually increase overall acid production. The good news is that most ulcers can be cured, making antacid use unnecessary.

The New Ulcer Cure

Most peptic ulcers are now believed to be caused by bacteria called *Helicobacter pylori*. Antibiotics can cure the bacterial infection and, as a result, cure the ulcer. Antibiotic treatments change rapidly. Your doctor will prescribe the treatment that is most current and suited to your own needs. A typical current antibiotic treatment for ulcers is as follows:

Tetracycline: 500 mg four times per day

Metronidazole (Flagyl): 250 mg three times per day

Pepto-Bismol: 2 tablets four times per day

A two-week treatment cures ulcers in the vast majority of cases.

Time for a Change

Turn on your television for a couple of hours in the evening. Notice the commercials for laxatives, antacids, fiber-supplemented products, weight-loss programs, and arthritis medicines. Imagine what would happen if people were to embrace the power of healthful eating. If children grew up eating from the New Four Food Groups, there would be lots of empty television airtime. And there might be fewer of us watching TV anyway. If arthritis, diabetes, constipation, food poisoning, and ulcers become less common, more of us will be on the dance floor, tennis court, golf course, or in the pool, enjoying our healthy bodies.

6

The New Four Food Groups
and How They Work

When the Physicians Committee for Responsible Medicine proposed the New Four Food Groups in April 1991, *Tonight Show* host Johnny Carson gave his own idea for the four food groups: cheeseburgers, fries, ketchup, and Coke.

Well, it is true that the New Four Food Groups are a departure from the diet on which most of us were raised. Years ago, when I decided to swap my North Dakota diet of pork chops and roast beef for a healthier menu, I was not so sure how to go about it, nor did I have any idea how wonderful this switch would turn out to be.

What kinds of foods can be made from grains, vegetables, fruits, and legumes? The most delightful menu you can imagine. In the Georgetown district of Washington, D.C., a Middle Eastern restaurant brings the patron a feast of fifteen different plates of exquisite tastes, from exotic salads to delicately spiced vegetables, spreads, and entrees. In a family-owned restaurant on Italy's Mediterranean coast, fresh linguine is combined with a hearty marinara sauce, with a selection of vegetables and breads. By a lake shore in Switzerland, the sidewalk cafés outside luxury hotels turn green beans, carrots, endive, and broccoli into tastes befitting such a wonderful place. These masterpieces were made from grains, vegetables, fruits, and legumes, not because the foods are the very basis of healthful eating but because they delight the palate.

You do not have to be a gourmet chef to make these foods. In Chapter 8 you will find menus and recipes that translate the New Four Food Groups into delicious meals.

The New Four Food Groups are grains, vegetables, fruits, and legumes. Together, they are a much more powerful menu than previous dietary plans.

Although the old nutritional food groups crowded vegetables and fruits into one group, we have given them separate categories because both are so important.

What is most noteworthy, of course, is that two of the old food groups—meat and dairy—have been dropped: Meats—all meats, poultry, and fish—contain cholesterol and saturated fat, and all meats are totally devoid of fiber and contain virtually no complex carbohydrates. So there is no meat group in the New Four Food Groups. Likewise, dairy products contain fat, cholesterol, lactose, and allergenic proteins, and have no fiber or complex carbohydrates. So there is no longer a recommendation that dairy products be included in the diet.

Now, you may be saying, can I get enough protein without animal products? Can I get calcium? The answer is yes, and in this chapter we will look at these and other common questions. The New Four Food Groups are the Clark Kents of the nutrition world. Their modest and unassuming nature hides extraordinary strength. If your goal is to reverse heart disease, the old food groups were simply too weak to help you. Cholesterol is found only in animal products, and most meat-eaters eat hundreds of milligrams of cholesterol every day. But there is not a speck of cholesterol in the New Four Food Groups because they are 100 percent plant derived. The New Four Food Groups are also dramatically lower in fat than any cut of meat or poultry. And they contain generous amounts of soluble fiber, which adds to their cholesterol-lowering power. Together, they are enormously helpful for anyone who wants to reverse or prevent heart problems.

If you would like to lose a few pounds (or more than a few), the New Four Food Groups are more effective than any commercial diet. They help you to stay slim (or to get there) with no calorie restrictions and no limit on portion sizes.

The New Four Food Groups can also greatly reduce your risk of the most common forms of cancer. Cancers of the breast, colon, prostate, and other organs are less common in populations whose menus approximate these food groups. It is not just that the foods are low in fat. It is the combined effect of less total fat, no animal fat, fewer contaminants, more fiber, more cancer-fighting vitamins and minerals, and other factors that are being discovered on a fairly regular basis.

Surprisingly, calcium balance is *improved*. As noted in Chapter 1, diets that are high in protein, particularly animal protein, tend to cause calcium to be lost from the body. This has been shown in numerous experiments in which volunteers eat meat meals and the calcium that is lost in their urine is measured. But when animal protein is replaced with plant protein, the body maintains a healthy calcium balance with less calcium intake.[1] In a recent experiment in which meat protein was replaced with soy protein, subjects maintained good calcium balance with a calcium intake of only 457 mg per day—about half the Recommended Daily Allowance of 800 mg.

It is not a coincidence that the United States, a heavy meat-consuming country, would set such a high RDA for calcium. Evidence suggests that meat-eaters are busy losing calcium in their urine, and nutritionists are busy promoting greater calcium ingestion to attempt to make up for it. Comparisons of people in various countries show that those whose diets are plant-based generally maintain their bone strength better, even if they consume more modest amounts of calcium. The World Health Organization recommends a lower protein intake than is recommended by the U.S. government, and a lower calcium intake as well—between 400 and 500 mg per day. Calcium is abundant in green, leafy vegetables and beans. Without the protein overdose, calcium has an easier time remaining in the bones.

The New Four Food Groups

- *The Whole-Grain Group.* Beyond the obvious whole wheat bread, oatmeal and other breakfast cereals, and corn, the grain group also includes pasta. An Asian invention, perfected in Italy, pasta comes in every shape and variety, from linguine to spaghetti, vermicelli to rotini.

Exquisite rice dishes transform the staple food of Asia into curries, pilafs, and Latin American specialties, using its many varieties, which differ in taste and texture, with centuries-old combinations of spices.

What's in them nutritionally? Lots of fiber, complex carbohydrates, important vitamins, and a healthful amount of protein—not too much and not too little. They fit easily under the 10 percent fat limit used in Dr. Ornish's study of reversal of heart disease described in Chapter 2, and contain no cholesterol.

- *The Vegetable Group.* Vegetables have become all too unfamiliar on the American plate. Former President George Bush declared that he did not like broccoli and made no secret of his taste for pork rinds. And Vice-President Quayle had trouble spelling *potato*. But it seems that a week does not go by without another discovery that a naturally occurring chemical in vegetables helps fight cancer or boost immunity. Broccoli and other green vegetables are loaded with calcium, complex carbohydrates, fiber, and vitamins. Vegetables tend to be very low in fat and, like all plant foods, contain no cholesterol.

• *The Fruit Group.* Fruits range from apples, bananas, oranges, and other familiar foods to kiwis from New Zealand, cherimoya from Ecuador and Peru, and carambola (starfruit) from southern China. They are rich in vitamins, carbohydrate, and soluble fiber—powerful artillery against heart disease, cancer, and weight problems. Fruit is great as a dessert, as a breakfast, or as a major part of any meal.

• *The Legume Group.* The term refers to beans, lentils, and peas. Americans are familiar with navy beans and a few other varieties, but many cultures have made skillful use of the full range of legumes. Lentils are turned into delicious soups or curries. Chickpeas are pureed with garlic and scallions to become Middle Eastern hummus (a dip for pita bread) or formed into a patty for a spicy falafel. Black beans, gently flavored with tomatoes, peppers, and onions, are a savory staple of Latin American cuisine.

These foods are rich in protein, carbohydrate, fiber, and minerals, and, of course, they are low in fat and have no cholesterol, and are a good source of stable omega-3 fatty acids.

You may be wondering why beef, poultry, dairy products, and oils are included in nutrition guidelines issued by the federal government and health groups but not in the New Four Food Groups. Part of the reason is intense promotional campaigns. The Beef Check-Off program spends $45 million a year to promote and research just one product: beef. Dairy subsidies average more than a half-billion dollars per year. The Department of Agriculture is required by federal law to promote agricultural commodities, even if they are at odds with your health.

The influence of the meat industry is widespread and sometimes hidden. When the New Four Food Groups were unveiled by the Physicians Committee for Responsible Medicine, the American Medical Association issued a press release criticizing the plan. In July 1991, *The Veal Checkoff Report,* a newsletter from the National Live Stock and Meat Board, carried a story entitled "Why Didn't the Industry Respond?" which stated that the Meat Board decided not to fight the New Four Food Groups because they could arrange for the AMA to do that for them:

> *"The Meat Board prepared no formal release nor issued any statement to the press, but instead chose to do a lot of work behind the scenes," says BIC Public Relations Chairman Ivan Kanak. "By working closely with other organizations, such as the American Medical Association (AMA)*

and the American Dietetic Association, we were able to get a responsible, credible message to consumers." ... *"That's the kind of response the meat industry could not deliver to consumers with the same impact and believability,"* says [*Meat Board director of public relations Donna*] *Schmidt.*

Unfortunately, there does not appear to be an end in sight to the influence of such groups on nutritional information. And we see the results everywhere in the enormous U.S. rates for obesity, heart disease, cancer, diabetes, and other health problems.

Meal Planning

What kinds of meals come from grains, vegetables, fruits, and legumes? Breakfast might start with fresh fruit: melon, grapefruit, oranges, bananas, pineapple, or any other variety you like. Fruit can be your entire breakfast or just the beginning.

Let's add some hot cereal: old-fashioned rolled oats, cream of wheat, or in the quintessential Southern breakfast, grits (ground corn hominy). Hot cereals offer particular advantages. They are usually made from whole grains and are enjoyable without milk. There are new and delicious varieties on the shelves at health food stores. Creamy rice cereals are especially tasty. Let's top them with cinnamon or strawberries, raisins, or other fresh fruit.

For those who are trying to break a sausage habit, new and delicious nonmeat selections will ease the transition. At health food stores or the gourmet or dietetic sections of supermarkets, look for nonmeat sausages or bacon that taste like the real thing. They are available canned or refrigerated. Most of them should not be part of your permanent breakfast, though. Although they are lower in fat than meat products, most are not as low as whole grains, fruits, beans, and vegetables.

For lunch, let's start with some minestrone, split pea, or lentil soup. Add a bean burrito, a hummus sandwich, or a cucumber, lettuce, and tomato sandwich with a little mustard. For dessert, enjoy an apple, orange, pear, banana, or any other fresh fruit.

For dinner, how about angel hair pasta with a delicate basil sauce, spaghetti marinara, mushroom stroganoff (yes, you can make it without sour cream), or rice pilaf? Look especially for whole-grain pastas, as opposed to traditional white varieties that lack fiber, and avoid egg noodles. And do try spinach pasta.

As an alternative, couscous and other grains are now available in the boxed rice section of many grocery stores. They are a snap to make and extremely versatile. Follow the serving suggestions on the package or see the recipes in Chapter 8.

Let's add a spinach and endive salad, and generous portions of broccoli, carrots, green beans, or sweet peas.

The variety of healthful and delicious foods is endless. In Chapter 8 you will find menus and recipes, both for people who are in a hurry and do not like to spend time in the kitchen and for people who love to cook.

QUANTITIES AND PROPORTIONS

General guidelines for food group proportions follow. Keep in mind that these are broad guidelines. A 200-pound athlete will need to eat more than a 120-pound student. Your own appetite will tell you when you have had enough, and you have nothing to fear from your appetite. When you eat from the New Four Food Groups, you may eat whenever you want and as much as you want, assuming you are not stuffing yourself in response to emotional stress.

You do not need to have all four food groups in the same meal. The number of servings given is general, for the long run. You may wish to eat foods at different times of the day. Some people, for example, like to have fruit in the morning rather than later in the day, and that is perfectly fine.

Daily Servings

- *Grains:* Five or more servings (1 serving = ½ cup hot cereal, 1 ounce dry cereal, 1 slice of bread, ½ cup cooked rice)

- *Vegetables:* Three or more servings (1 serving = 1 cup raw or ½ cup cooked vegetables)

- *Fruits:* Three or more servings (1 serving = 1 medium piece of fruit, ½ cup fruit juice)

- *Legumes:* Two to three servings (1 serving = ½ cup cooked beans, 8 fluid ounces soymilk)

There is also no need to "complement" proteins, as we will see shortly.

Unprocessed, whole-grain products (e.g., brown rice, whole-grain cereals, corn kernels) are preferable to grains that have been ground up into flour or stripped of their bran. In the process of refining the bran is discarded, so brown rice becomes white rice, and flour that would have yielded whole wheat bread now results in white bread.

When many of us think of grains, we think of wheat. But it is a good idea to acquire a taste for other grains, such as brown rice, which are nutritious, less frequently allergenic, and may be more helpful in terms of mineral absorption.

Most Americans are not big rice eaters, but I strongly suggest that you learn the simple recipe for brown rice on page 252. It is a great start for those working on losing weight or lowering their cholesterol.

Some people think of bean dishes as the replacement for the steak they are no longer eating, and so they take huge servings of beans. I recommend a greater emphasis on grains, vegetables, and fruits, with a more modest quantity of legumes.

Most people do not need to measure serving sizes, but nutritionists may wish to do so in menu planning. For such purposes, recommended daily quantities are listed.

MEAL-PLANNING EXAMPLES

Let's see how different people might put together a healthful meal.

Andy is a college student who has a half-hour for lunch. He stops into a taco shop and orders a bean burrito and rice, with an apple for dessert. There is no vegetable within 100 yards of the place, so unfortunately, he doesn't have one. He will have vegetables at dinner, however, and fruits between meals.

Bob starts with a chickpea salad, followed by mushroom stroganoff. On the side is broccoli and green beans. Dessert is fresh peaches.

Carla goes out to dinner with her boyfriend at a Chinese restaurant. She empties her bowl of rice onto her plate, and tops it with portions of the two entrees they share: broccoli in garlic sauce and home-style bean curd (tofu mixed with vegetables). Dessert is orange slices.

Diane is cooking for a group of neighborhood children. Dinner is spaghetti with tomato sauce, with salads of chickpeas and greens. After dinner, they have apple slices.

Diane got stuck cooking for the kids two nights in a row. Tonight the menu is green salad, savory baked beans, cornbread, and fresh fruit for dessert.

As for myself, I travel frequently and often eat at restaurants, particularly Italian, Mexican, Chinese, and Indian. When I am home, I prefer to eat very simply. When I plan a meal, half the plate will be a grain, usually short-grain brown rice. About one-quarter to one-third will be vegetables—and there will usually be two different kinds, such as broccoli and carrots. The remaining quarter will be beans, such as black beans, chili, or a curry. Fruit, for me, is usually a dessert or a between-meal snack. Sometimes, I substitute a potato or other starch for the grain.

Foods to Avoid

When the Physicians Committee for Responsible Medicine proposed the New Four Food Groups, the idea was that grains, vegetables, fruits, and legumes should be the foundation of the meal. Clearly, meat, dairy, oils, nuts, seeds, alcohol, and so on should not be the main part of the diet. The next question is, should they be consumed at all?

There is a great deal of scientific evidence that meat and dairy should be left out completely. And vegetable oils are not exactly health foods, either. When you make these part of your routine, you are on your own. Let's look at the reasons why:

MEAT, POULTRY, AND FISH

All meats contain saturated fat. This is especially true of "red meat" and poultry, and even a significant portion of fish fat is saturated. In addition, all meats contain cholesterol, and it is mainly in the lean portion. Even the "leanest" meats contain cholesterol and fat.

This is not just a theoretical problem. Researchers have studied people who eat lean meats and compared them to vegetarians. The vegetarians have a decided advantage in terms of lower cholesterol levels and lower risk of heart problems.

Several studies have shown that people with heart disease who follow a diet of lean meat, chicken, and fish continue to get worse over time. When Dr. Dean Ornish managed to shrink the plaques in patients with heart disease, he could not do it with such a diet. Fish, chicken, and lean meats are too weak to do the job. He used a much more powerful program: a vegetarian diet plus other life-style changes, as described in Chapter 2.

When it comes to cancer prevention, how much fiber is there in meats? Zero. That goes for all animal products. And there are virtually no complex carbohydrates either, and no vitamin C. What this means is that animal products tend to displace these vital nutrients from the plate.

Livestock producers describe their products as sources of protein, vitamins, and minerals, but the fact is, these nutrients are available in healthier forms from plants. Meat actually contributes too much protein, as noted in Chapter 1, which causes calcium to be lost from the bones, aggravates kidney problems, and may even increase the risk of certain forms of cancer.

The vitamin content of meat is more than counterbalanced by its load of fat and cholesterol. Researchers at the State University of New York at Buffalo[2] found that, although meats contain vitamin A—a chemical which theoretically helps protect against some forms of cancer, such as cancer of the esophagus and lung—people who consume meats have higher risks of these cancers, not lower. The form of vitamin A meat contains (preformed vitamin A, rather than its precursor beta-carotene) lacks some of beta-carotene's anticancer and immune-boosting effects, and the fat in meat and its lack of fiber contribute to cancer risk. The bottom line is that, even with their vitamins and minerals, meats increase—not decrease—the risk of disease.

It is easy to forget that meats are muscles. Their purpose in nature is to move a cow's leg, a chicken's wing, or a fish's tail, and for those purposes they are perfect. But just as Goodyear does not build vitamin C into its tractor tires, nature does not pack fiber and vitamin C into a chicken's leg muscles. Muscles are designed to move body parts around, not to be ideal nutritional supplements.

To build muscle, your body does not need to eat some other animal's muscles. Bulls, stallions, elephants, and gorillas get their massive strength from eating vegetation.

Do not think that chicken and fish will give you a health food diet. Chicken's cholesterol content is the same as for beef, about 100 mg in every four ounces, and the fat in chicken is only slightly less than in beef and is still typical artery-clogging animal fat. And in addition to all the above problems, one in three chicken packages at the retail store contains live salmonella bacteria, which can cause a flulike illness, not to mention thousands of deaths every year.

There are some special concerns about fish. Contamination has become a very serious problem. Take PCBs, for example. PCBs are industrial chemicals used in electrical equipment, hydraulic fluid, and carbonless carbon paper. When you eat fish or other animals contaminated with PCBs, the chemical accumulates in your body and stays there. PCBs are the uninvited guests who showed up at your biological party and don't know when to leave. They are linked to cancer, and spell big trouble for a developing fetus. *Consumer Reports* found PCBs in 43 percent of salmon, 50 percent of whitefish, and 25 percent of swordfish.[3]

Another problem with fish is mercury. The metal settles in rivers and oceans, and according to *Consumer Reports* tests, is in 90 percent of swordfish. A typical can of tuna contains about 15 mcg of mercury. Is that safe? The government says you should feel comfortable eating up to 30 mcg of mercury. Personally, I do not feel so comfortable with even that level of exposure, particularly for pregnant women and children. Fish also contain pesticides of all sorts. Half the flounder sampled in New York contained pesticides.

Why are fish so dirty? They live in what has become civilization's sewer— the inland waterways and oceans. After all, when water drains from pesticide-covered farm fields, city sewers, or factories, pollutants of all kinds are escorted into the chemical cornucopia of rivers and streams, and eventually to the oceans. Contaminants are absorbed by fish as water passes over their gills, and because fish are carnivorous, the contaminants in smaller fish become concentrated in larger fish. Some fish are also migratory; you don't know where they've been.

As noted in Chapter 5, fish often carry contaminants with them from polluted waterways to the fish counter at the grocery store, where about 40 percent of fish samples have so much bacterial contamination that they have already begun to spoil before they are sold.

Filth is not the only reason to skip fish. Many have promoted fish as a replacement for other meats, but it is completely out of the league of the New Four Food Groups. All fish contain cholesterol and fat, including saturated fat. As noted in Chapter 1, the fish oils that were once in vogue have been found to actually encourage the production of cancer-causing free radicals.[4,5]

DAIRY PRODUCTS

Many Americans still consume large amounts of dairy products. Some even force themselves to drink milk because they believe it will help prevent osteoporosis. But dairy products are not included in the New Four Food

152

Groups, and here are ten reasons, summarized from previous chapters, why you will want to take them off your menu:

1. Dairy products are not the solution to osteoporosis. As noted in Chapter 1, milk is largely ineffective in slowing bone loss. The high occurrence of osteoporosis has more to do with the excess of protein Americans eat, along with a sedentary life-style and tobacco and alcohol use, than with any "deficiency" of cow's milk.

2. Dairy products contribute cholesterol and fat. The fat in dairy products is animal fat—i.e., mostly saturated. This problem alone rules out virtually all dairy products except skim milk, some yogurts, and a very few other nonfat dairy products. Studies comparing the cardiovascular status of lacto-ovo-vegetarians and vegans clearly give the edge to the latter, as we saw in Chapter 2.

3. Insulin-dependent diabetes is linked to dairy products. Comparisons of various countries show a strong correlation between the use of dairy products and the incidence of insulin-dependent diabetes. Confirmatory research has shown that antibodies to cow's milk protein destroy the insulin-producing cells of the body, as was detailed in Chapter 5.

4. There are difficulties from lactose intolerance. Many people, particularly those of Asian and African ancestry, are unable to digest the milk sugar, lactose. Diarrhea and gas can result.

5. Milk is one of the most common food allergies. Respiratory problems, canker sores, skin conditions, and other subtle and not-so-subtle allergies can be caused by dairy products. The sad fact is that many people never know they have a dairy sensitivity; they thought their problems were "normal." If they had given themselves a break from dairy, they might get a very pleasant surprise. Asthmatics, in particular, should give themselves a long vacation from dairy products to see whether their condition improves.

6. Chemicals anyone? Like other products from animals, dairy products contain frequent contaminants, from pesticides to drugs. According to recent studies, about one in every three cartons of milk at the retail store contains some of the antibiotics that were fed to the dairy cow. Twenty different antibiotics and thirty-three other drugs are legal for use in dairy cows. Although farmers are supposed not to sell milk from medicated cows, the regulatory system is a clear failure.[6]

    Dairies add vitamin D to milk, but do so in a haphazard way that is poorly regulated. Vitamin D is poisonous—and potentially fatal—in overdose,[7] yet recent testing of 42 milk samples found only 12 percent within the expected range of vitamin D content. Testing of ten samples of infant formula revealed that all had more vitamin D than they were supposed to. Seven had more than twice the vitamin D content reported on the label, one of which had more than four times the label amount.[8]

7. About one in five babies develops the digestive irritability called colic. It has long been known that eliminating cow's milk formulas often solves the problem. However, researchers were surprised that some breast-fed babies also developed colic. In the April 1991 issue of *Pediatrics,* researchers reported a surprising finding. Although it had been believed that the antibodies in milk are completely broken down in the process of human digestion, some of the antibodies can actually pass into the mother's bloodstream and enter her own breast milk, where they are then passed along to her nursing baby.[9] So the solution to colic is not only to take the child off cow's milk, but to take the nursing mother off it as well.

8. Although iron deficiency is a less common problem among American adults than iron excess, dairy products make a deficiency more likely. First, cow's milk products are very low in iron,[10] containing only about one-tenth of a milligram per eight-ounce serving. This makes milk particularly risky for small children. To get the U.S. Recommended Daily Allowance for iron, which is 15 mg per day for infants less than a year of age, an infant would have to drink more than thirty-one quarts of milk per day.

The iron-deficiency associated with milk is not simply due to milk's low iron content and its tendency to displace iron-rich foods. Milk can also cause the loss of blood from the intestinal tract, which over time reduces the body's iron stores. It is not yet certain how cow's milk causes blood loss, but researchers speculate that the culprit may be bovine albumin, a protein present in milk, and that it may elicit an immune reaction that leads to blood loss.[11] Pasteurization does not eliminate the problem. Researchers from the University of Iowa recently wrote in the *Journal of Pediatrics*: "In a large proportion of infants the feeding of cow milk causes a substantial increase of hemoglobin loss. Some infants are exquisitely sensitive to cow milk and can lose large quantities of blood."[11] The American Academy of Pediatrics recommends that infants under a year of age not receive unmodified cow's milk because it is deficient in iron and other nutrients.[12]

In addition, dairy products interfere with the body's absorption of iron. Milk or cheese with a meal will reduce the amount of iron absorbed by about half.[13] Calcium supplements do the same thing. Many women, particularly pregnant women, take calcium and iron supplements, unaware that calcium inhibits the absorption of iron. All forms of calcium supplements[14] cut in half the amount of iron absorbed with meals. (Women for whom iron and calcium supplements are prescribed will absorb more iron if the supplements are taken between meals.)

This is not to say that reduced iron absorption is always a bad thing, since iron has toxicities in addition to its benefits for the body. But iron deficiency is risky for children, and when it occurs, dairy products are often the culprit.

9. Ovarian cancer is linked to dairy consumption, as described in Chapter 3.
10. In a similar way, cataracts are also linked to dairy products, as we noted in Chapter 1.

Now, many people anticipate that a dairyless existence will mean waking up in the night screaming for a cheese pizza. But the desire for dairy products soon passes. And once you get away from this culinary wrong turn, you may wonder who ever got the idea to consume milk from a cow in the first place.

VEGETABLE OILS

There is a small amount of oil inherent in grains, beans, vegetables, and fruits, and small amounts are needed by the body for a variety of functions. But in excess, vegetable oil may contribute to cancer risk, as animal fat does. And all forms of fat and oil, whatever the source, contribute to weight problems. It is advisable to keep nuts, seeds, and cooking oils to a minimum, and to avoid fried foods, oil, salad dressings, margarine, and fatty baked goods. Ideally, fats and oil should contribute roughly 10 percent of the calories in the foods you eat.

Protein and Other Myths
about Vegetarian Foods

Even though people who eat according to the New Four Food Groups live years longer than those on the typical American diet, have dramatically lower risks of heart disease, cancer, and diabetes, and tend to stay slimmer, it is still common to hear people ask whether it is *safe* to eliminate meat and dairy products. Because questions about protein and calcium, in particular, are raised so frequently, it is necessary to dispel some myths.

First, *protein.* It was once thought that people who avoided meat products had to be very careful about what they ate in order to get enough protein. But it has turned out to be very easy. If you had the idea that plant foods have to be carefully combined in order to get complete proteins, you can relax. According to the American Dietetic Association and others, you will get more than enough protein as long as you eat a variety of plant foods.[15,16] There is no need to carefully "complement your proteins," nor do you have to have foods from all four groups at every meal.

Unfortunately, the worry about getting enough protein has led to an overemphasis on high-protein foods that are also high in fat and cholesterol. Americans consume more than twice the amount of protein they need. A high-protein intake is detrimental to bone strength and overworks the kidneys.

Second, *calcium.* The key to bone strength is not to maximize calcium intake but to minimize calcium loss. A plant-based menu is far superior to meat diets in this respect. The best calcium sources are green leafy vegetables and beans. If you choose to supplement, calcium-fortified orange juice is a good choice. For more details, see Chapter 1.

Some ask whether plant-based diets can provide adequate *iron.* The answer is yes, although the factors that enter into the discussion are complex. The form of iron found in meats is more easily absorbed than that in plants. This has turned out to be a liability, because meats apparently contribute to iron overload, which is common in American adults. The New Four Food Groups allow the body to regulate its iron absorption more effectively, and provide plenty of iron without the excessive iron of meat products. According to research studies, populations that consume little or no animal products actually have equal or greater iron intake than meat-eaters,[17,18,19] although slightly less of it is absorbed. Iron absorption can be increased by vitamin C.

Zinc is provided by grains such as rice, corn, and oats, as well as by peas, potatoes, spinach, and other foods. Recent research shows that, while adequate intake is important to health, overingestion can be damaging to the immune system.[20,21] The best advice is to obtain zinc naturally from foods rather than from supplements.

Finally, *riboflavin*. I know the reader has not lost much sleep over riboflavin, but it is the subject of occasional discussion among nutritionists. Diets based on plant foods are somewhat low in riboflavin. However, researchers now believe that riboflavin needs may be lower than previously thought.[22] The China Health Study has found that low riboflavin intake may not be associated with clinical deficiency symptoms. Riboflavin is provided by broccoli, asparagus, Brussels sprouts, spinach, and other green leafy vegetables.

VITAMIN B_{12}, A GENUINE BUT SIMPLE ISSUE

There is one vitamin, called vitamin B_{12}, which does present a genuine nutritional issue, although one that is easily solved. B_{12} is important for maintaining healthy blood and healthy nerves. The vitamin is not produced by plants or animals, but rather by bacteria and other one-celled organisms. The body needs only about 1 mcg per day.[23] Since the body can store this vitamin, there is no need to have a source of B_{12} every day, but you should include B_{12} at least every few days.

There have traditionally been vegetarian sources of vitamin B_{12}. Some evidence suggests that bacteria in the soil can contribute traces of B_{12} to root vegetables, and Asian foods such as miso and tempeh are loaded with the vitamin, due to the bacteria used in their production. But improved hygiene, careful washing, and modern processing destroy the bacteria that make B_{12}. Spirulina, which is often sold at health food stores, is not a consistent source of true B_{12}.

Some packaged foods, particularly breakfast cereals, are enriched with B_{12}, as you will see on their labels. Nearly all common multivitamin tablets, from Flintstones to One-A-Day to StressTabs, also contain B_{12}. Health food stores carry vegetarian B_{12} supplements, usually made from algae. Look for the words *cobalamin* or *cyanocobalamin* on the label, which are the chemical terms for vitamin B_{12}.

Those who consume animal products still get plenty of B_{12}, because the bacteria in the animals' digestive tracts produce the vitamin, although, as you know, these foods are not recommended.

Deficiencies are quite rare, and you should certainly not include animal products in your diet to get B_{12}. But you do need to include a source of B_{12} in your diet. A deficiency is usually manifested by anemia and neurological problems, such as weakness, tingling in the arms and legs, and a sore tongue. Some people experience digestive disturbances. Findings can be subtle. Medical evaluation is essential because problems with B_{12} absorption—which is a digestive tract problem having nothing to do with the amount of the vitamin in your diet—are much more common than a dietary deficiency.

Special Considerations for
Pregnancy and Nursing

When one body builds another, it needs more nutrients. Pregnant women need roughly 300 more calories a day, which means an extra cup and a half of rice or corn, or a cup of baked beans or chickpeas, or three large apples, over and above their usual eating habits. This added food naturally brings protein along with it, which the body also needs.

They also need more iron, mainly in the second half of the pregnancy. Many women have adequate iron stores without supplementation, and some recent reports have suggested that iron supplementation can cause slightly prolonged pregnancies and a slightly higher rate of complications.[24] However, many women do not have enough stored iron and need about 30 mg of supplemental iron per day, or twice that amount for women who are large, anemic, or have twin fetuses. A history of poor eating habits or iron deficiency also calls for supplementation. The most prudent course may be to have an iron blood test, called a ferritin test, at the beginning and middle of the pregnancy. It allows your doctor to begin supplementation only when needed. If such testing is not done, then most authorities agree that supplemental iron is, on balance, a good idea.

Pregnant and nursing women should be sure to include a source of B_{12}, such as an enriched cereal, traditionally manufactured miso or tempeh, or a supplement (5 mcg per day is sufficient).

For calcium, have plenty of green leafy vegetables such as broccoli or kale. The calcium from green vegetables is actually more absorbable than the calcium in milk.

Plant-based diets provide a good balance of nutrients to support a healthy pregnancy and are superior to diets containing milk or other animal products.[25,26] Whole grains, vegetables, beans, and fruits give both mother and baby the nutrients they need. Support for a vegan diet during pregnancy comes from a study of 1,700 pregnancies at The Farm, a large vegan community in Tennessee. The study showed a record of safety that would delight obstetricians. Only one in a hundred delivered by cesarean section. And in twenty years, there was only one case of preeclampsia, a syndrome of hypertension, fluid retention, urinary protein loss, and excessive weight gain, that occurs in at least 2 percent of pregnancies in the United States overall. Other studies have found similar results.[27]

Some things to avoid are fatty, sugary, and refined junk foods, as well as alcohol entirely. Children born to drinking women are at risk for low birth weight, small head circumference, mental retardation, and abnormalities of the face, heart, and extremities. While one sometimes hears rationalizations for drinking during pregnancy, it is never advisable.

Dairy products should be avoided, during both pregnancy and nursing. Cow's milk proteins can cross the placenta and even enter a woman's breast milk. These proteins are believed to spark the production of antibodies that leads to insulin-dependent diabetes.

Also, it is a good idea to stop eating fish years before you plan to become pregnant. As noted earlier, PCB and mercury contamination are common in fish. PCBs can remain in your body for decades. According to a study at Wayne State University, women who consumed fish regularly—even years before getting pregnant—had a disproportionately high incidence of children who were sluggish at birth, had a small head circumference, and showed various developmental problems.

A vegan menu is preferred for nursing women, too. A plant-based diet reduces levels of environmental contaminants in breast milk, compared to that of meat-eaters.[28] The reason for this probably relates to the concentrations of chemical contaminants in animal tissues. And, as noted, antibodies can pass from cow's milk into a milk-drinking woman's bloodstream and ultimately into her breast milk, where they can cause colic. So steering clear of animal products benefits both mother and baby.

Special Considerations for Children

The New Four Food Groups are great for kids. Vegetarian children grow up to be slimmer and healthier, and to live longer than their meat-eating friends.

Breast-feeding is nature's way of meeting the infant's nutritional needs, and also helps boost the infant's immunity, not to mention its psychological benefits. When breast-feeding is not possible, commercial soy formulas are nutritionally adequate. There is no need for infants to be raised on cow's milk formulas.[29] Aside from the colic-inducing proteins that bother many children on cow's milk formulas, cow's milk is a common cause of allergies. Immune responses to milk proteins are implicated in insulin-dependent diabetes and even in sudden infant death syndrome. Soy formulas are commonly used in all hospital nurseries, although they can occasionally be allergenic as well. Soymilk sold in grocery stores is not the same as soy baby formula, however, and is not adequate for infants.

Babies are usually born with rather high iron levels. During the first three months of life, iron supplementation should be avoided unless prescribed by your pediatrician. There is evidence that overly high iron intake can disrupt immune function and make infection more likely. However, this soon changes. Growing children need iron. A variety of beans and green leafy vegetables help meet the body's needs. The vitamin C in vegetables and fruits enhances iron absorption. Iron is another reason to avoid cow's milk. As noted above, cow's milk is very low in iron, and can induce a mild, chronic blood loss from the digestive tract.

Calcium is supplied by beans, green leafy vegetables, enriched flour, and, if desired, fortified orange juice; and excluding animal proteins helps the body retain calcium.

Children need protein to grow, but they do not need high-protein foods. A varied menu of grains, beans, vegetables, and fruits supplies plenty of protein. The "protein deficiencies" that our parents worried about in impoverished countries were the result of starvation or diets restricted to very few food items. Protein deficiency is extremely unlikely on a diet drawn from a variety of plant foods.

Very young children may need a slightly higher fat intake than do adults. Soybean products may be helpful for this purpose. Tofu hot dogs and seasoned tempeh burgers, for example, are very well accepted. However, do not take the need for fat in the diet too far. American children very often have the beginnings of heart disease before they finish high school. In contrast, Japanese children in decades past grew up on diets that were much lower in fat than those which are common in America, and there is every indication that they were better off for it.

Vitamin B_{12} is plentiful in many commercial cereals. Children who do not eat these supplemented products should have a B_{12} supplement of 3 mcg per day. Common children's vitamins contain more than enough B_{12}.

Children also need sunlight, which allows the body to make vitamin D. Children in latitudes with diminished sunlight may need the vitamin D in a typical multivitamin supplement.

Perhaps the most important consideration for children is this: Childhood is the time when dietary habits are established—habits which exert a life-long effect. Children who acquire a taste for chicken nuggets, roast beef, and french fries today are the cancer patients, heart patients, and weight-loss clinic patients of tomorrow. Children who are raised on the New Four Food Groups will have a lower risk of heart disease and cancer, compared to their counterparts raised on the average American diet. They will also tend to stay slimmer and to live years longer.

Some studies suggest that the growth of vegetarian children is more gradual—that is, a bit slower at first, but then catching up later on.[25,30] Final heights and weights are comparable to those of meat-eating children.[31] Interestingly, breast-fed babies also grow more slowly than bottle-fed babies. It may well be that nature designed the human body to grow up more gradually, to reach puberty later, and to last longer than happens for most of us raised on omnivorous diets.

In a 1980 study in Boston, researchers measured the IQs of vegetarian children.[32] Some of the children were following a macrobiotic diet, a few were Seventh-day Adventists, and the rest were from families that had simply decided to go vegetarian. On intelligence testing, the kids were considerably above average. The average IQ was 116. Now the diet probably had nothing to do with their intelligence. Rather, these vegetarian families were better educated than the average meat-eating family, and it is probably the parental education, rather than a dietary effect, that was reflected in their children's measured intelligence. On the other hand, this study should help reassure vegetarian parents who wonder whether there is something in animal products that is needed for brain development. There isn't.

As noted in Chapter 1, evidence indicates that diet can affect the age of puberty, and it may well be that parents of vegetarian children sleep better at night, knowing their children are not dating earlier than they otherwise might.

In the next chapter, we look at the process of change, and how to make it stick.

7
Getting Started

We are creatures of habit, and food habits are among those most dearly held. By the time children start school they have very strong food preferences, and they fly into near panic with any violation of them. They do not want to try new foods, not even a little bit. And even foods they do like had better not touch each other on the plate. Once learned, our food preferences are resistant to change.

It is not just food. We have a hard time breaking any habit: alcohol, tobacco, and drugs, of course, but also work habits, our behavior with friends and family, and just about every other aspect of our lives. Newlyweds soon learn how upsetting it can be when their toothpaste tubes, toilet seats, and laundry no longer conform to their accustomed habits.

Food habits may actually have a biological value. Thousands of years ago, when one of our ancestors reached to pull a berry off a bush, there was some risk in being overly adventurous, and some reassurance in sticking to the tried-and-true. This same culinary conservatism is observed in other animals. As chimpanzee toddlers put every new and shiny fruit to their lips, their mothers will flick away any foods that are not part of the chimp culture in that area. A few miles away, a different group of chimps will have a different set of dietary traditions and will rigidly adhere to those as well.

Now, of course, we recognize a need to break some habits. Healthful eating is a significant departure from the standard American diet. It has to be, because the standard diet makes us fat, gives most of us either heart disease or cancer, and measurably shortens our lives.

Kicking animal products and other greasy foods off the menu does lead to a period of missing them. This is to be expected, since most of us became used to eating these foods in earliest childhood. Breaking any habit requires an adjustment period. Happily, food habits are among the easiest to change. For example, it is much easier to become a vegetarian than it is to quit smoking. I can say this as one who has done both. For smokers, there really is no substitute for tobacco, and they simply learn to forget about it, a process which often takes a long time. When it comes to food, the situation is much easier. New foods substitute very well for old foods and lead your tastes in a new direction. You will develop a palate for new and delicate flavors. Like the traveler enjoying the simple delights of a light *potage de legumes* on the Côte d'Azur, or a spiced pasta with wine on the coast of Italy, new and wonderful foods await you.

When we break food habits, what we are actually doing is *replacing* them with new ones. I suggest that you begin this program in this way: Try the 21 Day Meal Plan of simple and delicious menus in Chapter 8. It will help you adapt your tastes and learn about some new foods, new ways to select, and new ways to prepare food. You can, if you wish, add any of the other recipes and food ideas in Chapter 8, or add any other foods, so long as they come from grains, vegetables, fruits, or legumes. Eliminate animal products and keep vegetable oil to an absolute minimum.

Be strict for twenty-one days. Then size up how you feel. The goal is not to lose fifty pounds in three weeks or to lower your cholesterol level from 300 to 150 immediately. The goal is to start the ball rolling. The next step is to do the same for another three-week period.

Breaking the process of change into three-week blocks helps you give the program your best effort without feeling any pressure of a long-term change.

Different People, Different Needs

Everyone has different needs. Some have family members to help them. Others find family members offer more hurdles than help. Some people have struggled with diets for many years, while others have never given foods any thought at all. See if you find yourself described here. The New Four Food Groups are for everyone, but you may have special considerations in the process of change.

A person not well currently. If you have existing heart disease, diabetes, a weight problem, cancer, or other serious problem, this is not a time to flirt with dietary change. This is the time to commit to an optimal menu. Grains, vegetables, fruits, and legumes are a much more powerful regimen than most old-fashioned diets, and I recommend sticking very closely to these foods. Having said that, the information in this book cannot take the place of individualized treatment by your doctor, so be sure to discuss your dietary needs and plans with your health professional. Food changes can affect medical decisions—for example, they may lower your need for insulin, blood pressure medications, or cholesterol-lowering drugs. Moreover, you may have specific needs that cannot be addressed here.

A healthy young adult. Your biggest vulnerability is thinking that you can put off changing your diet. Now is the time when foods begin to cause cancer and heart disease. These conditions often start years before they are diagnosed. You may already have started to pay attention to your weight. This is a perfect time to build a solid healthful menu. I hope you will become familiar with all sections of this book, including those that do not seem to apply to you at the moment.

A chronic dieter. If you have been dieting to lose weight, set aside your calorie charts. Allow yourself to have generous portion sizes. Be sure not only to eliminate animal products but keep vegetable oil to an absolute minimum. If you are overeating for emotional reasons, use this book in conjunction with Overeaters Anonymous, as described in Chapter 4. If you have been on a very low calorie diet, do not increase your exercise level until after you have increased your calorie intake.

A family member. If you are married, have children, or have other loved ones living with you, you will want your family to change with you. Suggestions follow.

A businessperson or frequent traveler. If you eat in the office or at restaurants several days a week, it is hard to be the master of your cuisine. See the tips that follow on travel and restaurants.

A person with a sweet tooth. If you are eating occasional sugar candies without fat in them, then enjoy them and stop feeling guilty. However, if sweets lure you to fatty foods such as pies, cookies, cakes, and chocolate, give yourself a clean break from these foods. Do not tease yourself. The same applies if you are eating huge amounts of sugary foods.

Do you need transition foods? Some people use vegetarian hot dogs, soymilk, etc. to help them make the move away from fat and cholesterol. If you would like to do so, your local health food store or gourmet aisle will feature many of these. Some of these transition foods are listed in Chapter 8. Be on the lookout for fat content, though, because some are not much better than the foods they replace. Gradually phase them out in favor of grains, vegetables, fruits, and legumes.

Exploring New Foods

Look over the menus and recipes in Chapter 8, along with tips on modifying existing recipes. These are all you need to get started, but eventually you will want more. One of the most rewarding parts of changing your diet is exploring the world of healthful foods. Learning about new foods is like visiting interesting shops, with lots to see and try. Take advantage of the chance to try enticing new foods.

• Check the cookbook section of your local library or bookstore. Look at the enormous variety of vegetarian and international cookbooks. Try out the recipes that appeal to you. Experiment, and assume that some new recipes will be terrific and others will be duds. That is what experimentation is all about. Every healthful new recipe that suits your taste is going to help save your life. But you do not need to have hundreds of recipes and a gourmet certificate on your wall. Most people eat from relatively few recipes and are happy with them. You need only find about a half-dozen recipes that you really like. You will modify your list of favorites as time goes on.

• When you dine out, explore international restaurants for healthful food ideas. Italian pastas, Chinese vegetables, Japanese miso soup and vegetarian sushi, Indian curries, Mexican beans, tortillas, and rice, and many other ethnic cuisines make healthy eating a joy.

• Today's health food stores are wonderful places for America's favorite pastime—shopping. Not so many years ago, health food stores were dingy places with dusty shelves and never-ending folk music. Well, those days are gone. Beautiful new shops have opened up to display their wares, meeting the demand for healthy and delicious foods. Organic produce, vegetarian pizza, quick and easy soups, meatless burgers, nondairy "ice creams," tasty milk substitutes, and chemical-free frozen vegetables are only the beginning. There is a world of healthful eating in bright, colorful packages within anyone's reach. They also carry low-sodium varieties of canned foods.

- Take another look at your local grocery. The produce selection is more varied every year. The aisle that used to stock plain spaghetti and instant mashed potatoes now has an endless array of packaged dinners, from curried rice to tabouli, that are delicious and very easy to make. In the gourmet aisle, you will find interesting and exotic condiments to spice up your foods: elegant chutneys, mustards, and so on. Some groceries carry low-fat soymilks on shelves formerly reserved for canned condensed milk, and some have nonfat salad dressings, meatless hot dogs, and other unusual foods in the "dietetic" aisle. There are also healthful new soups, such as lentil, minestrone, and ramen noodle.

One suggestion: Do not go shopping on an empty stomach. Your stomach will override your judgment, and you will end up buying all kinds of things that will gather dust on the shelf.

The Process of Change

In my practice, I have helped patients deal with all kinds of destructive habits, from tobacco and alcohol to cocaine and heroin. The force of habit is tremendously powerful. The key is to get the force of habit working *for* you instead of against you. A person who is trying to stop smoking is set back by having an occasional cigarette. But every day without tobacco helps build a new habit: the habit of being a nonsmoker.

Similarly, you are not building a healthful habit if you are teasing yourself with fried chicken once a week and an occasional hamburger; doing so only reinforces your taste for greasy foods. So don't tease yourself. Get some distance from offending foods, and get the force of a new habit working for you. Every day that you don't eat animal products or added oils makes these products less likely to show up on your plate in the future. In the process, you are also resetting your taste for fat at a new lower level.

Now, I know what you are thinking. Most of us feel daunted by long-term commitments. A lifetime without pork chops or hamburgers may seem a harsh thing. The solution is to think short-term. Anyone can make a dramatic change for a few weeks. Resolve to change your menu completely, but only for three weeks. At the end of that time, decide if you would like to continue for another three weeks. Notice how your weight has changed. Have your cholesterol and blood pressure checked, if you like. You may be surprised at the improvement. Making a complete break from the offending old foods is so rewarding that most people want to stick with the new winning formula. Halfway measures give few rewards and make it all the harder to stick with dietary changes.

You won't need any calorie charts or food scales. The New Four Food Groups are low in fat, modest in calories, and contain no cholesterol, so you can eat generous amounts anytime you want. If you are measuring calories, fat content, or protein intake, there is something wrong with the foods you are eating.

Handling Slips and Cravings

When people change any habit, sometimes there is a period of uncertainty and cravings. Eventually a feeling of success takes its place. But initially you may find yourself window-shopping at a fast-food restaurant, thinking maybe just one burger can't do that much harm.

It takes most people anywhere from three weeks to two months to really get used to a new way of eating. It helps to anticipate that and to know that before long you will be totally comfortable with your new way of eating. Think of any habit you ever changed. When people quit smoking, for instance, they think about cigarettes after meals and during every lull in a conversation, and this goes on for several days. Cravings become less and less frequent, and the new nonsmoker often actually comes to dislike the smell of smoke and to be annoyed with smokers who bring their odors too close.

Food habits are much, much easier to break than tobacco habits, but something similar happens. For a while you may crave greasy foods, but this does not last. Very soon you may find that your taste for fat starts to diminish, and you may actually become annoyed when a waiter butters your toast or puts an egg sauce all over your broccoli.

You may have an occasional slip. You are at a Christmas party, and in all the excitement, you somehow polished off a cheese omelet with gravy. You can almost hear your coronary arteries complaining, chanting in protest like prisoners behind bars: How could you abuse us this way? OK, relax. Forgive yourself. The real danger of a slip is using it as an excuse to abandon your new way of eating. As you get back in gear with your healthful way of eating, you will find that slips are less and less likely.

A good way to handle cravings is to eat something healthful. Don't get judgmental about whatever craving you have had; just eat something healthful and as hunger dissipates, cravings tend to be forgotten, too.

It helps to get offending foods out of the house. This means animal products and oily foods. Throw them away or give them away, but get rid of the temptation. Restock with healthful foods so when snack time hits you have something good on hand. Fresh fruit, toast, cereal, air-popped popcorn, soymilks, bread, dried fruit, and instant soups make great snacks, and you will find endless other possibilities.

FAMILY ON YOUR SIDE

Our families eat with us. We share similar tastes, and we share all the family times when food plays a central role. As you redesign your menu, it helps to involve your family and friends, for two reasons. First, you need their support. Starting new habits is much easier with their help, and more difficult if they give you a hard time. Second, they need your help in changing their diets, too. If you don't help them improve their diets, you may wish you had. Don't think they can't change. Everyone is rethinking food choices now that the links with serious illness have become so clear. Just as smokers' families do them no favors by keeping quiet, people who watch their spouses or children eat the standard Western diet day after day may see them pay a very high price before long.

When loved ones don't care about their health (or yours), you have a problem, but one that can be solved. People who persist in unhealthful eating habits may simply be showing a lack of knowledge of the health risks, a lack of experience with healthy and tasty foods, or just plain denial.

Let's face it. Any change causes reactions in people around us. A woman who has had long hair all her life and decides to cut it short will encounter resistance from her family. A man who after several years shaves off his beard will elicit mixed reactions from family and friends. Dietary changes encounter the same expressions of surprise. Although you may be tempted not to "rock the boat," a little boat rocking may be a good idea if the boat is headed for the reefs. In the long run, you will be very happy that you've changed the way you eat, and so will your family.

When you talk about healthful eating, family members may react with jokes about "eating rabbit food," or with "bargaining," such as the statement, "I had a healthy breakfast so I can have fried chicken for dinner."

These statements, annoying as they may be, are actually very good signs. Why? Because they show—in spades—something that psychologists have studied for many years. The process of accepting new ideas occurs in stages. Denial, ridicule, and even anger are predictable events that occur early in the process of change. Elisabeth Kübler-Ross wrote of the stages of acceptance of death, and the "deaths" of outmoded ideas follow a very similar series: denial, then anger, followed by bargaining, depression, and ultimately acceptance, In other words, we first try to push away the need to change the way we eat, sometimes using jokes or ridicule. If that fails, we naturally become annoyed. We try to "bargain" so as to make as few changes as possible, counting the number of eggs we down in a week or which part of the chicken we ate. If we have the opportunity to learn why halfway changes are not much use, we come to the depressing realization that we have not done much for ourselves. Ultimately, we accept the need to change and begin to take steps to accomplish it. And the rewards follow. So do not despair when family members are resistant. Psychiatrists know that when patients begin to express their resistance to new ideas the process of resolving the resistance can begin.

So what are the best strategies for coping with family obstacles? People in the denial phase just need more information. Give them a book from the lists on pages 305–6. If reading is not their strong suit, try a tape. If you are in charge of the kitchen, ignore the resistance and prepare healthful meals. The palate can often be seduced even while the mind resists.

People in the anger phase simply need to be humored or ignored because they will pass into the next stage on their own. Those who are stuck in the bargaining stage need more information. They need to learn why a chicken salad sandwich will not clean out their coronary arteries or why their weight-loss diet did not work.

Some people will not change despite your best efforts. Human lethargy can be a powerful force, and sometimes the most you can do is not let someone else's resistance affect your own eating habits. And sometimes even the most reluctant family members will surprise you and suddenly want to improve their diets.

A word about guilt. People often feel terribly guilty about their dietary indiscretions. Family members may feel that you are slinging guilt if you even mention food. As the health-conscious member of the family, you may end up being regarded as everyone else's culinary conscience. People begin apologizing to you for something they ate, or they may start hiding things in the back of the refrigerator in hopes that you will not notice. This is not a role you asked for; it just seems to happen. I suspect that people tend to feel guilty about food issues because of the ways food was used in their earliest family interactions, with all the rules and demands that went with it. An uneaten portion was a snub to the cook. A spilled water glass aggravated an already strained young family. The dinner table is a place where family rules and traditions play a big role. Is it any surprise that discussions of food later in life can bring rules and guilt to mind?

Of course, there are moral issues that relate to eating. Anyone who has a spouse or a child needs to try to stay healthy. Those who neglect their own health are not doing their dependents any favors. Also there are moral issues in the experience of the billions of animals that are processed through livestock industries every year, and the use of millions of acres to grow feed crops for animals and the environmental damage that results from it. Even so, I try to provide information and to steer clear of guilt. If a family member feels that your insistence on healthful eating is sanctimonious, it is a good time to remind them, "I just love you and I want you to be around forever, or as close to it as possible."

If you are concerned that your new eating habits may present added burdens to others, don't worry. Even dining at restaurants and the family reunion barbecue can be a snap using the tips that follow for special situations.

It is easy to bring the chance to taste new foods to your family. Just pick out some recipes from this book or any of the huge variety of vegetarian cookbooks now available, and try some out. The transition foods can be very helpful. Nonmeat hot dogs and burgers are often indistinguishable from the artery-clogging varieties, especially after the ketchup and mustard are added. A trip to the health food store will supply you with lots of things to try out. No need for a lot of fanfare. My mother used to say, "Don't tell your father that the egg salad is really tofu." It tasted as good or better than the high-cholesterol variety.

Children are the truest traditionalists. They do not trust new foods, and may frustrate parents' hopes for variety in their diets. On the other hand, kids like to help out preparing new recipes. Children often like soymilks, which are widely available in a range of flavors and are very nutritious. When other children come over for dinner or a birthday party, try spaghetti instead of quinoa salad.

Don't be daunted by a loved one who seems not to care about health or denies the health risks. Education and the chance to taste new foods can overcome even dinosaur-size habits. Meat-eaters today are like smokers in the 1950s. They may not have stopped yet, but they know they cannot keep it up forever. That knowledge is half the battle.

DIGESTIVE PROBLEMS

A change in diet is always a temporary challenge for the digestion. This is true both for those who adopt a healthful menu and for those who slip from a healthful diet to a traditional one. But rest assured, the effect is usually short-lived.

Beans and some vegetables may cause gas for some people, some varieties more than others. Pinto beans, for example, seem to cause more gas than black beans. Try to pin down what is the dietary problem for you: cabbage, broccoli, orange juice, or whatever. Limit beans to moderate amounts, and include generous amounts of grains, such as rice. Most people find that, when they have adapted to a higher fiber diet, gassiness goes away.

Special Situations

DINING OUT

You are planning a night on the town, or maybe your boss asks you to lunch. No need to worry. Simply suggest a restaurant. Italian restaurants are everywhere. Spaghetti with tomato sauce or *pasta e fagioli* (pasta and bean soup) are healthful and taste terrific. Or how about Chinese? The menu of every Chinese restaurant has a vegetable section. These are not side dishes; they are entrees, usually served with rice. Delicate vegetables, sometimes combined with spiced tofu, are served with rice and various exotic teas. At Mexican restaurants, have a bean burrito with rice. Larger cities have Indian restaurants, with any number of delicious curries combining spinach, potatoes, chickpeas, cauliflower, and other vegetables with carefully combined spices, served with rice or exotic breads. Thai, Japanese, Vietnamese, Middle Eastern, and many other cuisines bring delicious and healthful cuisine. It is still important to be selective, however, because even many ethnic restaurants use excessive amounts of oil. Mexican restaurants may cook beans with lard. Look for menu items that are low in oil. Steamed, baked, or boiled foods are usually better than fried. When in doubt, ask.

At American-style restaurants, do not hesitate to ask for a vegetable plate, salad bar, or pasta dishes. They nearly always have them. At salad bars, skip fat-laden macaroni or potato salads and bacon bits, and favor bean salads or chickpeas prepared without oil, along with fresh vegetables and greens. Instead of dressing, try a sprinkle of lemon or lime juice, or enjoy the taste of salad with no dressing at all.

In 1991 the National Restaurant Association asked all its members to feature vegetarian entrees, because at that time about one in five diners was looking for them. If you don't see vegetarian dishes on the menu, by all means ask. Nowadays, that is a routine request.

Many people believe that they must stick to the menu. Don't. Restaurants are usually quite happy to leave the bacon off the spinach salad, to provide a tomato sauce instead of meat sauce for the spaghetti, or to bring you a hot vegetable plate.

Invited to a Dinner Party?

When I am invited to dinner or to a party at a friend's house, I find that the following simple strategy always allays any problem. At the time of the invitation, or as soon thereafter as I remember to do so, I call and say that I try to stick to vegetarian foods, and would like to bring something, like a meatless spaghetti sauce or hummus. Invariably, the hosts will say that there is no reason to worry—there will be plenty to eat. Whatever they were really thinking, they now will be sure to include something healthful, and I've just given them two suggestions. The risk of not telling them is that they will either be surprised when you avoid eating what they prepared or, if you do eat it, they will feel guilty later.

If the party is a backyard barbecue, bring along some tofu hot dogs, vegetable shish kebobs, or baked potatoes in foil. Your hosts will be delighted that you added something a little different to the party.

Travel

Travel does not have to mean giving up on healthy eating. All airlines now offer vegetarian meals if you ask for them in advance. The demand for these foods has led some to offer them as part of their in-flight routine. On the road, fast-food restaurants now offer baked potatoes and salad bars, and all taco restaurants have bean burritos (hold the cheese). In the car, bring along some fruit, and sandwiches filled with hummus, lettuce, tomato, and cucumber. Soups travel well in a thermos bottle. Stock up on some instant soups at your local health food store—restaurants along the way will be glad to give you some hot water. In some parts of the world, such as Eastern Europe, vegetarian cuisine has not yet made many inroads, and even fruits and vegetables may be scarce. When I am traveling to such places, I check the local phone book for a vegetarian restaurant or society and ask the hotel management for restaurant suggestions. I often bring along some emergency instant soups in my luggage, too.

I find that my own dietary habits continue to evolve. As I visit new places, I continually develop new tastes and find new and interesting food products. I hope you enjoy the same continuing exploration of healthful foods.

8
Menus and Recipes

This chapter will provide you with practical information about selecting and preparing the foods of the New Four Food Groups, including planning ideas and guidelines for modifying your own favorite recipes. You will discover that cooking from the New Four Food Groups opens up a world of exciting new flavors. Many of the recipes are based on the cuisine of other cultures, where the diet naturally tends to emphasize these foods. You will be amazed and delighted at how much more interesting and varied your diet becomes as you prepare these new recipes.

Getting to Know the Foods of the New Four Food Groups

As you begin the transition to a more wholesome diet, remember that tastes for food are learned. Just as you have learned to like high-fat, sugary, salty foods, your taste buds can be retrained to appreciate the fresh, full taste of nourishing, wholesome food. Recognizing, however, that some time may be required for your taste buds to adjust, a number of transition foods—foods which simulate the taste and texture of meat and other familiar foods—are listed in Table 9. Although these transition foods are generally lower in fat and sodium than their meat-based counterparts, they are still higher than is optimal. For this reason they should be used as a bridge between your old way of eating and your new, and eventually be phased out by the exciting new flavors of the New Four Food Groups.

Grains, Breads, and Pastas

Almost every culture has a staple grain around which its cuisine is centered. In the United States, that grain tends to be wheat, which is ground into flour and made into bread and other baked goods. To a lesser extent, we use rice, corn, and oats. Yet the array of grains presently available is practically endless, as a trip to your local health food store will show you. From kasha and quinoa to millet and polenta, grains offer a remarkable diversity of delicious tastes and textures. They can be used to prepare salads, pilaf, casseroles, and desserts. They are delicious in soups, and of course are an ideal food for breakfast.

In addition to being inexpensive and easy to prepare, grains are nutritious; they are rich in complex carbohydrates, fiber, and many vitamins and minerals. They are good sources of protein and are very low in fat. Whole grains should become the mainstay of your diet; plan your meals with grains at the center.

Grains that have been refined, such as white flour and white rice, have lost important vitamins, minerals, and fiber. Keep these to a minimum in your diet. Whole grains, on the other hand, retain their full nutritive value. They have more texture and are more filling. A diet based on whole grains is one of the best ways to reach and maintain your ideal weight because whole grains fill you up with fewer calories.

When purchasing bread, be sure to select a whole-grain bread, which provides fiber as well as important vitamins and minerals. By reading the label, you can determine if the bread you are buying is whole grain. The first ingredient should be a *whole*-grain flour such as "whole wheat flour." Don't be fooled by labels that list "wheat flour" (actually white flour) in an attempt to mislead you.

Pasta is another delicious way to enjoy grains. A wide variety of pastas, in different shapes and flavors, is available in health food stores and most supermarkets. In addition to traditional wheat-based pastas, you can find pastas made from corn, quinoa, spelt, and Jerusalem artichoke. Experimenting with these different pastas will add interest and variety to your meals. Look for pastas made without eggs. These are available in health food stores and most supermarkets. For a quick dinner simply top cooked pasta with a commercially prepared marinara sauce (be sure to choose a low-fat or fat-free variety). Add a green salad or cooked vegetable and whole-grain bread, then relax and enjoy the feast.

Some other whole grains that will add taste and variety to your diet include:

Barley. Many people are familiar with barley only as an addition to vegetable soup—and a delicious addition it is! Yet barley has many other possibilities. Its mellow sweet taste and satisfying texture make it a terrific breakfast cereal, and it can also be used as an addition to casseroles, pilaf, and salads. Pearl barley, which is more commonly available, has been refined. Look for unrefined, whole barley in health food stores.

Buckwheat. Often associated with Eastern European cuisine, buckwheat has a unique, robust flavor that goes well with onions, mushrooms, and cabbage. Its assertive flavor makes it a grain that people either love or hate. Toasted buckwheat, called kasha, has a stronger flavor than raw buckwheat groats. Both forms are sold in health food stores. Cook buckwheat over very low heat to keep it from becoming mushy.

Corn. Indigenous to the Americas, corn may be finely ground into cornmeal, or coarsely ground into grits or polenta. Use cornmeal for cornbread and as an addition to other breads and baked goods. Polenta, which is a staple in northern Italy, is delicious served with marinara or any spicy vegetable sauce.

Millet. This ancient grain of Asia and North Africa is rich in vitamins and minerals. Toast it in a dry skillet before cooking to help it retain its shape and add a delightful toasty flavor. Millet makes a delicious stuffing for vegetables, and is also good in pilaf, breads, and burgers.

Oats. When you mention oats, most people think oatmeal. If you are not an oatmeal fan, you might want to try steel-cut oats, which are chewy and much less mushy than rolled oats. I personally enjoy rolled oats prepared as müesli, a breakfast cereal of Swiss origin. The recipe is on page 215. Rolled oats can also be added to baked goods and used to thicken soups and sauces.

Quinoa. Originating in South America, quinoa (pronounced *"keen-wah"*) is high in protein and calcium. It cooks quickly and has a light, fluffy texture. Use it in salads and pilaf. Quinoa should be rinsed thoroughly before cooking to remove its bitter-tasting coating called saponin, which is believed to be the plant's naturally occurring protection from insects.

Rice. If instant-cooking rice is the only kind you've ever eaten, you are in for a treat as you discover the many varieties of rice available to you. To begin with, rice comes in white and brown versions. Choose brown rice whenever possible, as it is unrefined and retains all of its vitamins, minerals, and fiber. Long-grain brown rice is light and fluffy, and is probably the best initial substitute for the white rice you may be used to. Short-grain brown rice has a heartier texture and a nutlike flavor, which makes it an excellent addition to any meal. Basmati rice (which is available in both white and brown versions) is highly aromatic and flavorful.

Although brown rice takes about thirty minutes to cook, once it's been started it pretty much takes care of itself. I usually cook two or three times as much as I need and keep it on hand in the refrigerator or freezer. Reheating it takes just a matter of minutes in the microwave or in a nonstick pan on the stovetop. Several companies, including Arrowhead Mills, Uncle Ben's, and Fantastic Foods, make quick-cooking brown rice that cooks in just ten to fifteen minutes. Look in your health food store or the grain section of your supermarket.

Quick-cooking rice pilafs are also available in a variety of flavors in health food stores and supermarkets. These are great time-savers, but be sure to read the label to make sure they do not contain MSG, animal products, or artificial flavors. The instructions for many of these products call for added margarine or oil, but these can be omitted with no loss of flavor.

Wheat, bulgur, couscous. Wheat is the grain that most Americans are familiar with, though usually in its refined, white flour form. When wheat is processed to make white flour, the bran and germ portions are removed, and vitamins and minerals as well as protein and fiber are lost. Whole wheat flour retains all these nutrients, and should be used whenever possible. You will find that products made with whole wheat flour have more texture and are more filling than their white flour counterparts. For cookies, muffins, and quick breads where a lighter texture is desired, use whole wheat pastry flour, a whole-grain flour ground from a softer variety of wheat.

Bulgur is made from whole wheat kernels that have been cracked and toasted. It has a delicious, nutty flavor and is ready in just fifteen minutes. It is delicious as a breakfast cereal as well as in pilaf, salads, and stuffings.

Couscous is made from durum wheat that has been ground, steamed, and dried into small pieces. It is light, fluffy, and fun to eat. Because it can be prepared in just five minutes, it is a perfect addition to last-minute meals and for light meals on hot summer days. Whole-grain couscous is available in many health food stores, and is nutritionally superior to white couscous.

Most grains are cooked in the following manner: Bring water to a boil and add the grain. Allow water to return to a simmer, then cover and cook without stirring for the specified amount of time. One exception is cornmeal, or polenta, which is cooked uncovered and stirred frequently while it cooks. Use the following table to determine the cooking times for various grains.

Grains (1 cup dry)	Amount of Water	Cooking Time	Yield
Barley	3 cups	1¼ hours	3½ cups
Brown rice	3 cups	30 minutes	3 cups
Buckwheat	2 cups	15 minutes	2½ cups
Bulgur (cracked wheat)	2 cups	15 minutes	2½ cups
Couscous	1½ cups	10 minutes	1½ cups
Millet	3 cups	20 minutes	3½ cups
Polenta	4 cups	15 minutes	4 cups
Quinoa	1½ cups	15 minutes	4 cups
Whole wheat berries	3 cups	2 hours	2½ cups

Tips for Cooking Grains

- Lightly roasting grains in a dry skillet before cooking enhances their nutty flavor and gives them a lighter texture. The flavor of millet is particularly enhanced by roasting.

- With few exceptions, grains should not be stirred during cooking. Stirring tends to make most grains sticky. They will be fluffier if you leave them alone while they cook.

- When cooking grain for a meal, make more than you need. Refrigerate or freeze the extra in usable portions. Leftover grain is a great time-saver when preparing future meals.

- Fine-textured grains like couscous and bulgur are actually fluffier when they are not cooked. Simply pour boiling water over the grain, then cover and let stand for 15 to 20 minutes. Fluff the grain with a fork before serving.

LEGUMES

Beans may be purchased dried, canned, and in some cases, frozen or dehydrated. Good selections of beans may be found in supermarkets as well as in health food stores. Dried beans are very inexpensive and simple to cook. If you don't have the time to cook dried beans, canned beans are a good alternative. Kidney beans, chickpeas, pinto beans, black beans, and many others are available, including some in low-sodium varieties. For an even quicker meal, try vegetarian baked beans, chili beans, and refried beans—all available in the canned food section of most supermarkets.

Several varieties of beans, including pinto beans, black beans, split peas, and lentils, are available precooked and dehydrated. These cook in just ten to fifteen minutes, and are delicious. Check your local health food store.

• *Cleaning.* Dried beans may contain dust or small stones. Pinto beans and black beans are particularly notorious. For this reason, they should be picked over and washed thoroughly.

• *Soaking.* All beans, with the exception of lentils and split peas, should be soaked before cooking. Soaking beans improves digestibility and decreases cooking time. To decrease the gas-producing tendency of beans, soak them at least four

Cooking Beans

Beans (1 cup dry)	Amount of Water	Cooking Time	Yield
Aduki (azuki, adzuki) beans	3 cups	1½ hours	2¼ cups
Black beans	3 cups	1½ hours	2¼ cups
Black-eyed peas	3 cups	1 hour	2 cups
Chickpeas (garbanzos)	4 cups	2–3 hours	2½ cups
Great northern beans	3½ cups	2 hours	2 cups
Kidney beans	3 cups	2 hours	2 cups
Lentils	3 cups	1 hour	2¼ cups
Lima beans	2 cups	1½ hours	1½ cups
Navy beans	3 cups	2 hours	2 cups
Pinto beans	3 cups	2½ hours	2¼ cups
Red beans	3 cups	3 hours	2 cups
Soybeans	4 cups	3 hours	2½ cups
Split peas	3 cups	1 hour	2½ cups

hours, then pour off the soaking water and begin cooking the beans in fresh water.

• *Cooking.* Place soaked beans in a pot with fresh water and bring them to a simmer. Loosely cover the pot. Cook for the amount of time specified in the table on page 179, or until completely tender. Check occasionally to make sure there is sufficient water, adding extra if needed.

FRUITS AND VEGETABLES

I think of fruits and vegetables as beautiful gifts of stored sunshine. They are rich in vitamins, minerals, and fiber, and provide a tremendous variety of tastes and textures. Whenever possible, choose fresh fruits and vegetables in season. They taste better, are more nutritious, and cost less. Foods out of season must be stored in expensive warehouse space under refrigeration, and important vitamins are lost while they sit in storage. Other out-of-season fruits and vegetables are grown outside the United States. Pesticides which have been outlawed in the United States, such as DDT, are still used in many countries that supply produce to the United States.

Local farmers' markets are excellent sources of fresh, seasonal produce.

Tips for Cooking Beans

• Salt toughens the skins of beans and increases their cooking time. If you are adding salt, wait until the beans are tender.

• A crockpot is an ideal way to cook beans. The slow, even heat ensures thorough cooking and reduces the chance of scorching. If you add the beans to the crockpot with boiling water, and use the high setting, they will cook as quickly as on the stove. With cold water they take longer.

• Using a pressure cooker to cook beans is fast and efficient. Be sure to follow the instructions that come with the cooker.

• Beans, unlike other vegetables, should be very thoroughly cooked. It is better to err on the side of overcooking.

• Cooked beans keep in the refrigerator for up to a week. They also freeze well. You can save time by cooking extra and freezing them in airtight containers for later use.

The selection is usually more diverse than that found in supermarkets, and many items are organically grown. When shopping for produce at a supermarket, the items most abundant and lowest in price are usually those that are in season.

If fresh vegetables are unavailable, choose plain frozen vegetables prepared without sauce. If you cannot get fresh fruit, choose fruit canned in water or fruit juice. Avoid fruit canned in heavy syrup. Some fruits, especially berries, are available frozen. Read the label to be sure that they do not contain a lot of added sugar.

Transition Foods

Health food stores and some supermarkets carry a variety of products that will help you make the transition to a more healthful diet while still enjoying the familiar tastes of meat dishes. These transition foods, ranging from burgers to "ribs," are delicious stand-ins when you find yourself craving a burger, hot dog, or some other old favorite. They can also be useful for family members who are resistant to changing to a more healthful diet or fearful that they will no longer be able to eat the way other people do. Transition foods are also perfect for those special occasions, like company picnics, when you'd like to have something to throw onto the grill.

Soybeans are used to make a variety of products, including tofu burgers, seasoned tempeh burgers, and tofu hot dogs. Wheat gluten is used to make burgers and sliced "meats." Some of these products are higher in fat than is optimal, and you will probably want to phase them out over time, or reserve them for special occasions. See Table 9 for a list of these foods.

Table 9   *Transition Foods*

Product Name	Fat Content (% of calories)
Vegetarian Burgers	
Lightlife American Grill (soy)	26%
Lightlife Barbecue Grill (soy)	41%
Lightlife Lemon Grill (soy)	33%
Meat of Wheat Burger (wheat)	9%
Soy Deli Tofu Burger (soy)	56%
Stow Mills Tofu Burger (soy)	45%
White Wave Meatless Tofu Steaks (soy)	48%
White Wave Tempeh Burger (soy)	25%
White Wave Teriyaki Burger (soy)	25%
Worthington Vegetarian Burger (wheat)	25%
Yves Veggie Burgers (soy, wheat)	26%
Vegetarian Hot Dogs	
Lightlife Smart Dogs (soy, wheat)	0%
Lightlife Tofu Pups (soy)	53%
SoyBoy Not Dogs (soy)	49%
Yves Veggie Tofu Wieners (soy)	40%
Deli Meat Substitutes	
Heart & Soul BBQ Whibs (wheat)	13%
Heart & Soul Trim Slice Roast Beef Style (wheat)	19%
Heart & Soul Trim Slice Turkey Style (wheat)	11%
Lightlife Fakin' Bacon (soy)	29%
Lightlife Foney Baloney (soy)	53%
Lightlife Lean Links (soy)	39%
Loma Linda Little Links (wheat)	56%
Meat of Wheat Sausage Style (wheat)	11%
SoyBoy Vegetarian Breakfast Links (soy)	53%
Yves Veggie Deli Slices (soy)	26%
Other Meat Substitutes	
Meat of Wheat Chicken Style (wheat)	17%
Meat of Wheat Hearty Original (wheat)	9%

Stocking Your Pantry for Healthful Eating

By keeping a selection of the following items on hand, you can prepare a healthful meal on a moment's notice. Some of the items are ingredients that show up frequently in recipes. Others are healthful, quick-to-prepare alternatives for those days when there just isn't time to cook.

Produce

Yellow onions
Garlic
Carrots
Celery
Potatoes: russets and red
Raisins
Frozen strawberries
Frozen bananas

Grains

Pasta (fettuccine, spaghetti, lasagne noodles)
Bulgur (toasted cracked wheat)
Rice: basmati, white, and brown
Couscous
Polenta or other cornmeal
Rolled oats
Unbleached all-purpose flour
Whole wheat pastry flour
Whole wheat flour

Legumes

Dried lentils
Dried split peas
Dried pinto beans
Canned kidney beans
Canned chickpeas
Canned black beans
Dehydrated pinto beans
Dehydrated black beans

Nuts and Seeds

Peanut butter
Tahini (sesame seed butter)

Convenience Foods

Unsweetened apple butter
Fruit preserves, unsweetened or sweetened with fruit juice
Pancake mixes
Breakfast cereal
Fantastic Foods Tofu Scrambler
Ramen soups
Vegetarian soup cups
Canned soups
Dehydrated soup mixes
Canned tomatoes
Canned tomato sauce
Canned pumpkin
Quick-cooking brown rice
Burger mix: Fantastic Foods
Falafel mix
Canned vegetarian refried beans
Vegetarian baked beans
Dehydrated pinto beans, black beans
Spaghetti sauce: Healthy Choice, Newman's Own
Salsa
Aseptically packaged tofu (keeps unrefrigerated for 6
    months to 1 year)
Tortillas (these can be frozen)
Pita bread (this can be frozen)

Transition Foods

Baked tofu
Vegetarian hot dogs
Tofu burgers, tempeh burgers, veggie burgers

Snack Foods

Fat-free crackers: Health Valley, RyKrisp
Rice cakes, popcorn cakes
Fat-free tortilla chips: Barbara's Basically Baked

Pretzels
Popcorn (for air-popping)

Miscellaneous

Vegetable broth (powder or cubes)
Vegetable oil spray (optional)
Seasoned rice vinegar
Cider vinegar
Soy sauce
Stone-ground mustard
Nayonnaise (eggless mayonnaise made from tofu)
Salt substitutes: Mrs. Dash, Parsley Patch
Non-aluminum baking powder: Rumford
Hot beverages: herbal teas, Cafix, Postum, Pero

Modifying Your Own Recipes

The recipes in this chapter provide a wide variety of delicious low-fat foods. In addition, your own recipes can be made more healthful by using the following guidelines:

REDUCING FAT

Small changes in cooking techniques can reduce fat significantly with little or no effect on the final flavor of the dish.

- Steam or bake food instead of frying. Avoid deep-fried foods.
- Use nonstick pots and pans, which allow foods to be prepared with little or no added fat.
- Instead of sautéing vegetables in oil, braise them: Heat approximately ½ cup of liquid (water, vegetable stock, wine, dry sherry) in a large pot or skillet. Add the vegetables to be sautéed, then cover and cook over medium heat, stirring occasionally, until the vegetables are tender. This normally takes about five minutes. Add small amounts of additional liquid if the vegetables begin to stick.
- When absolutely necessary to sauté or fry in oil, nonstick vegetable oil sprays allow you to do so with a fraction of the fat.
- Use a steamer rack to cook vegetables, and a steamer or microwave oven to reheat foods that would otherwise stick to the pan.

- Use a fat-free dressing on salads. Several commercial varieties are available, or try the recipes beginning on page 233. Seasoned rice vinegar and lemon juice are also good on salads.

- Try eating cooked vegetables plain, or with a bit of seasoned rice vinegar or lemon juice, instead of olive oil or butter. Fat-free salad dressings are also delicious on cooked vegetables.

- Oil in salad dressing recipes can be replaced with vegetable stock or water. You can also use seasoned rice vinegar (mild and slightly sweet) to replace the oil. Add it to the recipe in addition to any other vinegar. For a thicker dressing, the oil may be replaced with a cornstarch and water mixture as follows: Whisk 1 tablespoon cornstarch with 1 cup water. Heat in a small saucepan, stirring constantly, until thick and clear. Refrigerate. Use in place of oil in any salad dressing recipe. May be kept refrigerated for up to three weeks.

- Cream soups are usually prepared with heavy cream or with butter-based sauces. A fat-free alternative for making soup thick and "creamy" is to add a potato. For soups that will be pureed, simply cook and puree the potato along with the other soup ingredients. For other soups, cook a scrubbed and diced potato in enough water to cover it. When the potato is fork-tender, puree it in its cooking water in the blender and add it to the soup.

- Sauces are traditionally prepared with fat, flour, and liquid. To omit the fat, toast the flour in a dry pan over medium heat until it is lightly browned. Add the liquid and any seasonings. Whisk to remove all lumps, then cook over medium heat, stirring constantly until thickened.

- Avocados and coconut should be regarded as practically pure fat and consumed in very limited quantities, if at all.

- Nuts and seeds are 80 to 90 percent fat. Omitting them from recipes will eliminate significant fat. When you remove nuts, you lose texture as well as flavor. Try replacing them with a crunchy vegetable or fruit to add texture to the dish. In some baking recipes, Grape-Nuts cereal may be substituted for nuts.

- When you are craving ice cream, consider fruit sorbet or one of the low-fat nondairy frozen desserts listed on page 276. Or try one of the recipes in this book.

- The amount of fat in recipes for baked goods is sometimes arbitrary and can easily be reduced. For example, most carrot cake recipes call for 1 cup of oil, yet this amount can be reduced to ⅓ or ½ cup with no noticeable effect on the cake.

- Eliminating fat completely from baked goods may affect the texture and will require some experimentation. In some recipes, the fat can be removed with no other modification. In other recipes, applesauce, mashed banana, or canned pumpkin may be substituted for all or part of the fat.

- Prepare pies with a single crust to reduce fat and calories (about 100 fewer calories per serving). Crumb crusts may be prepared with less fat than traditional flour-based crusts, or try the Fat-Free Pie Crust on page 286.

REPLACING EGGS

Omitting eggs from baked goods will reduce the fat and cholesterol significantly. If the recipe calls for one or two eggs, just leave them out, adding a couple of extra tablespoons of water for each egg to maintain the intended moisture content. If more than two eggs are called for, substitute one of the following for each egg:

- 1 ounce (2 tablespoons) pureed soft tofu
- ½ banana, mashed
- ⅓ cup applesauce or canned pumpkin
- 1 tablespoon flaxseeds pureed in a blender with ¼ cup water
- 1 heaping tablespoon soy flour mixed with 2 tablespoons water
- 2 tablespoons cornstarch
- Ener-G egg replacer—a mixture of potato starch, flour, and leavening—is available at most health food stores. Use according to directions.

To replace eggs that are used for binding, such as in burgers or loaves, try:

- Mashed potato
- Quick-cooking rolled oats
- Cooked oatmeal
- Fine bread crumbs
- Tomato paste

REPLACING MEAT

Several commercial products substitute nicely for meat in recipes. In addition to the suggestions below, see the section on Transition Foods (pages 181–82) for other substitutes.

- *Texturized vegetable protein (TVP)*. TVP is made from soybeans, and has a texture and taste much like ground meat. Use it in spaghetti sauce, sloppy joes, or chili. Available at health food stores.
- *Seitan ("say-tan")*. Also known as wheat meat, this is a chewy meat substitute made from wheat protein. It is delicious in stir-fries, stroganoff, or stews, or wherever strips or chunks of meat would be used. Seitan is usually sold marinated

with soy sauce and spices in plastic tubs in the refrigerator case of your health food store.

- *Tempeh ("tem-pay").* A fermented soybean product with a unique flavor and a texture similar to very tender meat, it can be marinated, then barbecued or grilled. It can also be cubed for kabobs or stews. Tempeh is available in a variety of styles, mixed with various vegetables and grains. Each has a unique flavor, so experiment to determine your favorite. Tempeh is also available as ready-to-heat burgers. Check the refrigerator or freezer sections of your health food store.

REPLACING MILK

There are several excellent options for replacing cow's milk in your diet.

- *Soymilk.* Available in several flavors, soymilk can be used as a beverage, on cereal, or in cooking to replace dairy milk or cream. There are many different brands, each with its own unique taste, so experiment to find one that you like. The original soymilks were quite high in fat (50% of calories from fat). However, many companies are now making low-fat and fat-free versions.
- *Rice milk.* The most widely marketed brand of rice milk is Rice Dream, which is available in a variety of flavors at most health food stores. Made from brown rice, Rice Dream is lighter in color and milder in flavor than soymilks. Fifteen percent of its calories come from fat. Like soymilk, it can be used as a beverage, on cereal, or in cooking.
- *Fruit juice.* While the idea may sound strange at first, fruit juice is a delicious substitute for milk on cereal. Fruit juice may also be substituted for milk in many baked goods.

REPLACING CHEESE

A sprinkle of nutritional yeast can lend a cheeselike taste to pizza, spaghetti, or casseroles without the high fat and cholesterol of cheese. Nutritional yeast flakes are available in health food stores. Be sure to purchase *nutritional yeast,* not baking yeast.

Another alternative is Cashew Cheese (page 243), which has the appearance and taste of a mild cheddar cheese sauce, and can be served on macaroni. This is a transition food, and is fairly high in fat (59% of calories from fat).

REDUCING SALT

The desire for salty foods is an acquired taste, and your taste buds can be retrained to appreciate the true flavors of food without the overbearing flavor of salt. Begin by progressively decreasing the amount of salt you use in cooking. For example, if a recipe calls for 1 teaspoon of salt, reduce it to ¾ teaspoon, then to ½ teaspoon, and so forth. As you gradually reduce the amount of salt you add to cooked foods, your taste for salt will diminish quite painlessly.

A number of sodium-free seasoning mixes are available to help you add flavor without adding salt. These come in shaker bottles, ready to put on the table in place of the salt shaker. Try Mrs. Dash or Parsley Patch for a variety of delicious flavors. Many unsalted snack foods are available, though you should be sure your selection is also low in fat. Guiltless Gourmet and Basically Baked tortilla chips are both fat-free and salt-free. Snyder's makes unsalted pretzels with no added fat.

Menu Planning

In this section you will find breakfast, lunch, and dinner menus for three weeks, based on recipes that are low in fat, high in fiber, and contain no cholesterol. These will help you get started with planning and shopping for a week's worth of meals at a time.

You may be most comfortable following the menus as written, or you may wish to pick and choose among the various menus and create your own. Don't hesitate to change the order of the menus or use ones you particularly like as often as you wish. Also, any fruits or vegetables that are specified in the menus may be replaced by others you prefer or that are in season.

Each of the menus contains several items to provide variety and plenty of food for people who are active. If you find this to be too much food, just omit an item. Do not, however, restrict calories in an attempt to hasten weight loss. Doing so will tend to lower your metabolism and ultimately slow weight loss.

A few of the menus use transition foods in order to familiarize you with these products. As mentioned earlier, these foods tend to be higher in fat than is optimal in the long run, and they may be omitted if desired.

Although the 21-Day Meal Plan in this chapter indicates a different menu for each meal, you will probably need fewer menus than this because leftovers will often provide a second meal. Dinner leftovers make wonderful lunches, or can be used for a second dinner. Remember, leftovers are a time-saving ally. For this reason, you may want to prepare double batches of recipes (cooking a double batch does not take twice as long, yet it provides twice as many meals). If the food will be used within a week, simply store it in airtight containers in the refrigerator. If you have more than a week's worth, divide it into usable portions and freeze it in airtight containers. I can't begin to tell you how welcome this "already ready" food will look after a long day at work.

Soups and stews make particularly good leftovers. They keep well in the refrigerator or freezer, and in many cases their flavors actually improve with reheating. I generally prepare a large pot of soup once or twice each week. I serve it for dinner the night I prepare it, along with bread and a green salad. Then I use it for lunches or as a main or side course for future dinners.

Salads based on grains or legumes also keep well and make an excellent second meal, especially in the summer when it is too hot for soup. Try serving Fiesta Salad (page 238) with sourdough French bread and melon wedges for a satisfying summer meal.

A variation on the leftover theme is to prepare foods that are eaten one way the first meal and modified for their next appearance. For example, adding a few chopped vegetables, seasonings, and some extra water to the Middle Eastern Lentils (page 270) produces a great lentil soup. Leftover Chili Beans (page 266) can be used to make Tamale Pie (page 267) with a minimum of effort and time.

Use the menus on pages 192–213 and 288–293 to plan a week's worth of meals. Convenience foods can easily be incorporated into the menus. Feel free to substitute a can of minestrone or a convenient package of vegetarian chili for the recipes in this section. After you have selected your menus for a week, turn to the recipes and make a list of ingredients that you will need. You'll also want to take a survey of the pantry (see Stocking Your Pantry for Healthful Eating, page 183) to determine what staples you might need— breakfast cereals, bread, soymilk, canned beans, and so on. Add some extra fresh fruits and vegetables to the list for snacks and fillers, and you're off to the store. By picking up a week's worth of groceries in a single shopping trip, you will save an incredible amount of time.

The 21-Day Meal Plan has been designed to make your meal preparation as quick and easy as possible. Although you will probably spend more time in the kitchen at first, as you become familiar with the ingredients and preparation techniques, the time you spend will decrease. By following the 21-Day Meal Plan you will:

- Become familiar with the flavors and textures of truly healthful foods
- Readjust your tastes to a lower amount of fat
- Readjust your tastes to a lower amount of salt
- Learn time-saving techniques for preparing delicious, nourishing meals

If you want a snack between meals, choose from grains, vegetables, or fruit. You may consume these foods in unlimited quantities as long as you are not adding fats or oils, and are not stuffing yourself for emotional reasons.

In addition to the 21-Day Meal Plan, I have included a menu and recipes for a holiday feast and for a summer barbecue. The question of how to deal with these traditionally meat-centered occasions is one that frequently arises. My solution is to present an array of such beautiful and bountiful food that the high-fat fare will not be missed.

Summary of Menu-Planning Tips

- Plan and shop for a week's meals to save time and money.
- Plan leftovers into your menus as time-savers.
- Substitute packaged foods for the recipes if desired.
- Use transition foods to satisfy the urge for old familiar fare.
- Repeat favorite menus as often as you wish.
- Modify the menus to fit your needs.

21-Day Meal Plan   Day 1

Breakfast

Whole Wheat Pancakes (page 217)

Maple syrup

Banana slices

Stewed Prunes (page 215)

Lunch

Pita Pizzas (page 259)

Tossed green salad with Mustard Vinaigrette (page 233)

Orange wedges

Dinner

Black Bean Chili (page 268)

Brown Rice (page 252)

Salsa Fresca (page 246)

Berry Cobbler (page 282)

21-Day Meal Plan   Day 2

Breakfast

Scrambled Tofu (page 216)
Cottage Fries (page 216)
Whole-grain toast with fruit preserves
Grapefruit

Lunch

Pasta Salad (page 239)
Banana Oat Muffins (page 220)
Melon slices with lime juice

Dinner

Lasagne (pages 262–63)
Italian Green Beans (page 248)
Garlic Bread (page 223)
Green salad with Balsamic Vinaigrette (page 233)
Fruit Gel (page 279)

21-Day Meal Plan   Day 3

Breakfast

Cold cereal with soymilk, rice milk, or fruit juice
Sliced banana
Fresh berries

Lunch

Missing Egg Sandwich (page 244)
Tomato Bisque (page 228)
Quick and Easy Brown Bread (page 223)

Dinner

Tofu Tacos (page 271)
Spicy Bulgur Pilaf (pages 256–57)
Green Salad with Piquant Dressing (pages 236–37)
Baked Apples (page 279)

21-Day Meal Plan   Day 4

Breakfast

Apple Oat Muffins (page 221)
Fruit Smoothie (page 219)

Lunch

Split Pea Soup (pages 230–31)
Antipasto Salad (page 240)
Whole-grain bread
Cantaloupe slices

Dinner

Simply Wonderful Vegetable Stew (pages 226–27)
Spinach Salad with Orange Sesame Dressing (page 236)
Quick and Easy Brown Bread (page 223)
Poached Pears (page 280)

Breakfast

Hot cereal with soymilk or rice milk

Whole-grain toast with apple butter

Grapefruit

Lunch

Tofu, Lettuce, and Tomato Sandwich (page 244)

Chinese Noodle Salad (page 237)

Red flame grapes

Dinner

Pasta with Broccoli and Pine Nuts (page 261)

Mixed greens with Mustard Vinaigrette (page 233)

Herb and Onion Bread (page 222)

Strawberry Freeze (page 277)

21-Day Meal Plan

Day 6

· ·

Breakfast

Cold cereal with soymilk, rice milk, or fruit juice

English muffin with fruit preserves

Orange wedges

Lunch

Pasta Salad (page 239)

Italian Green Beans (page 248)

Roasted Garlic (page 242)

French bread

Dinner

Chili Beans (page 266)

Cornbread (page 224) or warm corn tortillas

Green Salad with Piquant Dressing (page 236)

Pumpkin Spice Cookies (page 284)

Breakfast

French Toast (page 218)

Maple syrup

Fruit Smoothie (page 219)

Melon slice

Lunch

Minestrone (page 225)

Mixed greens with Balsamic Vinaigrette (page 233)

Herb and Onion Bread (page 222) or whole-grain bread

Dinner

Baked Falafel (pages 258–59)

Tabouli (page 241)

Cucumber Salad (page 234)

Middle Eastern Date and Banana Dessert (page 280)

21-Day Meal Plan

. . . .

Breakfast

Scrambled Tofu (page 216)
Pumpkin Raisin Muffins (pages 220–21)
Banana Shake (page 219)
Orange slices

Lunch

Antipasto Salad (page 240)
Tomato Bisque (page 228)
Herb and Onion Bread (page 222) or sourdough French bread

Dinner

Tamale Pie, using leftover Chili Beans (page 267)
Green Salad with Piquant Dressing (page 236)
Broccoli with Sun-Dried Tomatoes (page 251)
Melon slice

Breakfast

Müesli (page 214) with apple juice
Whole-grain toast with fruit preserves
Blueberries

Lunch

Minestrone (page 225)
Whole-grain bread
Steamed Cabbage (page 250)
Apple slices

Dinner

Vegetarian hot dogs
Oven Fries (page 254)
Curried Spinach Salad (page 235)
Prune Pudding (page 278)

21-Day Meal Plan   Day 10

Breakfast

Whole Wheat Pancakes (page 217)

Berries and banana slices

Stewed Prunes (page 215)

Lunch

Mock Tuna Salad Sandwich (page 243)

Curried Rice Salad (pages 240–41)

Red flame grapes

Dinner

Refried Beans (page 269)

Brown Rice (page 252) or Spicy Bulgur Pilaf (page 256)

Salsa Fresca (page 246)

Whole wheat tortillas

Green Salad with Piquant Dressing (page 236)

Banana Cake (page 284)

Breakfast

Hot cereal with soymilk or rice milk

Whole-grain toast with apple butter

Orange slices

Lunch

Lentil Barley Soup (page 232)

Green salad with Balsamic Vinaigrette (page 233)

Quick and Easy Brown Bread (page 223)

Dinner

Pasta with Peanut Sauce (page 262)

Steamed broccoli

Spinach Salad with Orange Sesame Dressing (page 236)

Poached Pears (page 280) with Vanilla Rice Dream

21-Day Meal Plan

Day 12

Breakfast

Banana French Toast (page 218)

Fresh blueberries

Orange juice

Lunch

Green Velvet Soup (page 226)

Baked yams or sweet potatoes

Whole-grain bread

Pear slices

Dinner

Red Lentil Curry (page 275)

Curried Rice Salad (pages 240–41)

Mushrooms in Spicy Tomato Sauce (page 274)

Apple Chutney (page 247)

Gingerbread (page 283)

21-Day Meal Plan   Day 13

Breakfast

Hot cereal with soymilk or rice milk
Whole-grain toast with fruit preserves
Stewed Prunes (page 215)

Lunch

Golden Mushroom Soup (page 229)
Butter Lettuce with Apples and Walnuts (page 234)
Banana Oat Muffins (page 220)

Dinner

Tofu Burgers (page 272)
Broiled Red Potatoes (page 253)
Chinese Noodle Salad (page 237)
Baked Apples (page 279)

21-Day Meal Plan   *Day 14*

· ·

Breakfast

Cold cereal with soymilk or rice milk
Toasted bagel with sliced banana
Applesauce (page 215)

Lunch

Pasta Salad (page 239)
Creamy Garbanzo and Cabbage Soup (page 227)
Tomato slices
Whole-grain crackers

Dinner

Middle Eastern Lentils (page 270)
Collard Greens (page 249)
Middle Eastern Date and Banana Dessert (page 280)

Breakfast

French Toast (page 218)
Maple syrup
Strawberries

Lunch

Fiesta Salad (page 238)
French bread or Cornbread (page 224)
Broccoli with Vinaigrette (page 248)
Melon slice

Dinner

Spicy Vegetable Soup with Black Beans (page 230)
Brown Rice (page 252)
Mixed greens with Raspberry Vinaigrette (page 233)
Fresh Peach Cobbler (page 281)

21-Day Meal Plan   Day 16

· ·

Breakfast

Scrambled Tofu (page 216)

Cottage Fries (page 216)

Whole-grain toast

Mixed fresh fruit

Lunch

Pita Pizzas (page 259)

Roasted Garlic (page 242)

Green salad with Mustard Vinaigrette (page 233)

Dinner

Buckwheat Pasta with Seitan (pages 260–61)

Steamed Cabbage (page 250)

Spinach Salad with Orange Sesame Dressing (page 236)

Pumpkin Raisin Muffins (page 220)

21-Day Meal Plan   *Day 17*

Breakfast

Polenta (page 253)
Applesauce (page 215)
English muffin with fruit preserves

Lunch

Chili Potato Soup
Green salad with Balsamic Vinaigrette (page 233)
Cornbread (page 224) or whole-grain bread
Red flame grapes

Dinner

Bean Burrito with Salsa (page 258)
Spicy Bulgur Pilaf (pages 256–57)
Broccoli with Vinaigrette (page 248)
Chocolate Pudding (page 278)

21-Day Meal Plan   Day 18

Breakfast

Cold cereal with soymilk or rice milk
Whole-grain toast with apple butter
Grapefruit

Lunch

Chickpea Pâté (Hummus) (page 242) with pita bread
Tabouli (page 241)
Cucumber Salad (page 234)
Red flame grapes

Dinner

Simply Wonderful Vegetable Stew (pages 226–27)
Quick and Easy Brown Bread (page 223)
Butter Lettuce with Apples and Walnuts (page 234)
Banana Freeze (page 277)

21-Day Meal Plan

....

Breakfast

Hot cereal with soymilk or rice milk

English muffin with fruit preserves

Melon slice

Lunch

Tofu, Lettuce, and Tomato Sandwich (page 244)

Curried Spinach Salad (page 235)

Orange slices

Dinner

Mushroom Marinara with Pasta (page 263)

Green salad with Balsamic Vinaigrette (page 233)

French bread

Apple Cranberry Crisp (pages 282–83)

21-Day Meal Plan   *Day 20*

· ·

Breakfast

Oatmeal Waffles (page 217)

Maple syrup

Sliced bananas

Fresh berries

Lunch

Golden Mushroom Soup (page 229)

Butter Lettuce with Apples and Walnuts (page 234)

Rye bread

Dinner

Zucchini Pockets (page 260)

Collard Greens (page 249)

Corn on the cob

Chocolate Pudding (page 278)

21-Day Meal Plan

. . . .

Breakfast

Whole Wheat Pancakes (page 217)

Hot Applesauce (page 215)

Fruit Smoothie (page 219)

Lunch

Tofu, Lettuce, and Tomato Sandwich (page 244)

Curried Spinach Salad (page 235)

Orange wedges

Dinner

Lasagne (page 262)

Winter Squash with Peanut Sauce (page 251)

Butter Lettuce with Apples and Walnuts (page 234)

Poached Pears (page 280)

Holiday Menu

Stuffed Spaghetti Squash (page 264) or Stuffed Eggplant (page 265)

Wild Rice Dressing (page 255)

Bread Dressing (page 257)

Zesty Cranberry Sauce (page 246)

Mashed Potatoes and Mushroom Gravy (pages 254–55)

Yams with Cranberries and Apples (page 250)

Green Beans with Toasted Almonds (page 249)

Broccoli with Sun-Dried Tomatoes (page 251)

Herb and Onion Bread (page 222)

Poached Pears (page 280)

Pumpkin Custard Pie (page 285)

Cranberry Apple Punch (page 288), hot or cold

Summer Barbecue

Tofu Brochettes (page 273)

Tofu or Tempeh Burger (see Transition Foods, page 182)

Vegetarian Hot Dogs (see Transition Foods, page 182)

Oven Fries (page 254)

Corn on the cob

Roasted Garlic (page 242)

Curried Spinach Salad (page 235)

Chinese Noodle Salad (page 237)

Watermelon

Breakfasts

The best breakfasts are often the simplest: meals based on whole-grain cereals (hot or cold), or whole-grain breads and fruit. Quick-cooking cereals include rolled oats, buckwheat, millet, quinoa, and cornmeal. Leftover grains from previous meals can be reheated for a quick hot breakfast. When selecting cold cereals, read the labels to make sure they do not contain added fat or excessive sugar. If sugar is the first or second ingredient on the label, or if the label lists more than one type of sugar (honey, corn syrup, dextrose, malt), then sugar is a major ingredient. Soymilk, rice milk, and fruit juice are all tasty on cereal. Use low-fat soymilk, or make your own by diluting regular soymilk with an equal amount of water.

Whole-grain breads are another good breakfast alternative, as are muffins, as long as they're not loaded with fat and sugar. The muffins sold in many bakeries are so high in fat and sugar that they're really just a way for people to eat cake for breakfast without feeling guilty! This section contains recipes for three fat-free muffins you will find to be delicious, substantial, and nourishing.

For weekends, and those occasions when you wish for more elaborate breakfast fare, I have included recipes for pancakes, waffles, and French toast. Commercially available pancake and waffle mixes can also be prepared without eggs or milk. If you yearn for a "traditional American breakfast," consider Scrambled Tofu with Cottage Fries and one of the vegetarian breakfast links listed on page 182.

If you happen to be one of those people who enjoys nontraditional foods for breakfast, don't feel limited to recipes in this section. Black Bean Chili with brown rice and hot salsa is a favorite breakfast of mine, and I can highly recommend it as a real eye-opener!

Müesli

Makes 3 cups

Müesli is a breakfast cereal of Swiss origin, made of uncooked grains, nuts, and dried fruits. It may be eaten with hot or cold soymilk, fruit juice, or applesauce.

    2   cups rolled oats
    ½   cup chopped dried fruit (apples, figs, apricots, etc.)
    ½   cup raisins

Combine all ingredients. They may be left whole, or ground in a food processor until they are of a fairly fine, uniform texture. Store in an airtight container in the refrigerator.

Applesauce
Serves 8

Applesauce is delicious on toast, pancakes, and hot cereal. It is also good all by itself.

    6   large tart apples
    ½–1   cup undiluted apple juice concentrate
    ½   teaspoon ground cinnamon

Peel apples if desired, then core and dice into a large pan. Add apple juice concentrate to just cover bottom of pan, then cook over low heat until apples are soft and mushy. Mash slightly with a fork, if desired, then stir in cinnamon. Serve hot or cold.

Stewed Prunes
Serves 3 to 4

Prunes are a delicious source of vitamins, minerals, and fiber.

    1   cup dried prunes
    1   cup water

Combine prunes and water in a covered saucepan and simmer for 20 minutes, until prunes are tender. Serve hot or cold, plain or with soymilk.

Scrambled Tofu

Serves 2 to 3

Scrambled tofu tastes remarkably like scrambled eggs, without the saturated fat or cholesterol. The recipe that follows is basic and can be embellished with additional vegetables, such as sliced mushrooms and celery, diced zucchini, or grated carrot. Sauté these with the green onions.

2   teaspoons oil
2   green onions, chopped (including tops)
1   cup firm tofu, crumbled
¼   teaspoon turmeric (or enough to give it a nice yellow color)
¼   teaspoon garlic powder
⅛   teaspoon ground cumin
⅛   teaspoon black pepper
1   teaspoon soy sauce

Heat the oil in a skillet and sauté the green onions for 3 minutes, then add remaining ingredients and cook 3 to 5 minutes longer.

Cottage Fries

Serves 6

4   medium red potatoes
1   medium onion, chopped
1   green bell pepper, diced
1   tablespoon plus 1 teaspoon olive oil
1   teaspoon paprika
½–1   teaspoon salt
¼   teaspoon black pepper

Dice potatoes into generous bite-size pieces. Steam over boiling water until they are just tender when pierced with a fork, about 15 minutes. Do not overcook!

In a large skillet, sauté the onion and bell pepper in 1 teaspoon olive oil until the onion is soft, about 5 minutes. Transfer to a bowl and set aside. Add 1 tablespoon olive oil to the skillet and sauté the potatoes over medium-high heat until they are hot and lightly browned, about 5 minutes. Return the onion mixture to the pan, add remaining ingredients, toss to mix, and serve.

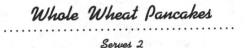

Whole Wheat Pancakes

Serves 2

1	cup whole wheat flour
¼	teaspoon salt
½	teaspoon baking powder
¼	teaspoon baking soda
1½	cups soymilk
1	tablespoon maple syrup
1	tablespoon vinegar

Stir flour, salt, baking powder, and baking soda together in a mixing bowl. Add soymilk, maple syrup, and vinegar, and stir just enough to remove the lumps. Preheat a lightly oiled or nonstick skillet or griddle. Pour small amounts of batter onto the heated surface and cook until the tops bubble. Turn with a spatula and cook the second sides until golden brown. Serve immediately.

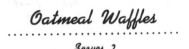

Oatmeal Waffles

Serves 2

Oatmeal waffles are substantial and slightly moist, a bit like eating oatmeal with a crunchy crust. They are easy to prepare and contain no added fat.

2	cups rolled oats
2	cups water
1	medium banana
1	tablespoon raw sugar or other sweetener
¼	teaspoon salt
1	teaspoon vanilla extract

Place all the ingredients in a blender and blend until smooth. Let stand a few minutes; if batter becomes too thick, add enough additional water to make batter easily pourable. Pour into a heated, oil-sprayed waffle iron. Cook for 10 minutes without lifting the lid.

French Toast

1 cup firm tofu
1 cup soymilk
2 tablespoons flour
2 tablespoons maple syrup
1 teaspoon vanilla extract
⅛ teaspoon ground cinnamon
⅛ teaspoon salt
8 slices bread

In a blender, process all ingredients except bread until very smooth. Pour into a flat, shallow dish and soak bread slices 1 minute on each side. Transfer carefully to a skillet that has been oiled or sprayed with nonstick vegetable spray. Cook first side until lightly browned, about 3 minutes, then turn and cook second side until browned. Serve with fresh fruit, fruit preserves, or maple syrup.

Banana French Toast

2 medium bananas
⅔ cup soymilk
2 tablespoons maple syrup
⅛ teaspoon ground cinnamon
4 slices bread

Blend bananas, soymilk, maple syrup, and cinnamon until smooth. Pour into a flat, shallow dish and soak bread slices 1 minute on each side. Transfer carefully to a skillet which has been oiled or sprayed with a nonstick vegetable spray. Cook first side until lightly browned, about 3 minutes, then turn and cook second side until browned. Serve with fresh fruit, fruit preserves, or maple syrup.

Fruit Smoothie

Serves 2

Try this smoothie with some müesli or muffins for a delicious and satisfying breakfast. The secret to its thick, creamy texture is frozen fruit. To freeze the strawberries, wash them and remove the stems. Place on a flat sheet in the freezer until frozen, then transfer to an airtight carton for storage. Peel and cut the bananas into 1-inch pieces. Place on a flat sheet in the freezer, then transfer to an airtight carton for storage. Bananas will keep in the freezer for about a month, strawberries for six months.

> 1 cup frozen strawberries
> 1 cup frozen banana pieces
> 1 cup unsweetened apple juice

Place all ingredients into blender and process on high speed until thick and smooth. You may have to stop the blender occasionally and move the unblended fruit to the center with a spatula in order to get the smoothie smooth!

Banana Shake

Serves 1

This thick "rich" shake is a real hit with children. Frozen bananas make it thick and creamy. To freeze bananas, peel and cut or break into 1-inch pieces. Place in freezer on flat tray until frozen, then transfer into airtight container for storage.

> 1 cup soymilk
> 1 cup frozen banana pieces

Place soymilk and banana pieces in blender and blend until thick and smooth.

Variation: For a sweeter shake, toss in 2 or 3 pitted dates.

Banana Oat Muffins

Makes 12 medium muffins

These quick and delicious muffins contain no added fat and no cholesterol.

2   cups flour (whole wheat pastry or unbleached all-purpose)
1½ cups quick oats or oat bran
1   teaspoon baking soda
2   ripe medium bananas, mashed
1½ cups soymilk
2   tablespoons vinegar
½   cup molasses
½   cup chopped dates or raisins

Preheat the oven to 375°F.

Mix the flour, oats, and baking soda and make a well in the center. Add the mashed bananas, the liquid ingredients, and the dates or raisins. Stir together just to mix. Spoon batter into nonstick or lightly oil-sprayed muffin tins and bake for 25 minutes, or until tops bounce back when pressed lightly.

Pumpkin Raisin Muffins

Makes about 15 muffins

These muffins are made with a flaxseed puree instead of eggs. Flaxseeds can be purchased in most natural food stores.

3   cups whole wheat pastry flour
4   teaspoons baking powder
1   teaspoon salt
1   teaspoon baking soda
1   teaspoon ground cinnamon
½   teaspoon grated nutmeg
1   cup raw sugar or other sweetener
4   tablespoons flaxseeds
1½ cups water
2½ cups solid-pack canned pumpkin (or cooked pumpkin)
1   cup raisins

Preheat the oven to 350°F.

Mix first 7 ingredients and set aside. Blend flaxseeds and 1 cup water in a blender for 1 to 2 minutes, until mixture is thick and has the consistency of beaten egg white. Add to the dry ingredients along with the pumpkin, additional ½ cup water, and raisins. Stir until just mixed.

Spoon the batter into nonstick or lightly oil-sprayed muffin tins. Bake 25 to 30 minutes, or until tops of muffins bounce back when pressed lightly. Remove from oven and let stand 1 to 2 minutes; this facilitates removal of muffins from the pan. Remove muffins and place on a rack to cool. Store in an airtight container.

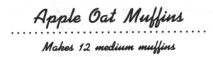

Apple Oat Muffins

Makes 12 medium muffins

    1½ cups whole wheat pastry flour
    1½ cups unbleached all-purpose flour
    1¼ cups quick oats or oat bran
    1   teaspoon ground cinnamon
    ½   teaspoon grated nutmeg
    ½   teaspoon salt (optional)
    2½ teaspoons baking soda
    2   large apples, finely chopped
    1   12-ounce can apple juice concentrate
    ½   cup raisins

Preheat the oven to 325°F.

In a large bowl, mix the flours, oats, spices, salt, and baking soda. Add the chopped apple along with the apple juice concentrate and raisins. Stir just enough to mix. Spoon batter into nonstick or lightly oil-sprayed muffin tins and bake for 25 minutes, or until tops bounce back when pressed lightly.

Breads

....

Herb and Onion Bread

....

Makes 1 loaf

Bake this quick yeast bread late in the day, and serve it warm with dinner. Its aroma is incredible! Although the recipe specifies the use of a heavy-duty electric mixer, the dough can be mixed by hand. Simply double the mixing time.

5–6	cups unbleached all-purpose or whole wheat flour (or a combination)
3	tablespoons raw sugar or other sweetener
2	teaspoons salt
2	packages (2 tablespoons) active dry yeast
½	teaspoon dried dill weed
1	teaspoon dried, crushed rosemary
2	cups hot water (105°F.–the temperature of a hot tub)
½	small onion, finely chopped

In a large bowl, thoroughly mix 2½ cups flour with the sugar, salt, yeast, and herbs. Stir in the hot water along with the chopped onion, and beat 2 minutes with a heavy-duty electric mixer. Scrape bowl occasionally during mixing.

Add small amounts of flour, beating well after each addition, until the batter pulls away from the sides of the bowl. It will be quite sticky. Beat 2 more minutes at medium speed.

Transfer the dough to an oiled bowl and put it in a warm place to rise until doubled, about 40 minutes.

Stir dough and beat vigorously for 30 seconds. Turn into a 5 × 10-inch (or two 4 × 8½-inch) nonstick or lightly oil-sprayed loaf pan and let rise in a warm place for 10 minutes. Preheat oven to 375°F.

Bake for 40 minutes. Loaf should be golden brown and sound hollow when tapped. Remove from pan and cool on a wire rack.

Quick and Easy Brown Bread

Makes 1 loaf

This bread, reminiscent of the Boston brown bread of my childhood, is sweet and moist without any added fat or oil. It can be mixed in a jiffy and requires no kneading or rising. It keeps well and makes wonderful toast.

1½	cups soymilk
2	tablespoons vinegar
2	cups whole wheat flour
1	cup unbleached all-purpose flour
2	teaspoons baking soda
½	teaspoon salt
½	cup molasses
½	cup raisins

Preheat the oven to 325°F.

Mix soymilk with vinegar and set aside. In a large mixing bowl, stir dry ingredients together. Add molasses, soymilk mixture, and raisins, and stir batter until thoroughly mixed. Do not overmix! Spoon batter into a nonstick or lightly oil-sprayed 5 × 9-inch loaf pan and bake for 1 hour, or until a toothpick inserted in the center comes out clean.

Garlic Bread

Use a fork to mash peeled cloves of Roasted Garlic (page 242) into a paste. Spread with a knife onto slices of French bread. Sprinkle with Italian seasoning if desired. Wrap tightly in foil and bake at 350°F. for 20 minutes.

Cornbread

. . . .

Serves 8

This cornbread, made without eggs, is delicious, and slightly more moist than traditional cornbread.

1½ cups soymilk
1½ tablespoons vinegar
1 cup cornmeal
1 cup unbleached all-purpose or whole wheat pastry flour
2 tablespoons raw sugar or other sweetener
¾ teaspoon salt
1 teaspoon baking powder
½ teaspoon baking soda
2 tablespoons oil

Preheat the oven to 425°F.

Combine soymilk and vinegar and let stand. Mix dry ingredients in a large bowl. Add the soymilk mixture and the oil, and stir until just blended. Spread the batter into a nonstick or lightly oil-sprayed 9-inch square baking dish, and bake for 25 to 30 minutes, or until a toothpick inserted in the center comes out clean. Serve hot.

Soups

. . . .

Soups are wonderful foods in so many ways. Nutritionally, soups retain all of the goodness of the vegetables from which they are prepared, and most are easily prepared without fat. Best of all, they practically cook themselves after just a bit of preparation. I frequently use a slow-cooker to cook soup, so that it can be simmering while I'm attending to other matters. There's nothing like coming home to the smell of hot, homemade soup!

Soups can play a central role in your menu planning, since they keep well and reheat easily. Put some of your leftover soup into individual serving containers which can be taken to work and reheated in the microwave. Use the remainder for another dinner.

For those occasions when you need an instant soup, there are many excellent canned and dehydrated soups available. Fantastic Foods and Nile Spice both make instant soup cups in an assortment of delicious flavors. All you add is hot water. These are perfect for keeping in a desk drawer at work, or on long airline flights as a hedge against the uncertainty of airline food. Health Valley, Progresso, and Hain offer a variety of instant canned soups.

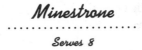

Minestrone

Serves 8

Serve with fresh-baked bread or muffins and a salad for a delicious and satisfying meal.

1	small onion, chopped
3½	cups water
3	cups tomato juice
1	garlic clove, minced
2	medium carrots, diced
1	stalk celery, diced
2	medium potatoes, diced
1	tablespoon chopped fresh parsley
1	teaspoon dried basil
1	medium zucchini, diced
½	cup pasta shells
1	cup cooked kidney beans, or 1 15-ounce can, drained
2½	cups chopped greens (spinach, collards, kale)
	Salt to taste

Heat ½ cup water in a large kettle. Add the onion and cook over medium-high heat, stirring frequently, until the onion is soft. Add the tomato juice, remaining water, garlic, carrots, celery, potatoes, parsley, and basil. Bring to a simmer, then cover and cook 20 minutes.

Add remaining ingredients except salt, then cover and simmer an additional 20 to 30 minutes. Additional tomato juice or water may be added if the soup is too thick. Add salt to taste.

Green Velvet Soup

Serves 8

This soup contains no added fat and is a delicious way to eat green vegetables.

1	medium onion, chopped
2	stalks celery, sliced
2	medium potatoes, scrubbed and diced
¾	cup split peas, rinsed
2	bay leaves
6	cups water or stock
2	medium zucchini, diced
1	medium stalk broccoli, chopped
1	bunch fresh spinach, washed and chopped
½	teaspoon dried basil
¼	teaspoon black pepper
	Pinch of cayenne
1½	teaspoons salt

Place onion, celery, potatoes, split peas, and bay leaves in a large kettle with water or stock and bring to a boil. Lower heat, cover, and simmer 1 hour.

Remove bay leaves. Add zucchini, broccoli, spinach, basil, black pepper, and cayenne, and simmer 20 minutes. Transfer to a blender in several small batches and blend until smooth, holding the lid on tightly. Return to kettle and heat until steamy. Add salt to taste.

Or to make in slow-cooker, place all ingredients into pot and cook on high for 4 to 6 hours. Puree as above and serve immediately.

Simply Wonderful Vegetable Stew

Serves 6 to 8

This stew has relatively few ingredients, is quick to prepare, and tastes wonderful. Who could ask for more? Serve it with a fresh green salad and bread or muffins.

2	medium onions, chopped
½	cup water

1   28-ounce can chopped tomatoes, with liquid
2   garlic cloves, minced
1   large green bell pepper, seeded and diced
6   medium red potatoes, unpeeled, cut into ½-inch cubes
1   teaspoon each dried basil and oregano
1   teaspoon mixed Italian herbs
½   teaspoon salt (optional)
1–2 cups green peas, fresh or frozen

Heat the water in a large kettle. Add the onion and cook over medium-high heat, stirring frequently until the onions are soft. Add all remaining ingredients except salt and peas and bring to a simmer. Cover and cook 20 to 25 minutes, or until potatoes are just tender. Add salt to taste. The amount you add will depend on the tomatoes you use. Some commercially canned tomatoes are very salty; if you use these, you may not need to add any additional salt. Stir in peas and continue cooking until heated through.

Creamy Garbanzo and Cabbage Soup

Serves 4 to 6

This soup is surprisingly quick to make. It is made with no added fat by braising the onion in water or stock in place of oil.

1   small onion, chopped
4½   cups water or stock
1   garlic clove, crushed
1   large tomato, diced
2   cups finely chopped cabbage
1   potato, diced
¼   cup finely chopped fresh parsley
2   cups cooked garbanzo beans
1   teaspoon paprika
1   teaspoon salt

In a large kettle, braise the onion in ½ cup water or stock until it is soft. Add remaining ingredients and simmer until potato and cabbage are tender, about 15 minutes.

Ladle approximately 3 cups of soup into blender and blend until smooth, being sure to hold the lid tightly and to start the blender on low speed. Return to kettle, stir to mix, and serve.

Tomato Bisque

Serves 6 to 8

Tomato soup is quick and easy using canned tomatoes, and oh so good on a cold winter day!

1	small onion, chopped
3	stalks celery, sliced
1	28-ounce can tomatoes, with liquid
2½	teaspoons raw sugar or other sweetener
½	teaspoon paprika
½	teaspoon dried basil
¼	teaspoon black pepper
2	tablespoons oil
3	tablespoons flour
2	cups water or stock
½	teaspoon salt

Place onion, celery, tomatoes, and seasonings in a kettle and simmer 15 minutes. Using a blender, puree until smooth. Do this in 2 or more small batches using only low speed. Hold the lid on the blender tightly to prevent the contents from exploding out the top.

At this point, you may strain the soup or not, depending on your taste. Left unstrained, it will contain small chunks of onion and celery as well as tomato seeds. If you want a perfectly smooth soup, use a strainer.

In the original kettle, whisk the oil and flour together. Cook 30 seconds, then whisk in 2 cups of stock or water until smooth. Stir in the blended tomato mixture, add salt to taste, and simmer until slightly thickened, about 5 minutes.

Golden Mushroom Soup

Serves 6 to 8

This is a rich-tasting soup, delicious with fresh baked bread and a green salad.

2 medium onions, chopped
2½ cups water or stock
1 pound fresh mushrooms, sliced
1½ teaspoons dried dill
1 tablespoon paprika
1 teaspoon caraway seeds (optional)
⅛ teaspoon black pepper
2 tablespoons soy sauce
2 tablespoons olive oil
3 tablespoons flour
1 cup soymilk
2 teaspoons lemon juice
2–3 tablespoons red wine (optional)

In a large pan, braise chopped onion in ½ cup water or stock until soft. Add mushrooms, dill, paprika, caraway, and pepper, and continue cooking for 5 minutes, stirring frequently. Add soy sauce and remaining water or stock, then cover and simmer for 15 minutes.

Lightly warm the oil in a saucepan, then add the flour. Cook 1 minute, stirring constantly, then whisk in the soymilk until smooth. Simmer over low heat, stirring constantly, until slightly thickened, then add to the mushroom mixture. Cover and simmer 15 minutes. Just before serving, whisk in the lemon juice and red wine.

Spicy Vegetable Soup with Black Beans

Serves 4 to 6

1 medium onion, chopped
4 large garlic cloves, minced
½ cup red wine, stock, or water
1 28-ounce can crushed tomatoes
4 cups water or stock
1 green bell pepper, diced
2 stalks celery, diced
2 cups sliced okra
2 teaspoons finely minced fresh ginger (don't leave this out)
1 teaspoon each dried oregano, dried thyme, paprika, and ground cumin
¼ teaspoon each black pepper and cayenne pepper
1 cup diced zucchini
1 15-ounce can black beans, with liquid
1–2 tablespoons soy sauce
4 cups cooked brown rice

Braise the onion and garlic in wine until onion is soft. Add tomatoes, water, green pepper, celery, okra, ginger, and seasonings; simmer for 15 minutes.

Add the diced zucchini and the black beans with their liquid, cover and cook until the zucchini is just tender, about 10 minutes. Add soy sauce to taste.

Serve over cooked brown rice.

Split Pea Soup

Serves 6 to 8

This extraordinary soup contains no added fat, and is easy to make on the stove or in a slow-cooker.

2 cups split peas, rinsed
6 cups hot water
1 cup sliced or diced carrots
1 cup sliced celery
1 medium onion, chopped

2 garlic cloves, minced
½ teaspoon dried marjoram
½ teaspoon dried basil
¼ teaspoon ground cumin
1 teaspoon salt
¼ teaspoon black pepper
Pinch of cayenne

Rinse the split peas, then place them in a large kettle with the remaining ingredients. Bring to a simmer, then cover loosely and cook until the peas are tender, 1 to 2 hours. Or, place all ingredients into a slow-cooker. Cover and cook on high for 3 to 4 hours, or until the peas are soft and the vegetables are tender.

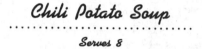

Chili Potato Soup

Serves 8

Here is a spicy alternative to traditional potato soup.

4 large russet potatoes, peeled and diced
3 cups water
1 tablespoon olive oil
1 large onion, chopped
1 teaspoon cumin
1 teaspoon basil
¼ teaspoon black pepper
2 garlic cloves, minced
1 large bell pepper, finely diced
1 4-ounce can diced Anaheim chilies
2 cups soymilk
1¼ teaspoons salt
2 green onions, finely chopped, including tops

Cook peeled, diced potatoes in water until tender, about 20 minutes. While the potatoes cook, sauté onions in the olive oil in a large pot for 2 minutes. Add the cumin, basil, black pepper, garlic, and bell pepper, and continue to cook until the onions are soft. When the potatoes are tender, mash them in their water, and add them to the onion mixture, along with the diced chilies and soymilk. Stir to blend, then heat gently until very hot. Add salt to taste. Sprinkle with chopped green onions and serve.

Lentil Barley Soup

....

Serves 12

Thick enough to be called a stew, this hearty soup is made in a single pot. Add more water or stock if you desire a thinner soup. The recipe makes quite a large quantity, so you can freeze half for later use.

2   cups lentils (about 1 pound)
¾   cup barley
8   cups water or vegetable stock
1   large onion, chopped
2   medium carrots, diced
2   stalks celery, sliced
½   teaspoon each dried oregano and ground cumin
¼   teaspoon dried red pepper flakes
¼   teaspoon black pepper
1½   teaspoons salt

Place all ingredients except salt into a large kettle and bring to a simmer. Cover and cook for 1 hour, stirring occasionally, until lentils and barley are tender. Add salt to taste.

Salads, Dips, Sandwiches, and Condiments
....

Traditional salad dressings are between 90 and 95 percent fat. A growing number of low-fat and fat-free alternatives are commercially available, but read the labels carefully. Many of the so-called lite or low-fat dressings are 80 to 85 percent fat, and some manufacturers label their products cholesterol free and saturated-fat free, which are not the same as fat-free.

To make your own fat-free dressing, replace the oil in the dressing with water, vegetable stock, or seasoned rice vinegar. Seasoned rice vinegar has a mild, slightly sweet flavor which cuts the sharpness of any other vinegar in the recipe.

The following recipe is a good everyday dressing. Based on seasoned rice vinegar, it has no fat and is simple to prepare. You can keep it in the refrigerator for two to three weeks. It is good on salad and also on cooked vegetables.

Mustard Vinaigrette

½ cup seasoned rice vinegar
1–2 teaspoons stone-ground or Dijon-style mustard
1 garlic clove, pressed

Whisk all ingredients together. Use as a dressing for salads and for steamed vegetables.

Balsamic Vinaigrette

Balsamic vinegar is a wine vinegar from Italy. It has a mellow, slightly sweet taste, and makes a delicious salad dressing.

2 tablespoons balsamic vinegar
2 tablespoons seasoned rice vinegar
2 tablespoons water
1–2 garlic cloves, crushed

Whisk all ingredients together.

Raspberry Vinaigrette

Raspberry vinegar has a mild fruity taste, well suited to salad dressing.

2 tablespoons raspberry vinegar
2 tablespoons seasoned rice vinegar
2 tablespoons water
¼ teaspoon crushed rosemary
¼ teaspoon dried tarragon

Whisk all ingredients together.

Butter Lettuce with Apples and Walnuts

Serves 6 to 8

Though this is a simple salad with just a few ingredients, the flavors are deliciously complementary. Try using a mixture of lettuces or a commercial salad mix for a variation in flavor.

1   bunch butter lettuce or a mixture of salad greens
1   large tart green apple
½   cup coarsely chopped walnuts
3–4 tablespoons seasoned rice vinegar

Wash and dry the lettuce, and tear it into bite-size pieces. Core and dice the unpeeled apple. Add it to the lettuce along with the walnuts.

Pour seasoned rice vinegar over the salad and toss gently.

Cucumber Salad

Serves 6 to 8

This salad is quick to make and keeps well. It is low in fat and calories, high in fiber, and tastes great!

3   large cucumbers
2   large tomatoes
½   small red onion
½   teaspoon dried basil
½   teaspoon dried dill
1   tablespoon chopped fresh parsley
     Apple cider vinegar

Peel the cucumbers, slice them in half lengthwise, and scoop out the seeds. Cut the cucumbers into bite-size pieces. Dice the tomatoes, and finely chop the red onion. Toss the vegetables together, then sprinkle with basil and dill and the fresh parsley. Add enough vinegar to coat all the vegetables, and toss. Chill before serving if possible.

Curried Spinach Salad

. . . .

Serves 6 to 8

This wonderful spinach salad has a multitude of flavors and textures. The recipe calls for golden raisins, which contain sulfites. If you are sensitive to sulfites, substitute coarsely chopped unsulphured dried apricots for the raisins.

1	bunch fresh spinach (about 1 pound)
1	tart green apple, diced
2	green onions, including green tops, finely sliced
¼	cup golden raisins or coarsely chopped dried apricots
⅓	cup roasted Spanish peanuts
1	tablespoon sesame seeds, toasted
3	tablespoons seasoned rice vinegar
3	tablespoons water
2	teaspoons stone-ground or Dijon-style mustard
1	teaspoon soy sauce
1	teaspoon raw sugar or other sweetener
½	teaspoon curry powder
¼	teaspoon black pepper

Wash the spinach thoroughly. The easiest way to do this is to swish it in a basin of cold water. Remove the spinach and replace the water. Repeat until no new grit shows up at the bottom of the bowl. Pat spinach dry and tear leaves into bite-size pieces. Add apple, green onions, and raisins or apricots.

To roast the peanuts and sesame seeds, place them in an ovenproof pan and bake at 350°F. for 10 to 15 minutes. Allow to cool, then add to the salad.

Combine the vinegar, water, mustard, soy sauce, sugar, curry powder, and black pepper. Whisk together. Pour over salad and toss to mix just before serving.

Spinach Salad with Orange Sesame Dressing

Serves 6

1 bunch fresh spinach
1 cup fresh mushrooms (buttons if possible)
1 orange, peeled and sliced
1 tablespoon sesame seeds
3 tablespoons seasoned rice vinegar
2 tablespoons orange juice

Wash the spinach carefully to remove all sand and dirt. Trim off the stems, and dry the leaves, then tear them into bite-size pieces.

Clean the mushrooms and slice into bite-size pieces if necessary. Add to the spinach along with the orange slices. Toast sesame seeds by placing in a dry skillet over medium heat until seeds begin to pop. Add toasted seeds to salad.

Mix rice vinegar and orange juice. Dress salad just before serving.

Green Salad with Piquant Dressing

Serves 8

This salad has a south-of-the-border flair. Serve it with Refried Beans (page 269) or Black Bean Chili (page 268).

1 bunch leaf lettuce
¾ cup cooked kidney beans, drained
1 avocado, diced (optional)
1 green bell pepper, diced
1 medium cucumber, sliced
1 medium tomato, diced
½ cup finely shredded red cabbage
2 tablespoons each seasoned rice vinegar, cider vinegar, water, and lemon juice
1 garlic clove, minced
½ teaspoon paprika
¼ teaspoon each dry mustard, dried oregano, and salt
⅛ teaspoon ground cumin
1 tablespoon ketchup

Wash and dry the lettuce, and tear it into bite-size pieces. Add the kidney beans along with the avocado, bell pepper, cucumber, tomato, and cabbage.

Whisk the remaining ingredients together, and pour over the salad. Toss gently to mix just before serving.

Chinese Noodle Salad

Serves 8

This salad is easy to prepare and keeps well. It is always a favorite at potlucks.

6–8 cups finely shredded green cabbage (or a mix of green and red)
½ cup slivered almonds, toasted
¼ cup sesame seeds, toasted
3–4 green onions, thinly sliced, or ¼ cup finely chopped red onion
1 package ramen noodle soup (see Note)
1 tablespoon toasted sesame oil
⅓ cup seasoned rice vinegar
2 tablespoons raw sugar or other sweetener
½ teaspoon black pepper
Cilantro (optional)

Place the shredded cabbage in a large salad bowl.

Toast the almonds and sesame seeds by placing them in an ovenproof dish and baking at 350°F. for 5 to 10 minutes, until lightly browned and fragrant. Add to the shredded cabbage, along with the green onions. Coarsely crush the ramen noodles and add them to the salad, uncooked, along with the packet of seasoning mix.

Mix the remaining ingredients together and pour over salad. Let stand 30 minutes or more before serving. The noodles become soft as the salad stands. Garnish with cilantro just before serving, if desired.

Note: Ramen noodle soups are available in natural food stores and most supermarkets. They contain noodles and a seasoning packet. Be sure the noodles are not fried, and that the seasonings do not include animal products or tropical oils.

Fiesta Salad

Serves 10

This salad is a celebration of color and taste. It may be made in advance, and keeps well for several days. If you are a cilantro lover, you may want to double the amount.

1½ cups dry black beans, or 3 15-ounce cans black beans
3½ cups water
2 cups frozen corn, thawed
2 large tomatoes, diced
1 large green bell pepper, diced
1 large red or yellow bell pepper, diced
½ cup chopped red onion
¾ cup chopped cilantro (optional)
2 tablespoons seasoned rice vinegar
2 tablespoons apple cider or distilled vinegar
1 lime or lemon, juiced
2 garlic cloves, minced
2 teaspoons ground cumin
1 teaspoon ground coriander
½ teaspoon crushed red pepper, or a pinch of cayenne
½–1 teaspoon salt

Sort through beans to remove any debris, then wash them and place them in a large pan or bowl with about 6 cups water. Soak overnight. Pour off soaking water and place in a kettle with the 3½ cups of fresh water. Bring to a simmer, and cook until the beans are just tender, about 45 minutes to 1 hour. (Although the beans should be thoroughly cooked, in this case they should not be overcooked.) Drain and cool the cooked beans. If you are using canned black beans, simply drain them and proceed.

When the beans are cool, combine them with the corn, tomatoes, bell peppers, red onion, and cilantro. Whisk together dressing ingredients and pour over the salad. Toss gently to mix.

Pasta Salad
. . . .
Serves 8 to 10

This pasta salad is delicious hot or cold. It is made without oil, and is lighter than traditional pasta salads. Artichokes packed without oil are available in cans and jars, and in the frozen food section of most supermarkets.

12	ounces pasta shells (about 2 cups)
1	jar water-packed artichoke hearts, drained and quartered
2–3	cups button mushrooms (about ½ pound)
¼	cup cider vinegar
⅓	cup seasoned rice vinegar
2	tablespoons fresh lemon juice (optional)
2	teaspoons stone-ground or Dijon-style mustard
½	cup chopped green onions
1	garlic clove
½	teaspoon each dried basil and oregano
½	teaspoon salt
¼	teaspoon black pepper
3	tablespoons water
3	tablespoons chopped fresh parsley
1	small red bell pepper, diced

Bring water to a boil in a large pot, then add the pasta. Cook until pasta is just tender. Rinse, drain, and place in a large bowl. Add the artichoke hearts and mushrooms.

In a blender, combine the vinegars, lemon juice, mustard, ¼ cup green onions, garlic, seasonings, and water. Process until smooth. Pour over pasta, and allow to marinate until pasta is cool. Add the remaining green onions, parsley, and red bell pepper and gently toss to mix.

Antipasto Salad

Serves 6 to 8

The vegetables in this salad are steamed until just tender, then marinated in a vinaigrette dressing. This salad is good hot or cold.

4 medium red potatoes, scrubbed
2 medium carrots, scrubbed or peeled
¼ pound fresh green beans
½ head fresh cauliflower, washed and broken into florets
1 cup green peas, fresh if possible (otherwise use frozen)
¼ cup cider or wine vinegar
2 tablespoons lemon juice
2 tablespoons seasoned rice vinegar
2 garlic cloves, crushed
2 teaspoons stone-ground or Dijon-style mustard
½ teaspoon salt
¼ teaspoon black pepper
1 red bell pepper, sliced

Cut the potatoes into 1-inch cubes. Cut the carrots on the diagonal into ½-inch-thick wedges. Steam over boiling water until just tender, about 10 minutes. Cut the green beans into 1-inch pieces. Steam over boiling water until just tender, about 7 minutes. Steam the cauliflower until just tender, about 8 minutes.

Gently combine all the vegetables. Mix the remaining ingredients except red pepper, then pour over the vegetables and toss gently. Serve immediately or refrigerate until thoroughly chilled. Add the sliced bell pepper just before serving.

Curried Rice Salad

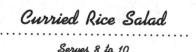

Serves 8 to 10

This salad is as colorful as it is delicious.

3 cups water
½ teaspoon salt
1 cup brown basmati rice
½ small red onion, finely chopped
1 small green bell pepper, diced
1 small red bell pepper, diced

  1 stalk celery, thinly sliced
  1 medium carrot, grated
  1 cup finely shredded green cabbage
  1 cup green peas, fresh or frozen
  ¼ cup balsamic vinegar
  ¼ cup seasoned rice vinegar
  2 teaspoons stone-ground or Dijon-style mustard
  2 teaspoons toasted sesame oil
  2 garlic cloves, minced or pressed
  1 teaspoon soy sauce
  2 teaspoons curry powder

Bring water to a boil, add salt and rice, then return to a simmer. Cover and cook until rice is just tender about 25 minutes. Drain off excess liquid. Cool.

Add vegetables to cooled rice and toss to mix. Combine vinegars and remaining dressing ingredients and mix well. Pour over salad and toss to mix.

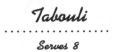

Tabouli
Serves 8

Tabouli is a Middle Eastern salad made with bulgur, which is cracked, toasted wheat. It is seasoned with typical Middle Eastern flavors: lemon, parsley, mint, and garlic.

  1 cup bulgur
  2 cups boiling water
  ½ cup chopped green onions
  ½ cup finely chopped fresh parsley
  3 tablespoons finely chopped fresh mint leaves
  3 medium tomatoes, diced
  ¼ cup lemon juice
  1 tablespoon olive oil
  1 teaspoon salt
  1 garlic clove, minced

Put bulgur in a large bowl and pour boiling water over it. Cover and let stand 30 minutes, until tender. Drain off any excess liquid, then, using a fork, gently fluff the bulgur. Add remaining ingredients, stir to mix, and adjust seasonings to taste. Chill 2 to 3 hours before serving.

Roasted Garlic

Roasted garlic makes a delicious appetizer or accompaniment to a meal. I place several heads on the table along with the meal, and let people pick off cloves, peel them, and discover the mild taste and creamy texture. Roasted garlic can also be used as a spread on bread, or in salads and dressings. Store it in a sealed container in the refrigerator for up to two weeks.

Start with a large, firm head of garlic. Place it into a small baking dish. Bake in a toaster oven or a regular oven at 375°F. until the cloves feel soft when pressed lightly, about 25 minutes.

Chickpea Pâté (Hummus)

Serves 6 to 8

Hummus (pronounced *HUMM-us*) is a Middle Eastern spread that is delicious with crackers, wedges of pita bread, or fresh vegetable slices. It also makes a delicious sandwich spread. It is very easy to make in a food processor—just add all the ingredients and process until smooth—or by hand. Store it in an airtight container in the refrigerator for up to a week for quick sandwiches and snacks.

2	cups cooked chickpeas, or 1 15-ounce can
1–2	garlic cloves, minced
¼	cup tahini (sesame seed butter)
2	tablespoons lemon juice
¼	teaspoon salt
1	tablespoon finely chopped fresh parsley
¼	teaspoon each ground cumin and paprika

Drain the chickpeas, reserving the liquid. Mash the beans, then add the remaining ingredients and mix well. The texture should be creamy and spreadable. If it is too dry, add enough of the reserved bean liquid to achieve the desired consistency.

Variation: For a fat-free version, replace the tahini with 1 finely grated carrot.

Cashew Cheese

Makes 2 cups

This sauce can be used as a topping on pasta or pizza, or as a dip for vegetables.

½   cup raw cashews
2   ounces pimientos
¼   cup lemon juice
3   tablespoons nutritional yeast flakes
1   teaspoon salt
½   teaspoon onion powder
¼   teaspoon garlic powder
1½ cups water

Place all ingredients in a blender and process until very smooth.

Mock Tuna Salad

Makes 4 sandwiches

This spread is delicious and easy to prepare, and you don't risk the mercury and other contaminants often found in tuna fish.

1   15-ounce can chickpeas, drained
1   stalk celery, finely chopped
1   medium carrot, grated (optional)
1   green onion, finely chopped
2   teaspoons eggless mayonnaise
1   tablespoon sweet pickle relish
¼   teaspoon salt (optional)

Mash the chickpeas with a fork or potato masher. Leave some chunks. Add the celery, carrot, green onion, mayonnaise, and relish. Add salt to taste.

Serve on whole wheat bread or in pita bread with lettuce and sliced tomatoes.

For a fat-free version, substitute 2 teaspoons of mustard for the 2 teaspoons of mayonnaise.

Tofu, Lettuce, and Tomato Sandwich

Makes 4 sandwiches

This sandwich is somewhat reminiscent of the classic BLT, without the fat, cholesterol, and nitrates of bacon! Here's what you need:

> 1 pound firm tofu
> Oil for sautéing
> Soy sauce
> 8 slices whole wheat or rye bread
> Eggless mayonnaise
> Stone-ground or Dijon-style mustard
> Lettuce
> Sliced tomato

Slice tofu into ¼-inch-thick slabs. You will need about 1½ slabs for each sandwich. Place a small amount of oil in a skillet (preferably nonstick), and fry the tofu on both sides until golden brown. Turn off the heat, sprinkle with soy sauce, and turn to coat both sides.

Spread the bread lightly with mayonnaise and mustard, and top with fried tofu, lettuce, and tomato.

Missing Egg Sandwich

Makes 4 sandwiches

This looks and tastes like egg salad, but without the cholesterol and saturated fat.

> ½ pound firm tofu, mashed
> 1 green onion, finely chopped
> 2 tablespoons eggless mayonnaise
> 1 tablespoon pickle relish
> 1 teaspoon mustard
> ¼ teaspoon each ground cumin, turmeric, and garlic powder
> Pinch of salt

Combine all ingredients and mix thoroughly. Serve on whole wheat bread with lettuce and tomato.

Tempeh Sandwich

Makes 6 sandwiches

Tempeh is a fermented soybean product available in natural food stores. It is high in protein and fiber, and has a more substantial texture than tofu. Guests will insist it must be chicken salad!

8 ounces tempeh
3 tablespoons eggless mayonnaise
2 teaspoons stone-ground or Dijon-style mustard
2 green onions, chopped (including green tops)
1 stalk celery, diced
1 tablespoon pickle relish
¼ teaspoon salt (optional)

Steam the tempeh in a vegetable steamer over boiling water for 20 minutes. Allow it to cool, then grate it and mix in the remaining ingredients. Cover and chill if time allows. Serve on whole wheat bread with lettuce and sliced tomatoes.

Tahini Sauce

Makes ½ cup

Serve with wedges of whole wheat pita bread, or as a topping for falafel.

¼ cup tahini (sesame seed butter)
1 tablespoon lemon juice
1 tablespoon soy sauce
1 tablespoon vinegar
1 garlic clove, pressed
2 tablespoons water or more as needed

Mix the tahini, lemon juice, soy sauce, vinegar, garlic, and water, using a fork or whisk to remove the lumps. Stir in additional water, 1 tablespoon at a time, if needed to make the sauce pourable.

Salsa Fresca
....
Makes approximately 2 quarts

A chunky, delicious salsa—just barely cooked. The recipe as written produces a very mild salsa. For more zip, add more crushed red peppers or cayenne.

1   medium onion, chopped
4   garlic cloves, minced
1   28-ounce can tomato sauce
¼   teaspoon crushed red pepper (add more for a hotter salsa)
1½ teaspoons ground cumin
2   tablespoons cider vinegar
1   bunch cilantro
1   small green bell pepper, chopped
4   cups chopped tomatoes, fresh or canned

Place onion, garlic, tomato sauce, red pepper, cumin, and vinegar in a kettle and simmer 10 to 15 minutes. Remove from heat.

Wash the cilantro and remove the stems. Chop the leaves and add to the salsa along with the chopped bell pepper and tomatoes.

Zesty Cranberry Sauce
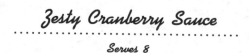
....
Serves 8

2   cups fresh or frozen cranberries
½   cup undiluted orange juice concentrate
2   ripe pears, finely chopped
1   medium apple, finely chopped
¼   teaspoon ground cinnamon
1   teaspoon grated orange rind
½   cup raw sugar or other sweetener

Combine all ingredients except sweetener in a saucepan, and bring to a simmer over medium heat. Continue cooking, uncovered, until cranberry skins pop and mixture is thickened slightly, about 10 minutes. Add sweetener to taste if desired.

Serve hot or cold.

Apple Chutney

·······························
Makes 3 cups

A chutney is a spicy relish, prepared from a variety of fruits and vegetables, served as a condiment with the meal. The following is a simple chutney made with apples. It takes about 1 hour to cook, and may be kept refrigerated for several weeks. It also freezes for longer storage.

1½   pounds tart apples (about 3 large apples)
1   medium garlic clove, minced
1   tablespoon chopped fresh ginger, or ½ teaspoon ground ginger
½   cup orange juice
1   teaspoon each ground cinnamon and cloves
½   teaspoon salt
1   cup raw sugar or other sweetener
1   cup cider vinegar
¼   teaspoon cayenne, or more to taste

Coarsely chop the apples, then combine them with all the remaining ingredients in a heavy saucepan. Bring to a boil, then lower heat and simmer uncovered, stirring occasionally, for 1 hour, until most of the liquid is absorbed.

Vegetables and Side Dishes

Broccoli with Vinaigrette

Serves 4 to 6

America's favorite vegetable is even better when it is served with this delicious fat-free dressing. It's easy to make, keeps well in the refrigerator, and is tasty on other vegetables as well.

1	bunch broccoli
½	cup seasoned rice vinegar
2	teaspoons stone-ground or Dijon-style mustard
1–2	garlic cloves, pressed or minced

Break the broccoli into bite-size florets. Peel the stems and slice them into ¼-inch-thick rounds. Steam until just tender, about 3 minutes.

While the broccoli is steaming, whisk the dressing ingredients in a serving bowl. Add the steamed broccoli and toss to mix. Serve immediately.

Italian Green Beans

Serves 6 to 8

1½	pounds fresh green beans, trimmed
1	tablespoon olive oil
2–3	large tomatoes, chopped
2	large garlic cloves, minced
1	tablespoon chopped fresh basil, or 1 teaspoon dried
	Salt and fresh ground black pepper to taste

Trim beans and break them into bite-size pieces. Steam until just tender, 5 to 10 minutes, then chill in cold water. Drain and set aside.

Heat oil in a large skillet, then add tomatoes and garlic. Simmer over medium heat 10 minutes. Add beans and basil and cook 10 minutes longer, stirring occasionally. Add salt and pepper to taste and serve.

Green Beans with Toasted Almonds

Serves 6

Toasted sesame oil, seasoned rice vinegar, and soy sauce give these green beans a tasty Asian flair.

> 1 pound fresh green beans, trimmed
> 1 medium onion, chopped
> ½ cup slivered almonds
> 1 tablespoon toasted sesame oil
> 1 tablespoon seasoned rice vinegar
> 1 tablespoon soy sauce

Cut ends off beans and break into bite-size pieces. Steam until just tender. Set aside.

In a large skillet, sauté the onion and slivered almonds in oil until onion becomes transparent. Lower heat, add vinegar, and continue cooking until onion starts to caramelize and almonds begin to brown, about 10 minutes. Stir in soy sauce and beans. Cook 1 to 2 minutes before serving.

Collard Greens or Kale

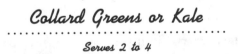

Serves 2 to 4

Collard greens and kale are wonderful sources of calcium, vitamin A, iron, and other nutrients. They can be steamed, like spinach, and their flavor is nicely complemented with the addition of garlic suggested below.

> 1   bunch (about 1 pound) collard greens or kale
> 2–3 garlic cloves, minced
> 1–2 teaspoons olive oil, or ½ cup vegetable stock

Wash the greens, then remove the stems and chop the leaves into ½-inch-wide strips. Sauté the garlic in the oil or cook it in the stock for 30 seconds (do not let it brown). Add the greens, toss to mix, then cover and cook over medium-low heat for 2 to 3 minutes. Add water, 1 tablespoon at a time, if necessary to keep the greens from sticking.

Steamed Cabbage

Serves 2 to 3

I owe my wonderful mother-in-law, Adrien Avis, an eternal debt of gratitude for this recipe. Cabbage was not a part of my childhood, and it was not until she introduced me to it, prepared in this manner, that I knew how delicious it could be.

> 2 cups green cabbage, coarsely chopped
> ½ cup vegetable stock
> Salt and fresh ground black pepper
> Caraway seeds

Cook cabbage over medium heat in vegetable stock until it is just tender, about 5 minutes. Sprinkle with salt and pepper to taste, and caraway seeds if desired.

Yams with Cranberries and Apples

Serves 8

A beautiful blend of sweet and tart flavors, this recipe is a perfect addition to any meal, Thanksgiving or otherwise. I buy extra cranberries when they are available in the fall and freeze them so I can make this dish year-round.

> 4 yams, peeled
> 1 large, green apple, peeled and diced
> 1 cup raw cranberries
> ½ cup raisins
> 2 tablespoons raw sugar or other sweetener
> ½ cup orange juice

Preheat the oven to 350°F.

Cut peeled yams into 1-inch chunks and place in a large baking dish. Top with diced apple, cranberries, and raisins. Sprinkle with sugar or other sweetener, then pour orange juice over all. Cover and bake for 1 hour and 15 minutes, or until yams are tender when pierced with a fork.

Winter Squash with Peanut Sauce
. . . .
Serves 8

Peanut sauce is a delicious complement to the slightly sweet flavor of winter squash. Cook the squash by baking or steaming.

1   medium winter squash (butternut, acorn, hubbard, kabocha, etc.)
⅓ cup peanut butter
½ cup hot water
1   tablespoon soy sauce
1   tablespoon vinegar (white wine vinegar works well)
2   teaspoons raw sugar or other sweetener
2   garlic cloves, minced
     Pinch of cayenne
1   green onion, finely chopped

Slice the squash in half lengthwise, and scoop out the seeds. To bake, place cut side down on a large baking dish in a 350°F. oven for 50 to 60 minutes, or until easily pierced with a fork. To steam, place on a vegetable steamer in a large kettle. Cover and steam until fork-tender, 40 to 60 minutes.

Whisk peanut butter with remaining ingredients except the onion in a small saucepan. Heat gently until the sauce is smooth and slightly thickened. Add more water if the sauce seems too thick. When the squash is tender, top with peanut sauce, sprinkle with chopped onion, and serve.

Broccoli with Sun-Dried Tomatoes
. . . .
Serves 6

The tangy flavor of sun-dried tomatoes is a wonderful complement to steamed broccoli. Be careful not to overcook the broccoli; it should be bright green and still slightly crisp.

1   bunch broccoli
5–6 sun-dried tomatoes in olive oil

Break or cut broccoli into florets; peel and slice stems into rounds. Steam over boiling water until just tender, 3 to 5 minutes. While the broccoli is cooking, cut the tomatoes into small pieces and place in a serving dish. When broccoli is tender, add to the tomatoes, toss, and serve.

Brown Rice

Makes 3 cups

By using extra water, and actually cooking rice like pasta, the grains end up separate and slightly crunchy. The liquid that is poured off can be added to soup if you like.

    1   cup short-grain brown rice
    3   cups water
    ¼   teaspoon salt (optional)
         Tamari or other soy sauce

Rinse rice in a saucepan of cool water, then drain off the water as thoroughly as possible. Put the saucepan on medium heat, stirring constantly until the rice dries, about 1 minute. Add water and salt, bring to a boil, then lower heat slightly, cover, and simmer 30 to 40 minutes, until the rice is soft but still retains a hint of crunchiness. Pour off any excess water. Season with soy sauce if desired.

Couscous

Makes 3 cups

Couscous is somewhat like bulgur, but made from a different type of wheat. It is delicious plain, as a pilaf, or topped with a vegetable sauce. It is one of the easiest grains to prepare: just add boiling water and let it stand. It is one of my favorites for camping and backpacking.

    ½   teaspoon salt
    1½   cups boiling water
    1   cup instant couscous

Bring salted water to a boil in a small pan. Stir in the couscous, then remove the pan from heat and cover it. Let stand 10 to 15 minutes, then fluff with a fork and serve.

Polenta

Makes 4 cups

Polenta, or coarse cornmeal, is a staple in northern Italy. It is delicious in place of pasta with marinara sauce, or with any spicy vegetable sauce. The technique for preparing it is much like cooking hot cereal: stir it into boiling water and cook until thickened. For a variation, the hot, cooked polenta can be poured into a bread pan and chilled. Once cold, it makes a solid loaf from which ¼-inch-thick slices can be cut and fried or broiled. Serve with the same sauces as above, or try it for breakfast with maple syrup or homemade applesauce.

  1 teaspoon salt
  4 cups water
  1 cup polenta or stone-ground yellow cornmeal
  ½ teaspoon crushed dried rosemary (optional)

  Bring salted water to a boil, then slowly pour in the polenta, stirring constantly with a whisk to prevent it from lumping. Lower heat and simmer, stirring fairly constantly until thick, about 10 minutes.

Broiled Red Potatoes

Serves 4

  4 medium red potatoes (about 1 pound)
  2 teaspoons olive oil
     Fresh or dried rosemary
     Salt
     Freshly ground pepper

  Preheat the oven to 450°F.
  Scrub the potatoes and cut them into ¼-inch-thick rounds. Place in a 9 × 13-inch baking dish and sprinkle with olive oil. Toss to distribute the oil, then sprinkle with rosemary, salt, and pepper. Bake for 15 minutes, then turn with a spatula. Continue baking about 20 more minutes, until tender when pierced with a fork.

Oven Fries

Serves 4

These baked french fries are always a hit.

> 2 large russet potatoes (about 1 pound)
> 1 tablespoon olive oil
> Paprika
> Herbs as desired
> Salt (optional)

Preheat the oven to 450°F.

Scrub potatoes, but do not peel. Cut into strips ¼ inch wide and the length of the potato. Place in a 9 × 13-inch baking dish and sprinkle with oil. Toss to distribute the oil, then sprinkle with paprika and other herbs if desired (I like to use fresh rosemary). Bake for 10 minutes, then loosen and turn with a spatula. Bake 20 to 30 minutes longer, turning once or twice, until insides are tender when pierced with a fork. Sprinkle with salt if desired, and serve.

Mashed Potatoes and Mushroom Gravy

Serves 6

American traditional cuisine at its finest. Serve with Tofu Burgers (page 272) or with other transition foods.

> 4   large potatoes, peeled and diced
> 1½   cups water
> ½   teaspoon salt
> ½   cup soymilk
> ½   cup chopped onion
> 1   cup sliced fresh mushrooms
> 2   tablespoons oil
> 2   tablespoons flour
> 2   teaspoons soy sauce
> ¼   teaspoon black pepper

Simmer potatoes in a kettle with water and ¼ teaspoon salt until tender, about 10 minutes. Drain and reserve liquid. Mash the potatoes, then add soymilk and salt to taste. Cover and set aside.

In a large skillet, sauté onion and mushrooms in oil until onion is soft and transparent. Stir in flour; the mixture should be quite dry. Whisk in cooking liquid from potatoes, stirring to dissolve any lumps of flour, then add soy sauce and pepper. Cook over medium-low heat until thickened. If a smooth gravy is desired, puree in a blender after adding the soy sauce and pepper, then return it to the pan and cook as above. Serve over mashed potatoes.

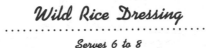

Wild Rice Dressing

Serves 6 to 8

This dressing is made with a combination of wild rice and brown rice. You could also substitute some of the specialty rices, such as wehani or basmati, for part of the brown rice.

    4 cups water
    ¾ teaspoon salt
    ¾ cup long-grain brown rice
    ¾ cup wild rice
    2 tablespoons olive oil
    1 small onion, chopped
    1 pound fresh mushrooms, cleaned and sliced
    ½ cup finely chopped fresh parsley
    1 cup sliced celery
    ¼ teaspoon crumbled sage
    ⅛ teaspoon each black pepper, dried marjoram, and dried thyme
    1 cup pecan halves, broken lengthwise

Bring water to a boil and add ¼ teaspoon salt and both varieties of rice. Lower to simmer, then cover and cook until rice is tender but still crunchy, 30 to 40 minutes.

Preheat the oven to 350°F.

In a large ovenproof skillet, gently heat the oil and sauté the onion and mushrooms until the onion is transparent. Add the parsley, celery, cooked rice, seasonings, and pecans. Add salt to taste. Stir to mix, then cover and bake for 15 minutes.

Curried Rice
....
Serves 6 to 8

Basmati rice imparts a wonderful flavor to this dish. It is available in Indian markets, natural food stores, and in many supermarkets.

2 cups basmati rice, white or brown
¼ teaspoon ground cinnamon
⅛ teaspoon ground cardamom (or seeds of 8 cardamom pods, crushed)
½ teaspoon turmeric
1 teaspoon salt
½ cup slivered almonds
½ cup raisins
4 cups boiling water
1 cup green peas, fresh or frozen

Toast the rice in a large skillet over medium heat until it starts to become opaque and somewhat chalky in appearance. Add remaining ingredients, except peas, and bring to a simmer.

Cover the pot, and cook until the rice is tender and all the water is absorbed (20 minutes for white rice, 60 minutes for brown rice).

Stir in the peas just before serving (a few minutes sooner if you're using fresh peas).

Spicy Bulgur Pilaf
....
Serves 4 to 6

Bulgur is whole wheat that has been cracked and toasted. It is available in health food stores, and many supermarkets carry it in the pasta and rice section. This Mexican pilaf is delicious with chili or refried beans and a green salad. The key to keeping the bulgur fluffy is to refrain from stirring it while the bulgur is cooking.

1 medium onion, chopped
1 tablespoon olive oil
2 garlic cloves, minced
1 cup bulgur
2 teaspoons chili powder
¾ teaspoon ground cumin

⅛   teaspoon celery seed
½   red bell pepper, finely diced
½   teaspoon salt
1¾   cups boiling water or vegetable stock

Sauté the onion in olive oil in a large skillet for 3 minutes. Stir in garlic and bulgur and continue cooking 2 minutes, then add the chili powder, cumin, and celery seed. Cook another 3 to 5 minutes, stirring frequently.

Add the red pepper and salt, then pour in the boiling water (or stock). Bring to a boil, then reduce to a simmer. Cover and cook, without stirring, until all liquid is absorbed, about 20 minutes.

To make in oven, prepare all ingredients as above, up to the addition of adding boiling water or stock. Preheat oven to 350°F. Place bulgur mixture into an ovenproof dish, pour in boiling liquid, cover with foil, and bake for 30 minutes, until all liquid is absorbed.

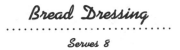

Bread Dressing

Serves 8

1   small onion, chopped
2   tablespoons oil
3   cups sliced fresh mushrooms
1   cup sliced celery
4   cups cubed bread
¼   cup finely chopped fresh parsley
¼   teaspoon each dried sage and thyme
⅛   teaspoon dried marjoram
⅛   teaspoon black pepper
½   teaspoon salt
1   cup (approximately) very hot water or vegetable stock

Preheat the oven to 350°F.

In a large kettle or skillet, sauté the onion in oil for 2 minutes, then add mushrooms and celery. Cook over medium heat until mushrooms begin to brown, then stir in the bread and seasonings. Lower heat, and continue cooking for 4 to 5 minutes, then stir in water or stock, a little at a time until dressing obtains desired moistness. Place in a nonstick or oil-sprayed 1-quart baking dish, cover, and bake for 20 minutes. Remove cover and bake 10 minutes longer.

Entrees

....

Bean Burrito with Salsa

....

Makes 6 burritos

1   15-ounce can refried beans
1   16-ounce jar salsa
1   package whole wheat tortillas

Heat the beans in one pan and the salsa in another. Heat a tortilla in a dry, heavy skillet over moderate heat until it is warm and flexible. Remove from pan and spread refried beans in a line down the middle of the tortilla. Fold in the ends, then starting at one side, roll up around the beans. Place on a plate, then spoon heated salsa over the top.

Baked Falafel

....

Serves 6 to 8

These spicy falafel patties are baked instead of fried.

1   medium potato, diced
1   15-ounce can chickpeas, drained
1   small onion, finely chopped
½   cup finely chopped fresh parsley
2   garlic cloves, minced
2   tablespoons tahini (sesame seed butter)
2   tablespoons soy sauce
½   teaspoon turmeric
½   teaspoon ground coriander
1   teaspoon ground cumin
⅛   teaspoon cayenne
6–8   pita breads
      Fillings: chopped lettuce, cucumber, tomato, green onions
      Tahini Sauce (page 245) or Salsa Fresca (page 246)

Preheat the oven to 350°F.

Cook the potato in a covered pan in a small amount of water until soft. Drain. Add the drained chickpeas and mash. Add remaining ingredients and mix well. Form into small patties and place on a nonstick or oil-sprayed baking sheet. Bake for 15 minutes, then turn with a spatula and bake an additional 15 minutes.

Warm the pita breads in a toaster oven or steam them briefly. Slice a bit off one side and split open to reveal pocket. Stuff 2 or 3 falafel patties into each pocket and fill with lettuce, cucumber, tomato, and green onions. Top with tahini sauce or salsa if desired.

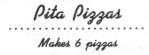

Pita Pizzas

Makes 6 pizzas

Whole wheat pita bread makes an ideal crust for individual pizzas. These are quick and easy to make, and may be baked in a toaster oven. You can use a commercial pizza sauce, or make your own with the following recipe.

1   15-ounce can tomato sauce
1   6-ounce can tomato paste
1   teaspoon each garlic powder and dried basil
½   teaspoon each dried oregano and thyme
6   pita breads
2   cups chopped vegetables: green onion, bell pepper, mushrooms, olives

Preheat the broiler.

Combine tomato sauce, tomato paste, and seasonings. This will make about twice as much sauce as you need. The extra may be refrigerated or frozen for future use.

To assemble the pizza, turn pita bread upside down so it looks like a saucer. Spread with tomato sauce, then top liberally with chopped vegetables. Place on a cookie sheet and broil about 5 minutes, or until the edges just start to get crisp. Or place individual pizzas in toaster oven and toast for 3 to 5 minutes.

Zucchini Pockets

Makes 4 pockets

2 medium zucchini
1 teaspoon olive oil
¼ teaspoon each dried basil, dried oregano, and garlic powder
1 medium tomato, diced
1 teaspoon soy sauce
2 whole wheat pita breads

Slice the zucchini into thin rounds and sauté in oil with the seasonings for 3 minutes. Add the tomato and soy sauce and stir to mix. Remove from heat. Warm pitas in a toaster oven or a steamer, then cut them in half and stuff halves with a generous serving of the zucchini mixture.

Buckwheat Pasta with Seitan

Serves 6

Seitan *(say-tan)* is a high-protein wheat product with a meaty taste and texture. In this recipe it is served with soba, Japanese buckwheat pasta. Look for seitan in health food stores. Soba is available in the Asian food section of many supermarkets and health food stores, as well as in Asian markets.

1 medium onion, chopped
2 tablespoons oil
3 cups sliced fresh mushrooms
8 ounces seitan, sliced
2 tablespoons flour
1½ cups cold water
2 teaspoons soy sauce
½ teaspoon garlic powder
¼ teaspoon black pepper
12 ounces soba noodles
1 teaspoon salt

Sauté the onion in a large skillet with the oil until transparent, then add the mushrooms. Cover and continue cooking until mushrooms are brown, then stir in the seitan.

Whisk flour and water together until smooth, then add to the skillet along with the soy sauce, garlic powder, and pepper. Cook, uncovered, over medium-low heat until thickened.

Bring water to boil in a large kettle. Add the soba and the salt and boil until al dente, about 8 minutes. Top with seitan mixture and serve.

Pasta with Broccoli and Pine Nuts

Serves 4

Perfect for a light supper on a hot summer evening. Serve with a crisp green salad.

12 ounces pasta (fettuccine, linguine, or other)
½ teaspoon salt
1 pound broccoli
3 large garlic cloves, finely chopped
¼ teaspoon dried red pepper flakes, or a pinch of cayenne
2 tablespoons pine nuts
1 tablespoon olive oil
1 28-ounce can chopped tomatoes

Begin heating water for pasta in a large kettle. When water is boiling add the pasta, along with salt, and cook until just tender. Drain.

Break or cut broccoli into florets, and slice stems into rounds. Steam over boiling water until just tender, about 3 minutes. Set aside.

Sauté garlic, red pepper flakes, and pine nuts in olive oil in a large skillet for 1 minute, then add tomatoes and cook over medium heat 5 to 10 minutes. Stir in the cooked broccoli.

Serve over cooked pasta.

Pasta with Peanut Sauce
....
Serves 4

Peanut sauce takes just minutes to prepare and gives pasta a whole new personality. Serve with an assortment of steamed vegetables for a complete and satisfying meal.

12 ounces pasta (spaghetti, linguine)
⅔ cup peanut butter
1 cup hot water
2 tablespoons soy sauce
2 tablespoons vinegar
1 tablespoon raw sugar or other sweetener
2–3 garlic cloves, minced
3 green onions, finely chopped
¼ teaspoon dried red pepper flakes, or a pinch of cayenne

Bring water to boil in a large kettle and cook pasta until just tender.

While the pasta is cooking, whisk together the remaining ingredients in a small saucepan. Heat gently until the sauce is smooth and slightly thickened. Add more water if the sauce becomes too thick.

When pasta is tender, drain and toss it gently with the sauce.

Lasagne
....
Serves 6 to 8

1 medium onion, chopped
1 medium carrot, grated
½ cup water or red wine
3 garlic cloves, minced
2 cups sliced fresh mushrooms
1 15-ounce can tomatoes, chopped with their juice
1 28-ounce can tomato sauce
1 teaspoon each dried basil and oregano
½ teaspoon each dried thyme and fennel seed
⅛ teaspoon cayenne
1 pound firm tofu, mashed
½ cup chopped fresh parsley
2 tablespoons soy sauce

1   10-ounce package frozen chopped spinach, thawed and squeezed dry
12 ounces lasagne noodles (about 10 noodles)

Braise the onion and carrot in the water or wine until soft, then add the garlic and mushrooms; continue cooking until mushrooms are brown. Stir in the tomatoes, tomato sauce, and seasonings and simmer 20 to 30 minutes.

Combine the tofu, parsley, and soy sauce in a bowl.

Preheat the oven to 350°F.

Spread about ½ cup of sauce over the bottom of a 9 × 12-inch casserole. Cover with a layer of uncooked noodles, then with half of the tofu mixture and half the spinach. Spread half the remaining sauce over this. Now make layers with the remaining noodles, tofu mixture, spinach, and sauce. Cover tightly with foil, and bake for 1 hour, or until the noodles are tender.

Let stand 10 minutes before serving to allow it to set.

Mushroom Marinara with Pasta

Serves 8

1   medium onion, chopped
½   cup red wine or water
2   garlic cloves, minced
3–4 cups sliced fresh mushrooms
1   15-ounce can chopped tomatoes
1   28-ounce can tomato sauce
1   teaspoon each dried basil, oregano, and thyme
⅛   teaspoon cayenne
½   teaspoon fennel seed (optional)
1   pound pasta (spaghetti, fettuccine)

Braise the onion for 2 minutes in the wine, then add the garlic and mushrooms. Continue cooking until the onion is soft and the mushrooms are light brown. Stir in the tomatoes, tomato sauce, and seasonings and simmer 20 to 30 minutes.

Cook pasta according to package directions and top with sauce.

Stuffed Spaghetti Squash

Serves 8 to 10

The texture and flavor of spaghetti squash are deliciously complemented with a fresh vegetable medley and white sauce.

1   medium-large spaghetti squash
1   medium onion, chopped
½   pound fresh mushrooms, washed and sliced
2   garlic cloves, minced
1   teaspoon dried basil
½   teaspoon dried oregano
¼   teaspoon dried thyme
1   tablespoon oil
4   large tomatoes, finely chopped
¼   cup chopped fresh parsley, plus additional for garnish
½   teaspoon salt
2   tablespoons margarine
2   tablespoons flour
1   cup soymilk
    Salt and black pepper to taste

Slice the squash in half lengthwise, and scoop out the seeds. Place on a vegetable steamer in a large kettle. Cover and steam until fork-tender, 40 to 60 minutes.

While the squash cooks, sauté the onion, mushrooms, garlic, and herbs in the oil. When the mushrooms are brown, add the tomatoes and parsley and simmer about 10 minutes, or until most of the liquid is evaporated. Add salt to taste.

In a separate pan, melt the margarine and stir in the flour. Cook 30 seconds, then whisk in the soymilk and cook over medium heat, stirring constantly until thickened. Keep warm.

Preheat the oven to 350°F.

When the squash is tender and cool enough to handle, place both halves in a baking dish. Sprinkle with salt and pepper. Divide the white sauce between the two halves and spread evenly, then top each with half the vegetable mixture. Bake for 20 minutes.

Place on a platter and garnish with parsley. To serve, use a large spoon to scoop squash and toppings out of the shell.

Stuffed Eggplant

Serves 3 to 4

One of my students was brave enough to try this recipe on her husband, a confirmed meat-eater and eggplant-hater. He declared it "the best meat he ever ate!" Serve with Brown Rice (page 252) or Wild Rice Dressing (page 255).

3	small eggplants
2	tablespoons olive oil
2	medium onions, chopped
2	garlic cloves, minced
2	green bell peppers, diced
1	teaspoon salt
3	tablespoons finely chopped fresh parsley
¼	teaspoon dried basil
1½	cups chopped tomatoes
½	cup wheat germ
½	cup chopped walnuts

Slice each eggplant in half lengthwise, and scoop out the insides, leaving a ¼-inch-thick shell. Set shells aside.

Coarsely chop the insides, then heat the oil in a large skillet, and add the chopped eggplant, onions, garlic, and bell peppers. Cook over medium heat, stirring often, until the eggplant begins to soften, about 10 minutes (add a small amount of water if necessary to prevent sticking). Add the salt, parsley, basil, and tomatoes and simmer until the eggplant is tender when pierced with a fork. Divide the mixture among the 6 eggplant shells.

Preheat the oven to 350°F.

Combine the wheat germ and chopped nuts, and sprinkle evenly over the eggplant shells. Place the shells in a nonstick or oil-sprayed baking dish and bake until the shells are tender, about 45 minutes.

Chili Beans

....

Serves 8

I often get sidetracked on my way to making chili beans. The pinto beans, cooking with cumin and garlic, smell so good that we often eat them as is, with a bit of salt added, over brown rice. A crisp green salad rounds out this meal beautifully.

The addition of tomato sauce, onion, bell pepper, and seasonings makes a great chili. If you have any left over, use it to make Tamale Pie (page 267), spicy chili beans with a golden cornbread crust.

3	cups dried pinto beans
8–9½	cups water
4	garlic cloves, minced
1	teaspoon ground cumin
2	medium onions, chopped
2	green bell peppers, diced
1	28-ounce can tomato sauce
2	cups corn kernels, fresh or frozen
1½	teaspoons chili powder
⅛	teaspoon cayenne
1	teaspoon salt

Wash the beans thoroughly, then soak overnight. Discard the soaking water. Place beans in a large kettle with 8 to 9 cups fresh water, garlic, and cumin and cook until tender, about 2½ hours.

When the beans are tender, braise the onion and bell pepper in remaining ½ cup water until the onion is soft, then add to the cooked beans along with the tomato sauce, corn, chili powder, and cayenne. Simmer at least 30 minutes. Add salt to taste.

....

Note: To prepare in a slow-cooker, begin cooking the beans in the morning, using hot water and the high setting on the pot. By mid- to late afternoon, the beans will be tender. Add the remaining ingredients (excluding the ½ cup water), and continue cooking on high until dinnertime.

Tamale Pie

Serves 8

Tamale Pie is my idea of comfort food. It is a simple, satisfying casserole with spicy beans on the bottom and cornbread on the top. It is especially good when made with the Chili Beans on page 266, and can also be made with commercial vegetarian chili.

2 cups soymilk
2 tablespoons vinegar
6 cups Chili Beans, with juice
2 cups cornmeal
2 teaspoons baking soda
½ teaspoon salt
2 tablespoons oil

Preheat the oven to 400°F.

Combine the soymilk and vinegar and let stand 5 minutes or more.

Heat the beans until very hot, then pour into a 9 × 12-inch baking dish.

Mix the dry ingredients in a large bowl, and add the soymilk mixture and oil. Stir just to mix, then pour over the hot beans, and bake until the bread is set and golden brown, about 30 minutes.

Beanburgers

Makes 6 patties

1 cup cooked chickpeas, coarsely mashed
1 cup cooked brown rice
½ cup rolled oats
1 teaspoon paprika
2 tablespoons soy sauce
¼ teaspoon black pepper
1 stalk celery, finely chopped
1 small onion, finely chopped
1 garlic clove, minced

Combine all ingredients and mix thoroughly. Form into patties. Fry in a nonstick or lightly oil-sprayed pan until lightly browned, about 3 minutes on each side. Serve on whole wheat buns.

Black Bean Chili

· ·

Serves 6 to 8

This chili can be cooked on the stovetop or in a slow-cooker. Serve with Brown Rice (page 252) or Spicy Bulgur Pilaf (pages 256–57) and a green salad.

2	cups dried black beans
6½	cups water
1	bunch cilantro, chopped (optional)
1	tablespoon cumin seed
1	tablespoon dried oregano
1	teaspoon paprika
½	teaspoon cayenne
1	large onion, chopped
1	green bell pepper, diced
2	garlic cloves, minced
1½	cups chopped tomatoes
½	teaspoon salt
¼	cup chopped green onion

Wash beans and place in a large pan or bowl with 4 to 6 cups water. Soak overnight. Pour off soaking water and place in a kettle with 6 cups fresh water. Add cilantro, if you wish to use it, then bring to a simmer, and cook until the beans are tender, about 2 hours.

In a small, dry skillet, heat the herbs and toast until fragrant. (Be careful not to inhale the fumes; the cayenne can be very irritating.)

In a larger skillet, braise the onion in ½ cup water for 2 minutes. Stir in the bell pepper, garlic, and herbs and cook until the onion is soft. Add to the beans when they are tender, along with the tomatoes. Simmer 30 minutes or longer if time allows (the flavor improves with longer cooking). Add salt to taste.

Serve in individual bowls, topped with chopped green onion. Pass the salsa!

· ·

Note: To use a slow-cooker, place washed, soaked beans in pot with boiling water, chopped cilantro, herbs, onion, bell pepper, and garlic. Cover and cook on high until beans are completely tender, about 3 hours. Add chopped tomato and salt to the cooked beans, and cook 1 hour more or longer.

Refried Beans

Serves 6

These tasty refried beans are made with much less fat than in more traditional recipes.

1½ cups dried pinto beans
4   cups water
4   garlic cloves, minced
1   teaspoon ground cumin
⅓   teaspoon cayenne
1   tablespoon olive oil, or ½ cup water
1   medium onion, chopped
1   15-ounce can tomatoes, chopped with their juice
¼   cup diced Anaheim chilies, canned or fresh
1–2 teaspoons salt

Pick the beans over, removing any stones or other debris. Wash thoroughly, then soak in 4 to 6 cups water for 8 hours. Discard water, rinse beans, and place in a kettle with 4 cups fresh water, 2 minced garlic cloves, cumin, and cayenne. Simmer until tender, about 3 hours.

In a large skillet, sauté the onion and remaining garlic in olive oil or water until the onion is golden. Stir in the tomatoes and chilies, then begin adding the beans, 1 cup at a time, mashing them as you add them. When all the beans have been added, stir to mix, then cook over low heat, stirring frequently, until the mixture is quite thick. Add salt to taste.

Middle Eastern Lentils

Serves 8

This is a traditional dish of the Middle East that is hearty and satisfying. As strange as it may sound, a green salad is served on top of the hot lentil mixture, and the combination is marvelous.

Lentils		
	2	large onions, coarsely chopped
	1	tablespoon olive oil
	¾	cup brown rice
	1½	teaspoons salt
	1½	cups lentils, rinsed
	4	cups water

Salad		
	1	bunch leaf lettuce
	2	medium tomatoes, diced
	1	medium cucumber, peeled and thinly sliced
	2	green onions, chopped
	1	bell pepper, green or red, diced
	1	avocado, sliced (optional)

Dressing		
	2	tablespoons olive oil
	2	tablespoons lemon juice
	½	teaspoon paprika
	¼	teaspoon dry mustard
	1	garlic clove, pressed
	¼	teaspoon salt
	½	teaspoon raw sugar or other sweetener

In a large kettle, sauté onions in olive oil until soft and golden. Add the rice and salt, and continue cooking over medium heat for 3 minutes. Stir in lentils and water. Bring to a simmer, then cover and cook until rice and lentils are tender, about 50 minutes.

While the lentil mixture cooks, prepare salad. Mix ingredients for dressing.

Toss salad with the dressing. To serve, place a spoonful of the lentil mixture on a plate and top with a generous serving of salad.

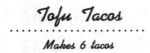

Tofu Tacos

Makes 6 tacos

Firm tofu makes a quick and delicious taco filling. You can also use frozen tofu in this recipe. Freezing tofu gives it a meaty texture. To use frozen tofu, first thaw it, then squeeze out the excess water in it by squeezing it just as you would squeeze a sponge. Then crumble the tofu and proceed with the recipe.

½ onion, chopped, or 1 tablespoon onion powder
2 garlic cloves, crushed, or 1 teaspoon garlic powder
1 small bell pepper, diced (optional)
1 tablespoon oil
½ pound firm tofu, crumbled (about 1 cup)
1 tablespoon chili powder
1 tablespoon nutritional yeast (optional)
¼ teaspoon each ground cumin and dried oregano
1 tablespoon soy sauce
¼ cup tomato sauce
6 corn tortillas

Sauté the onion, garlic, and bell pepper in oil for 2 to 3 minutes, then add tofu, chili powder, yeast, cumin, oregano, and soy sauce. Cook 3 minutes, then add tomato sauce and simmer over low heat until mixture is fairly dry.

Heat tortillas in a heavy, ungreased skillet, turning each from side to side until soft and pliable. Place a small amount of the tofu mixture in the center, fold the tortilla in half, and remove from heat. Garnish with lettuce, onions, tomatoes, salsa, and avocado if desired.

Tofu Burgers

Makes 6 to 8 burgers

These burgers are quick and easy to make. The ingredients can be mixed in advance and stored in the refrigerator for up to a week. Form and cook the patties as needed. Or you can make and cook all the patties at once, then store them in the refrigerator and reheat them in a toaster oven or microwave. For barbecued burgers, precook the patties as directed, then put them on the grill.

1   pound firm tofu, mashed
½   cup rolled oats
1   slice whole wheat bread, finely crumbled
½   cup finely chopped onion, or 2 tablespoons onion powder
1½   tablespoons finely chopped fresh parsley
3   tablespoons soy sauce
½   teaspoon each dried basil, dried oregano, and ground cumin
1   teaspoon garlic powder
     Whole wheat burger buns
     Lettuce
     Sliced tomatoes
     Red onion slices

Mix burger ingredients and knead for a minute or so, until mixture holds together. Shape into patties. Brown on both sides in a nonstick skillet or oil-sprayed skillet. Serve on a bun with lettuce, tomato, and red onion slices.

Variation: To bake burgers, place patties on a nonstick or oil-sprayed baking sheet. Bake at 350°F. for 25 minutes, or until lightly browned.

Tofu Brochettes

....

These are perfect for a barbecue or summer outing. Grill them and serve with cooked brown rice or bulgur.

1 pound firm tofu
2 teaspoons dried oregano
1 cup water
½ cup soy sauce
½ cup balsamic vinegar or wine vinegar
½ cup red wine (optional)
¼ teaspoon black pepper

Vegetables

Red onion
Green bell pepper
Red bell pepper
Button mushrooms
Japanese eggplant
Zucchini
Cherry tomatoes

Press the tofu to remove some of its moisture. Place on a cutting board or baking sheet and cover with a second cutting board or baking sheet. Put 2 or 3 heavy items (like cans of beans) on top of this and let it stand at least 30 minutes.

In the meantime, toast the oregano in a large, dry skillet over medium-low heat for 2 to 3 minutes. Add the remaining marinade ingredients and stir to mix. Remove from heat. Cut the pressed tofu into 1-inch cubes and add to the marinade. Allow the tofu to marinate for at least 1 hour, occasionally turning it gently.

Cut the onion into 1-inch chunks. Seed the peppers and cut them into large pieces. Clean the mushrooms. Slice the eggplant and zucchini into ½-inch-long pieces.

Place an assortment of vegetables and marinated tofu onto each skewer, and grill under a broiler or over coals, turning every few minutes to expose all sides to the heat. Cook 5 to 10 minutes, until vegetables are lightly browned and everything is hot.

Mushrooms in Spicy Tomato Sauce

Serves 8

The original version of this recipe called for 2 teaspoons of cayenne and was a real eye-opener. I have reduced the cayenne to ½ teaspoon; if it is still too hot for your taste, decrease to ¼ teaspoon. Serve with curried lentils and rice.

2	large onions, chopped
½	cup water
1½	tablespoons cumin seed
1½	pounds sliced fresh mushrooms
1	28-ounce can chopped tomatoes
2	cups cooked chickpeas, or 1 15-ounce can, drained
1	teaspoon turmeric
1	teaspoon ground coriander
½	teaspoon cayenne
½	teaspoon ground ginger
1	teaspoon salt

Braise the onions in water for 2 to 3 minutes, then add cumin seed and mushrooms. Continue cooking over medium heat until onions are soft and mushrooms are browned, about 5 minutes.

Add the tomatoes with their juice to the onions along with the chickpeas and spices. Cook 20 to 30 minutes, or longer if time allows, until the mushrooms are tender and most of the liquid has disappeared. Add salt to taste.

Red Lentil Curry

Serves 4 to 6

Red lentils are available in health food stores and markets that sell Indian foods. If you are unable to find red lentils, substitute yellow split peas. This dish is delicious with rice or Couscous (page 252) and Apple Chutney (page 247).

> 1 cup red lentils
> 3 cups water
> 1 tablespoon oil
> ¼ teaspoon each turmeric, ground cumin,
>   ground coriander, ground ginger
> ⅛ teaspoon cayenne
> 1 teaspoon mustard seeds
> ½ teaspoon salt

Sort through the red lentils and pick out any small pebbles, then rinse and put them in a kettle along with the water. Bring to a boil, then reduce heat and simmer until completely tender, 15 to 20 minutes (45 minutes if you are using yellow split peas).

Begin heating the oil in a large skillet, then add all the spices and cook over medium heat until the mustard seeds begin to pop. Slowly add the cooked lentils to the skillet, and stir to mix. Simmer gently, stirring often until thickened. Add salt to taste. Serve hot.

Desserts

. . . .

ICE CREAM SUBSTITUTES

A wide array of nondairy frozen desserts are now available, particularly in health food stores. Be sure to read the label to determine that the dessert is actually nondairy (contains no cream, milk, or milk products such as whey). Also check the fat content, as some of these products are notoriously high in fat.

- *Rice Dream.* In the process of fermenting rice, a thick, sweet liquid called *amasake* is produced. The inventors of Rice Dream reasoned that this liquid could be flavored and frozen to produce a naturally sweet, nondairy dessert. The result is a delicious frozen dessert, available in a variety of flavors, with fat ranging from 32 to 35 percent of calories.
- *Living Lightly.* This dessert is made from soybeans and has no added fat (except the nuts which are added to some flavors). With flavors like Mint Carob Chip and Espresso, you'll never miss ice cream. Fat ranges from 9 percent in some flavors to 32 percent in the flavors which include nuts.
- *Nouvelle Sorbet.* Although this product may be hard to find, it is well worth searching for (ask your health food store to order it). The ingredient list is short and simple—fruit, fruit juice, and fruit pectin—yet the flavors, ranging from apricot to raspberry to passion fruit, are smooth, varied, and delicious. Nouvelle Sorbet gets less than 1 percent of its calories from fat.

In addition to these commercial products, be sure to try the Strawberry Freeze and Banana Freeze (page 277) in this section. They are delicious and simple to make, fat-free, and significantly less expensive than the commercial counterparts.

Strawberry Freeze
. . . .
Serves 2

The ingredients for this delicious fat-free dessert and the one that follows are identical to those for the Fruit Smoothie and Banana Shake (page 219). The amount of liquid is decreased, resulting in a rich, thick, soft-serve dessert. To freeze strawberries and bananas, see page 219.

> 1 cup frozen strawberries
> 1 cup frozen banana chunks
> ½ cup unsweetened apple juice

Place all ingredients into blender and process on high speed until thick and smooth. You will have to stop the blender frequently and stir the unblended fruit to the center.

Banana Freeze
. . . .
Serves 1

> ½ cup soymilk or rice milk
> 1 cup frozen banana chunks

Place soymilk and banana in blender and blend until thick and smooth, stopping the blender occasionally to stir the unblended fruit to the center.

Variation: For a banana date freeze, add 3 pitted dates to the banana and soymilk, and process as above.

Chocolate Pudding

Serves 4

This delicious, old-fashioned pudding contains no eggs and no added fat.

1½ cups soymilk or rice milk
3   tablespoons cornstarch or arrowroot
¼   cup cocoa powder
⅓   cup maple syrup
¼   teaspoon vanilla extract

Whisk all ingredients together in a medium saucepan. Cook over medium heat, stirring constantly until pudding is thickened. Pour into individual serving dishes and chill for at least 1 hour.

Prune Pudding

Serves 3 to 4

Who ever dreamed that prunes could taste so good?

1   cup prunes
1   cup water
⅓   cup soymilk or rice milk
3   tablespoons carob powder
2   tablespoons maple syrup

Place prunes and water in a covered saucepan and simmer until tender, about 20 minutes. Allow to cool slightly, then transfer the prunes and any remaining liquid to a blender. Add remaining ingredients and blend until completely smooth. Spoon into small serving dishes and chill for at least 1 hour.

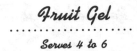

Fruit Gel

Serves 4 to 6

This natural, vegetarian version of Jell-O uses agar, a sea vegetable, which is available at health food stores and Asian markets.

4   cups fruit juice (I like to use strawberry-apple)
4   tablespoons agar flakes
1–2 cups fresh fruit

Combine fruit juice and agar in a saucepan. Bring to a boil over medium heat. Boil 3 minutes. Remove from heat and stir in fresh fruit. Pour into individual serving dishes and chill until firm, about 2 hours.

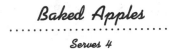

Baked Apples

Serves 4

This dessert contains no added sugar or fat, yet it is delicious and satisfying.

4   large, tart apples
3–5 pitted dates, chopped
1   teaspoon ground cinnamon

Preheat the oven to 350°F.

Wash apples, then remove core to within ¼ inch of bottoms. Combine dates and cinnamon, then distribute equally in the centers of the apples. Place in a baking dish filled with ¼ inch of hot water, and bake for 40 to 60 minutes. Serve hot or chilled.

Poached Pears

Serves 4

These are delicious, and deceptively easy to prepare.

    2   large ripe pears
    ½   cup apple juice concentrate
    ½   cup water
    ¼   teaspoon ground cinnamon
    ⅛   teaspoon ground cloves
        Vanilla nondairy frozen dessert

Peel pears, then slice in half and remove cores. Place in a saucepan. Mix the apple juice concentrate and water with the spices, then pour over pears. Bring to a simmer over medium heat, then cover and cook about 15 minutes.

Remove pears and place into individual serving dishes. Continue to simmer the juice until decreased by half, about 5 minutes. Pour over pears. To serve, top with a scoop of vanilla nondairy frozen dessert.

Middle Eastern Date and Banana Dessert

Serves 3 to 4

This simple dessert seems indulgent, almost decadent. Layers of bananas and dates are covered with a rich soy beverage. The liquid soaks into the fruit, and all the flavors meld beautifully.

    2   large ripe bananas, sliced
    2   cups pitted dates
    2   6-ounce packages Westbrae Vanilla Malted

Peel and slice the bananas. Cut the dates lengthwise into quarters. In a serving dish, make alternate layers of dates and bananas. Pour Westbrae Vanilla Malted over all. The fruit should be almost completely covered by liquid. Refrigerate for at least 3 hours before serving.

. . . .

Note: Westbrae Vanilla Malted is a sweetened soymilk sold in 6-ounce packages in health food stores. It is richer than regular vanilla soymilk, and is necessary in this recipe.

Fresh Peach Cobbler

. . . .

Serves 8

½   cup raw sugar or other sweetener
2   tablespoons cornstarch or arrowroot powder
4   cups fresh peaches, sliced
1   cup water
    Ground cinnamon
1   cup whole wheat pastry flour
2   tablespoons sugar
1½ teaspoons baking powder
¼   teaspoon salt
3   tablespoons margarine
½   cup soymilk or water

Combine sugar and cornstarch in a saucepan, then stir in the peaches and water. Bring to a boil, then boil 1 minute, stirring constantly. Pour into a 9-inch square baking dish, and sprinkle with cinnamon.

Preheat the oven to 400°F.

Combine flour, sugar, baking powder, and salt. Cut in margarine until mixture resembles cornmeal. Stir in soymilk until mixed, then drop by spoonfuls onto the hot fruit. Bake until golden brown, about 25 minutes.

Berry Cobbler
Serves 12

This cobbler is quick and easy to make and contains no added fat. I have sub-stituted fresh sliced peaches for the berries with excellent results.

- 1⅓ cups whole wheat pastry flour
- 1 cup raw sugar or other sweetener
- 1 tablespoon baking powder
- ½ teaspoon salt
- 1⅓ cups soymilk
- 4 cups berries (boysenberries, blackberries, raspberries)

Preheat the oven to 350°F.

In a mixing bowl, stir together the dry ingredients, then add the soymilk, and stir until batter is smooth.

Spread the berries and any juice evenly in a 9 × 13-inch baking dish. Pour in the batter. Bake for 45 minutes, or until lightly browned. Serve warm.

Apple Cranberry Crisp
Serves 8

This dessert is perfect for autumn, when cranberries are available and the apples are fresh, but you can make it at other times of the year if you buy extra bags of cranberries and freeze them. Brown rice syrup is available at health food stores.

- 2 large, tart apples, peeled and sliced
- ½ cup cranberries, fresh or frozen
- ¾ cup Grape-Nuts cereal
- ¾ cup rolled oats
- ½ teaspoon ground cinnamon
- ⅓ cup brown rice syrup
- ⅔ cup apple juice
- ¼ teaspoon cornstarch, or arrowroot

Preheat the oven to 350°F.

Arrange the apple slices in a 9-inch square baking dish, then sprinkle with cranberries. In a bowl, mix the Grape-Nuts, rolled oats, and cinnamon, then stir in the brown rice syrup. Spread evenly over apples. Mix the apple juice and cornstarch or arrowroot, then pour evenly over other ingredients.

Bake for 50 minutes, or until apples are tender.

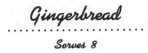

Gingerbread

Serves 8

This gingerbread contains no animal ingredients and no added fat, and is moist and delicious. Try serving it with hot applesauce for a real treat.

½   cup raisins
½   cup chopped pitted dates
1¾ cups water
¾   cup raw sugar or other sweetener
½   teaspoon salt
2   teaspoons ground cinnamon
1   teaspoon ground ginger
¾   teaspoon grated nutmeg
¼   teaspoon ground cloves
2   cups unbleached all-purpose or whole wheat pastry flour
1   teaspoon baking soda
1   teaspoon baking powder

Combine dried fruits, water, sugar, and seasonings in a large saucepan and bring to a boil. Continue boiling for 2 minutes, then remove from heat and cool completely.

Preheat the oven to 350°F.

When fruit mixture is cool, mix in dry ingredients. Spread into a nonstick or lightly oil-sprayed 9-inch square pan and bake for 30 minutes, or until a toothpick inserted into the center comes out clean.

Pumpkin Spice Cookies

. . . .

Makes about 36 cookies

These plump, moist cookies are made with a puree of flaxseed and water to replace the eggs called for in the original recipe. Flaxseeds are available in most natural food stores.

3	cups whole wheat pastry flour
4	teaspoons baking powder
1	teaspoon salt
1	teaspoon baking soda
1	teaspoon ground cinnamon
½	teaspoon grated nutmeg
1½	cups raw sugar or other sweetener
4	tablespoons flaxseeds
1½	cups water
1¾	cups solid-pack canned pumpkin
1	cup raisins

Preheat the oven to 350°F.

Mix the dry ingredients and set aside.

Blend flaxseeds and 1 cup water in a blender for 1 to 2 minutes, until the mixture has the consistency of beaten egg white. Add to the dry ingredients, along with the pumpkin, remaining water, and raisins. Mix until just combined.

Drop by tablespoonfuls onto a nonstick or lightly oil-sprayed baking sheet. Bake 15 minutes, or until lightly browned. Remove from baking sheet with a spatula, and place on a rack to cool. Store in an airtight container.

Banana Cake

. . . .

Serves 8

2	cups unbleached all-purpose or whole wheat pastry flour
1½	teaspoons baking soda
½	teaspoon salt
1	cup raw sugar or other sweetener
⅓	cup oil

4   ripe bananas, mashed (about 2½ cups)
¼   cup water
1   teaspoon vanilla extract
1   cup chopped walnuts

Preheat the oven to 350°F.

Mix flour, baking soda, and salt in a bowl.

In a large bowl, beat sugar and oil together, then add the bananas and mash them. Stir in the water and vanilla, and mix thoroughly. Add the flour mixture along with the chopped walnuts, and stir to mix.

Spread in a nonstick or lightly oil-sprayed 9-inch square baking pan, and bake for 45 to 50 minutes, or until a toothpick inserted into the center comes out clean.

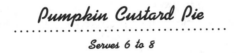

Pumpkin Custard Pie

Serves 6 to 8

Cornstarch is used as a thickener in place of eggs in this pie.

1½   cups soymilk
4   tablespoons cornstarch
1½   cups cooked pumpkin
½   cup raw sugar or other sweetener
½   teaspoon salt
1   teaspoon ground cinnamon
½   teaspoon ground ginger
⅛   teaspoon ground cloves
1   9-inch unbaked pie shell or prebaked Fat-Free Pie Crust (page 287)

Preheat the oven to 375°F.

In a large bowl, whisk together the soymilk and cornstarch until smooth, then blend in remaining ingredients. Pour into pie shell and bake for 45 minutes, or until firm. Cool before cutting.

Sweet Surprise Pumpkin Pie

Serves 6 to 8

No one will guess that the egg substitute in this pie is agar, a type of seaweed, available in health food stores.

        1½ cups soymilk
        3   tablespoons agar flakes
        1½ cups cooked pumpkin
        ½   cup raw sugar or other sweetener
        ½   teaspoon salt
        1   teaspoon ground cinnamon
        ½   teaspoon ground ginger
        ⅛   teaspoon ground cloves
        1   9-inch unbaked pie shell or prebaked Fat-Free Crust (below)

Preheat the oven to 375°F.

Combine soymilk and agar in a saucepan and let stand 5 minutes. Bring to a simmer over medium heat and cook 2 minutes, stirring constantly. Stir in remaining ingredients and blend well. Pour into pie shell and bake for 45 minutes. The filling will still be quite liquid, but will set as the pie cools. Cool before cutting.

Fat-Free Pie Crust

Makes one 9-inch crust

This recipe was developed by Mary McDougall, a pioneer of low-fat cuisine. I use it regularly as a substitute for crumb crusts, and often find it appropriate in place of a regular pastry crust. In addition to being fat-free, it is blessedly easy to prepare.

        1 cup Grape-Nuts cereal
        ¼ cup apple juice concentrate

Preheat the oven to 350°F.

Mix the Grape-Nuts and apple juice concentrate. Pat into a 9-inch pie pan. Bake for 10 minutes, then cool before filling.

Tofu "Cheesecake"

. . . .

Serves 8 to 10

This smooth and velvety "cheesecake" is delicious topped with a simple lemon glaze or with fresh fruit. Agar flakes, which are derived from seaweed, are used as a thickener. Look for them in your health food store.

    2   tablespoons agar flakes
    ⅔   cup soymilk
    ½   cup raw sugar or other sweetener
    ½   teaspoon salt
    2   teaspoons grated lemon rind
    4   tablespoons lemon juice
    2   teaspoons vanilla extract
    1   pound tofu
    1   9-inch prebaked crumb crust or Fat-Free Crust (opposite)

Lemon Glaze   ⅓   cup raw sugar or other sweetener
                 1½ tablespoons cornstarch or arrowroot
                 1½ tablespoons lemon juice
                 ½   teaspoon grated lemon rind
                 ⅓   cup water

Combine agar and soymilk and let stand 5 minutes. Add sugar and salt, and simmer over low heat, stirring often, for 5 minutes. Pour into a blender, add remaining filling ingredients, and blend until smooth. Spread evenly in crust and chill 30 minutes.

Combine all ingredients for glaze in a small saucepan and whisk until smooth. Heat, stirring constantly, until mixture thickens. Allow to cool, slightly, then spread over cheesecake. Chill an additional 2 hours.

Cranberry Apple Punch

Makes 6 cups

This beverage is delicious hot or cold. I serve it from my slow-cooker at winter parties in place of hot mulled cider. The tart cranberry tea is a perfect foil to the sweetness of the apple juice.

4½ cups water
8 Cranberry Cove tea bags (see Note)
1 12-ounce can apple juice concentrate
Orange or lemon slices (optional)

Bring water to a boil. Turn off heat and pour over tea bags. Allow to steep at least 15 minutes, then remove tea bags. Add apple juice concentrate and stir to mix.

For a hot beverage, heat in a slow-cooker or large kettle until steamy. Add a few orange and lemon slices for a garnish before serving.

For a cold beverage, chill thoroughly, then serve over ice.

Note: Cranberry Cove is a tea made by Celestial Seasonings, available in many supermarkets and at most natural food stores.

Super-Quick Meals for a Week

Day 1

Menu

Black Bean Chili

Spanish rice

Green salad

Warm tortillas

Shopping List

Fantastic Foods Instant Black Beans
Fantastic Foods Quick Brown Rice Pilaf
Whole wheat or corn tortillas
Lettuce, tomato, avocado, cucumber
Oil-free salad dressing
Salsa (optional)

Preparation

Prepare beans and rice according to package instructions. While they cook, prepare the salad. Heat the tortillas by zapping them quickly in the microwave or by flipping them in a hot, ungreased skillet on the stove. Dress the salad. Put a serving of beans, rice, and salad on each plate, along with a warm tortilla. Pass the salsa!

Day 2

Menu

Veggie burgers
Tabouli Salad
Broccoli

Shopping List

Nature's Burger or refrigerated tofu burgers
Whole wheat buns
Casbah Tabouli Salad
Broccoli

Preparation

Mix burgers according to package instructions; form patties, then fry in an oil-sprayed skillet or bake on an oil-sprayed cookie sheet at 375°F. for 20–25 minutes. Prepare tabouli according to package instructions. Steam the broccoli or cook it in the microwave.

Day 3

Menu

Meatless lasagne

Green salad

Garlic bread

Shopping List

Legume Lasagne (frozen food section)

Lettuce, tomato, avocado, cucumber

Oil-free salad dressing

Sourdough French bread

Jar of crushed garlic

Preparation

Heat lasagne according to package instructions. While it cooks, slice the bread and spread each slice lightly with crushed garlic. Wrap in foil and heat in 350°F. oven for 20 minutes. Assemble and dress salad.

Day 4

....

Menu

Not dogs

Baked red potatoes

Steamed cabbage

Shopping List

Yves Tofu Wieners (refrigerated or frozen)

Whole wheat hot dog buns

Mustard, ketchup, relish

Red potatoes

Salsa

Green cabbage

Preparation

Scrub the red potatoes and bake them at 350°F. until they are easily pierced with a fork, about 50 minutes, or cook them in the microwave. Cut in half and top with salsa. Slice the cabbage into thin strips. Place in a steamer and steam until tender, about 5 minutes. Sprinkle with salt and pepper. Heat the hot dogs in a steamer or in the microwave.

Day 5
....

Menu

Vegetarian beans
Couscous pilaf
Green salad

Shopping List

Heinz Vegetarian Beans
Casbah Couscous Pilaf
Lettuce, tomato, avocado, cucumber
Oil-free salad dressing

Preparation

Heat beans on stove or in microwave. Prepare pilaf according to package instructions. Assemble and dress salad.

Day 6
....

Menu

Ramen soup
Bread or muffins
Broccoli

Shopping List

Westbrae Natural Ramen (many flavors available)
Whole wheat bread, rolls, or muffins
Broccoli

Preparation

Prepare ramen according to package instructions. Steam broccoli or cook in microwave. Warm bread if desired.

Day 7

Menu

Lemon broil tempeh
Rozdali lentils and rice
Green salad

Shopping List

White Wave Lemon Broil Tempeh (deli case)
Rozdali
Lettuce, tomato, avocado, cucumber
Oil-free salad dressing

Preparation

Prepare Rozdali according to package instructions. Heat tempeh in oven or microwave. Assemble and dress salad.

You are beginning a whole new way of eating, and you deserve congratulations. You have in your hands a powerful program that can help keep you feeling good and looking good. And you will find that changing your diet is not a one-time event. You will keep learning new things about foods and health, and will find many more wonderful foods to try.

I hope you will have opportunities to share information with others. Unfortunately, not everyone yet has access to the vital information you now know. Federal nutrition guidelines still aggressively promote unhealthful foods, even as the evidence against them mounts higher.

Shortly after the Physicians Committee for Responsible Medicine unveiled the New Four Food Groups in 1991, the U.S. Department of Agriculture issued its own new plan, a pyramid that pictured grains, vegetables, and fruits at its broad base, indicating that these foods should be the main portion of the diet. Meat and dairy products were pictured at the upper, smaller portion of the pyramid, just under the most shunned foods: fats, oils, and sweets. The outraged meat and dairy industries forced the Department of Agriculture to reconsider the graphic, which delayed the release of the food guide for nearly a year.

The pyramid was a big improvement over the old depictions of the four food groups, which put meat and dairy on a par with grains, vegetables, and fruits. But even the new pyramid promotes two to three servings of meat and two to three servings of dairy products *every day,* which is more than most of us can take over the long run. The predictable result is obesity, high cholesterol levels and heart attacks, and ever-climbing cancer rates.

A pair of scissors provides you a solution. Simply cut along the line indicated in the diagram. Throw away the top portion, and save the bottom, which you now call the Food Guide Trapezoid. You can then, in good conscience, tape this to your refrigerator and mail copies to your friends.

Imagine what would happen if everyone were to follow the type of program you have read about in this book. As a group, we would manage to eliminate the majority of our heart disease risk, at least half of our risk of high blood pressure, and most of our cancer risk.

As America grapples with how to pay for its health-care costs, a big part of the solution is to reduce our need for medical care. If we avoid tobacco, our collective lung cancer bill, so to speak, will be cut dramatically. And those of us who are also sticking to a low-fat vegetarian menu will keep the need for doctors, drugs, and hospitalization to a minimum. Vegetarians use less medication; have fewer hospital stays, fewer operations, and X-rays; and spend far less of their time in doctors' offices.

One day insurance companies will offer lower premiums for vegetarians, as they now do for nonsmokers and safe drivers. As it stands, businesses pay enormous costs for medical insurance and pass them along to consumers. For instance, health-related costs add hundreds of dollars to the price of every new car sold in America. When a company sells a computer, or a long-distance service links up to a home, or a college enrolls students, the companies involved have to charge enough to cover all their costs. Those costs include health insurance for their employees and their employees' spouses and children, the costs of replacing workers who die or become disabled, and the costs of absenteeism owing to illness. Costs that should be small have become so great as to affect the competitiveness of U.S. products and services.

But the real issue is not economics. People on low-fat vegetarian diets are able to feel better, live longer, and enjoy life more. They have more power to keep serious illnesses at arm's length. And they are able to pass on a healthy life-style to the next generation.

If you would like to keep up to date on nutrition, I encourage you to join the Physicians Committee for Responsible Medicine. PCRM is a nonprofit organization that supplies information on nutrition, research, and other medical issues of interest to physicians and nonphysicians alike through a fascinating quarterly magazine called *Good Medicine.* Other PCRM programs include the Gold Plan, an innovative nutrition-education program for businesses, hospitals, and schools, and the New Four Food Groups curriculum for junior high students. PCRM also has lecturers and speakers for broadcast programs. The tax-deductible membership fee is $20. For information, write PCRM, Box 6322, Washington, D.C. 20015.

Let me also invite you to help spread the word by sending information to friends and family members, writing letters to the editors of newspapers and magazines, and suggesting topics for radio and television talk shows.

When I began my work in medicine, my goal was to help people stay healthy, both physically and mentally. Happily, I hear from a great many people, who tell me how much these dietary improvements have helped them. I hope you will let me know how this program works for you, and I wish you the very best of success!

Food Guide Pyramid

A Guide to Daily Food Choices

Fats, Oils, & Sweets
USE SPARINGLY

Milk, Yogurt,
& Cheese
Group
2-3 SERVINGS

Meat, Poultry, Fish,
Dry Beans, Eggs,
& Nuts Group
2-3 SERVINGS

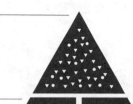

Vegetable
Group
3-5 SERVINGS

Fruit
Group
2-4 SERVINGS

Bread, Cereal,
Rice, & Pasta
Group
**6-11
SERVINGS**

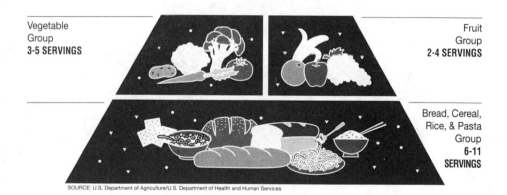

SOURCE: U.S. Department of Agriculture/U.S. Department of Health and Human Services

Appendix I

Use Your Body

Physical activity is great for your heart, your waistline, and your sense of well-being. Unfortunately, many people associate exercise with misery: jogging down a smoggy roadway at 6:00 A.M. or peddling on a stationary bike for as long as boredom will allow. Let's face it. These forms of exercise are not natural. Jogging is the physical equivalent of an instant diet shake—an unnatural compensation for an unhealthful life-style. People jog because they have forgotten more enjoyable ways of getting their bodies moving. Of course, some people do enjoy jogging, running, weight-lifting, or structured aerobics. If that includes you, then there is nothing wrong with those exercises, so long as you stay within the limits of safety. But my recommendation for most people is different.

Our bodies are designed for physical activity: walking, dancing, biking, games, and playing with children. These activities can get your heart moving and can burn a lot of calories. But we do them for fun, not to burn calories. Honeymooning couples do not, in the midst of afterglow, check their pulses and calculate calorie expenditure. The key is to remember what it was like to move your body—to enjoy a walk in the woods, a game of volleyball or touch football, a night on the dance floor.

For starters, I recommend something very simple. Just walk a half-hour per day, or 1 hour three times per week. This is easy, and it gives you plenty of exercise. And by all means smell the roses along the way. Pick a place to walk that is enjoyable for you, with interesting sights, sounds, and smells.

If you prefer, pick any other activity. To give you an idea of how quickly your body can part with calories, here are some activities people enjoy and the number of calories they burn per hour for a 150-pound adult:

· ·

Activity	Calories Burned per Hour
Bicycling	400
Canoeing	180
Cooking	180
Dancing, ballroom	240
Gardening	480
Golf	345
Jumping rope	570
Ping-Pong	285
Playing piano	165
Racquetball	615
Swimming	525
Tennis—doubles	270
Tennis—singles	435
Volleyball	330
Walking, brisk	360

· ·

Fun is the key. And bring a friend along.

A word of caution: Do not push yourself too hard. If you are over forty or have any history of illness, medication use, or joint problems, talk over your plans with your doctor before you begin.

Managing Stress

Reducing stress helps cut your risk of heart problems, strengthens your immune system, and reduces anxiety so you are more likely to stick to a healthful life-style and less likely to depend on sedatives or the daily Martini that many people use to deal with stress.

First, get plenty of sleep. You know the amount of sleep you need to feel well. And if you can spare the time, a short nap before dinner is a great stress reducer. At work, take a break every now and then to move around, take a deep breath, stretch, and have a big yawn.

Here are three simple exercises that melt away stress. These techniques work by turning off external stimuli and relaxing your muscles. When your body is relaxed, your mind tends to let go of tension, too. Twice a day, try any one of these for several minutes. They also help if you are having trouble falling asleep.

For each exercise, sit in a comfortable chair or lie on your back in a quiet room. Unplug the phone and use a DO NOT DISTURB sign. If you should happen to doze off, don't worry. That is a sign that your body wants more rest.

RELAXATION BREATHING

For about thirty seconds, simply relax with your eyes closed, thinking about nothing at all. Then start to pay attention to your breathing. Let your breathing slow down naturally, like a person sleeping. Feel the cool air come in through your nose with each inhalation, and feel your breath leave as you exhale. Imagine that tension is leaving your body with each exhalation.

Now imagine that, as you breathe in, the air comes into your nostrils and caresses your face like a gentle breeze. As you breathe out, the exhalation carries away the tension from your face. As you breathe slowly in and out, tension gradually leaves your body and you become more and more relaxed.

Now imagine that, as you breathe in, the gentle air enters your nose and spreads relaxation up over the top of your head. As you exhale, imagine the tension leaving this area and passing out of your body. Then imagine the next breath carrying relaxation over your face, your scalp, and both sides of your head. As you exhale, let the tension flow out easily.

If other thoughts come to mind, simply return to paying attention to your breathing. Your breathing is slow and easy, with no effort at all. Let your body relax.

Now let a breath carry relaxation to your neck. As you exhale, tension passes out of your neck and out of your body with the exhaled air. Then feel a breath carry relaxation to your shoulders. As you exhale, tension leaves your shoulders and passes out of your body.

Now, one breath at a time, focus your attention on each part of your body from the top down: your upper arms, forearms, hands, chest, stomach, hips, thighs, knees, calves, ankles, and feet. Imagine each breath of air carrying relaxation into each part of your body. As you breathe out, tension passes out through your nostrils.

This relaxing exercise will take several minutes, and you can do it at whatever pace is comfortable for you. When you have finished, allow yourself to sit quietly for two minutes or more.

MUSCLE RELAXATION SEQUENCE

As in the previous exercise, focus on one body part at a time from the top down. This time, tighten and release the muscles in each body part, one at a time. This allows the muscles to achieve a deep state of relaxation.

Start by sitting quietly for about thirty seconds. Allow your breathing to slow down naturally. Now gently raise your eyebrows for a second, and then relax. You may briefly feel tension in the front and back of your head, followed by relaxation. Breathe slowly in and out. Now gently tighten the muscles of your face into a slight grimace for about one second, then let them totally relax. Take a normal breath in and out, and feel your face relaxing. Then gently clench your jaw and release it. This tightens and then relaxes the muscles of the cheeks and above the ears.

Tighten the muscles of your neck and release them. After a moment, raise your shoulders and drop them. Let each body part relax in sequence. Take your time, and allow your body to completely relax after each tightening. Tighten and release the muscles of your upper arm, and then your forearm. Ball your hand into a fist for a moment and then release it. Feel the tension leave each body part. Continue slow and relaxed breathing.

Then briefly tighten and release, in succession, the muscles of your chest, your abdomen, your thighs, calves, and feet. When you are finished, notice whether tension remains in any part of your body. If it does, imagine that body part gradually releasing tension as you breathe slowly in and out.

Enjoy the feeling of relaxation for a few minutes before getting up.

LISTENING TO BREATHING

This exercise can be used anywhere, whether you are on a stage waiting to give a speech or tossing and turning in a hotel bed unable to unwind from the stresses of the day. It uses imaginary sounds with no meaning to focus your attention away from the events of the day.

Sit quietly or lie on your back. Listen to your breathing, and let your breathing slow down. Imagine that as you breathe in, the inhalation makes a sound like the word *so*. As you exhale, imagine that your breathing sounds like the word *hum*. You need not make these sounds; just imagine them as you inhale and exhale.

Let your breathing slow down a little more, and slowly imagine the word *so* with each inhalation. Slow and silently say *hum* to yourself as you slowly exhale. Repeat this for several minutes. If you find your mind drifting to something else, gently come back to listening to your breathing. You can also use this technique for just a few seconds, if you like, as a quick stress reducer.

Recommended Reading

General Books

Alabaster, Oliver. *The Power of Prevention*. Washington, D.C.: Saville Books, 1988.

Chopra, Deepak. *Perfect Health*. New York: Harmony, 1991.

Colbin, Annemarie. *Food and Healing*. New York: Ballantine, 1986.

Lauffer, Randall B. *Iron Balance*. New York: St. Martin's, 1991.

McDougall, John. *The McDougall Program*. New York: NAL Penguin, 1990.

McDougall, John and Mary. *The McDougall Plan*. Piscataway, N.J.: New Century, 1983.

Moran, Victoria. *The Love-Powered Diet*. San Raphael, Calif.: New World Library, 1992.

Ornish, Dean. *Dr. Dean Ornish's Program for Reversing Heart Disease*. New York: Random House, 1990.

Stamford, Bryant A. and Porter Shimer. *Fitness Without Exercise*. New York: Warner, 1990.

Swank, Roy L. *The Multiple Sclerosis Diet Book*. New York: Doubleday, 1987.

Weil, Andrew. *Natural Health, Natural Medicine*. Boston: Houghton Mifflin, 1990.

Cookbooks
....

Diamond, Marilyn. *American Vegetarian Cookbook*. New York: Warner, 1990.

Gelles, Carol. *Wholesome Harvest*. Boston: Little, Brown, 1992.

Katzen, Mollie. *Moosewood Cookbook*. Berkeley: Ten Speed, 1977.

Kushi, Aveline and Alex Jack. *Aveline Kushi's Complete Guide to Macrobiotic Cooking*. New York: Warner, 1985.

McDougall, Mary. *The Health-Supporting Cookbook, Vols. I & II*. Clinton, N.J.: New Win, 1985.

Pickford, Louise. *The Inspired Vegetarian*. New York: Stewart, Tabori, and Chang, 1992.

Thomas, Anna. *The Vegetarian Epicure*. New York: Vintage, 1972.

Wagner, Lindsay and Ariane Spade. *The High Road to Health*. New York: Prentice Hall, 1990.

References

....

Chapter 1

1. Hayflick L. The limited in vitro lifetime of human diploid cell strains. *Exp Cell Res* 1965;37:614–36.

2. Stanulis-Praeger BM, Gilchrest BA. Effect of donor age and prior sun exposure on growth inhibition of cultured human dermal fibroblasts by all trans-retinoic acid. *J Cell Physiol* 1989;139:116–24.

3. Gilchrest BA, Szabo G, Flynn E, Goldwyn RM. Chronologic and actinically induced aging in human facial skin. *J Invest Dermatol* 1983,80:81s–85s.

4. Kligman LH. Preventing, delaying, and repairing photoaged skin. *Cutis* 1988;41:419–20.

5. Sanford KK, Parshad R, Gantt R. Responses of human cells in culture to hydrogen peroxide and related free radicals generated by visible light: relationship to cancer susceptibility. In Johnson JE, Walford R, Harman D, Miquel J., eds. Free radicals, aging, and degenerative diseases. New York, Alan R. Liss, 1986.

6. Sistrom WR, Griffiths M, Stanier RY. The biology of a photo synthetic bacterium which lacks colored carotenoids. *J Cellular Comp Physiol* 1956;48:473–515.

7. Matthews-Roth MM, Pathak MA, Fitzpatrick TB, et al. Beta-carotene as a photoprotective agent in erythropoietic protoporphyria. *N Engl J Med* 1970;282(22):1231–34.

8. Matthews-Roth MM, Pathak MA, Fitzpatrick TB, et al. Beta-carotene therapy for erythropoietic protoporphyria and other photosensitivity diseases. *Arch Dermatol* 1977;113:1229–32.

9. Bendes JH. Heliotherapy in tuberculosis. *Minnesota Med* 1926;9:112.

10. Matthews-Roth MM, Pathak MA, Parris J, Fitzpatrick TB, Kass EH, Toda K, Clemens W. A Clinical trial of the effects of oral beta-carotene on the responses of human skin to solar radiation. *J Invest Dermatol* 1972;59(4):349–53.

11. Vahlquist A, Berne B. Sunlight, vitamin A and the skin. *Photodermatology* 1986;3:203–5.

12. Willett WC, Stampfer MJ, Underwood BA, Taylor JO, Hennekens CH. Vitamins A, E, and carotene: effects of supplementation on their plasma levels. *Am J Clin Nutr* 1983;38:559–66.

13. Niki E, Yamamoto Y, Komuro E, Sato K. Membrane damage due to lipid oxidation. *Am J Clin Nutr* 1991;53:201S–5S.

14. Frei B. Ascorbic acid protects lipids in human plasma and low-density lipoprotein against oxidative damage. *Am J Clin Nutr* 1991;54:1113S–18S.

15. Diplock AT. Antioxidant nutrients and disease prevention: an overview. *Am J Clin Nutr* 1991;53:189S–93S.

16. Odeleye OE, Watson RR. Health implications of the n-3 fatty acids. *Am J Clin Nutr* 1991;53:177–78.

17. Kinsella JE. Reply to O Odeleye and R Watson. *Am J Clin Nutr* 1991;53:178.

18. Lauffer RB. Iron balance. New York, St. Martin's Press, 1991.

19. Varma SD. Scientific basis for medical therapy of cataracts by antioxidants. *Am J Clin Nutr* 1991;53:335S–45S.

20. Jacques PF, Chylack LT Jr. Epidemiologic evidence of a role for the antioxidant vitamins and carotenoids in cataract prevention. *Am J Clin Nutr* 1991;53:352S–5S.

21. Robertson JM, Donner AP, Trevithick JR. A possible role for vitamins C and E in cataract prevention. *Am J Clin Nutr* 1991;53:346S–51S.

22. Garland D. Role of site-specific, metal-catalyzed oxidation in lens aging and cataract: a hypothesis. *Exp Eye Res* 1990;50:677–82.

23. Simoons FJ. A geographic approach to senile cataracts: possible links with milk consumption, lactase activity, and galactose metabolism. *Digestive Diseases and Sciences* 1982;27(3):257–64.

24. Couet C, Jan P, Debry G. Lactose and cataract in humans: a review. *J Am Coll Nutr* 1991;10(1):79–86.

25. Hamilton JB. Male hormone stimulation is prerequisite and an incitant in common baldness. *Am J Anat* 1942;71:451–80.

26. Adachi K, Motonari K. Adenyl cyclase in human hair follicles: its inhibition by dihydrotestosterone. *Biochem Biophys Res Comm* 1970;41:884–90.

27. Burke KE. Hair loss: what causes it and what can be done about it. *Postgraduate Medicine* 1989;85:52–77.

28. Bingham KD. The metabolism of androgens in male pattern alopecia: a review. *International J Cosmetic Sci* 1981;3:1–8.

29. Sawaya ME, Honig LS, Garland LD, Hsia SL. Hydroxysteroid dehydrogenase activity in sebaceous glands of scalp in male-pattern baldness. *J Invest Dermatol* 1988;91:101–5.

30. Cabanac M, Brinnel H. Beards, baldness, and sweat secretion. *Eur J Appl Physiol* 1988;58:39–46.

31. Meikle AW, Bishop DT, Stringham JD, West DW. Quantitating genetic and nongenetic factors that determine plasma sex steroid variation in normal male twins. *Metabolism* 1987;35:1090–95.

32. Meikle AW, Stringham JD, Bishop DT, West DW. Quantitating genetic and nongenetic factors influencing androgen production and clearance rates in men. *J Clin Endocrin Metab* 1988;67:104–109.

33. Hamalainen EK, Adlercreutz H, Puska P, Pietinen P. Decrease of serum total and free testosterone during a low-fat high-fiber diet. *J Steroid Biochem* 1983;18:369–70.

34. Hamalainen EK, Adlercreutz H, Puska P, Pietinen P. Diet and serum sex hormones in healthy men. *J Steroid Biochem* 1984;20:459–64.

35. Adlercreutz H. Western diet and Western diseases: some hormonal and biochemical mechanisms and associations. *Scan J Clin Lab Invest* 1990;50, Suppl 201:3–23.

36. Hill PB, Wynder EL, Garbaczewski L, Garnes H, Walker ARP. Diet and urinary steroids in black and white North American men and black South African men. *Cancer Res* 1979a;39:5101–5.

37. Hill PB, Wynder EL. Effect of a vegetarian diet and dexamethasone on plasma prolactin, testosterone and dehydroepiandrosterone in men and women. *Cancer Letters* 1979b;7:273–82.

38. Hill P, Wynder E, Garbaczewski L, Garnes H, Walker ARP, Helman P. Plasma hormones and lipids in men at different risk for coronary heart disease. *Am J Clin Nutr* 1980;33:1010–18.

39. Howie BJ, Shultz TD. Dietary and hormonal interrelationships among vegetarian Seventh-Day Adventists and nonvegetarian men. *Am J Clin Nutr* 1985;42:127–34.

40. Goldin BR, Gorbach SL. Effect of diet on the plasma levels, metabolism and excretion of estrogens. *Am J Clin Nutr* 1988;48:787–90.

41. Reed MJ, Cheng RW, Simmonds M, Richmond W, James VHT. Dietary lipids: an additional regulator of plasma levels of sex hormone binding globulin. *J Clin Endocrin Metab* 1987;64:1083–85.

42. Reinberg A, Lagoguey M, Chauffournier J-M, Cesselin F. Circannual and circadian rhythms in plasma testosterone in five healthy young Parisian males. *Acta Endocrinol* 1975;80:732–43.

43. Reinberg A, Lagoguey M, Cesselin F, et al. Circadian and circannual rhythms in plasma hormones and other variables of five healthy young human males. *Acta Endocrinol* 1978; 88:417–27.

44. Smals AGH, Kloppenborg PWC, Benraad Th J. Circannual cycle in plasma testosterone levels in man. *J Clin Endocrinol Metab* 1976;42:979–82.

45. Bellastella A, Criscuolo T, Mango A, et al. Circannual rhythms of plasma luteinizing hormone, follicle-stimulating hormone, testosterone, prolactin and cortisol in prepuberty. *Clin Endocrinol* 1983;19:453–59.

46. Randall VA, Ebling FJG. Seasonal changes in human hair growth. *Br J Derm* 1991; 124:146–51.

47. Kessels AGH, Cardynaals RLLM, Borger RLL, et al. The effectiveness of the hair-restorer "Dabao" in males with alopecia androgenetica: a clinical experiment. *J Clin Epidemiol* 1991;44:439–47.

48. Burton JL, Ben Halim MM, Meyrick G, Jeans WD, Murphy D. Male-pattern alopecia and masculinity. *Br J Dermatol* 1979;100:567–71.

49. Inaba M. Can human hair grow again? Tokyo, Japan, Azabu Shokan, Inc., 1985.

50. Lookingbill DP, Demers LM, Wang C, Leung A, Rittmaster RS, Santen RJ. Clinical and biochemical parameters of androgen action in normal healthy caucasian versus Chinese subjects. *J Clin Endocrinol Metab* 1991;72:1242–8.

51. Herrera CR, Lynch C. Is baldness a risk factor for coronary artery disease? A review of the literature. *J Clin Epidemol* 1990;43:1255–60.

52. Riggs BL, Wahner HW, Melton J, Richelson LS, Judd HL, O'Fallon M. Dietary calcium intake and rates on bone loss in women. *J Clin Invest* 1987;80:979–82.

53. Dawson-Hughes B. Calcium supplementation and bone loss: a review of controlled clinical trials. *Am J Clin Nutr* 1991;54:274S–80S.

54. Kolata, G. How important is dietary calcium in preventing osteoporosis? *Science,* 1986;233:519–20.

55. Mazess RB, Barden HS. Bone density in premenopausal women: effects of age, dietary intake, physical activity, smoking, and birth-control pills. *Am J Clin Nutr* 1991;53:132–42.

55A. Zemel MB, Schuette SA, Hegsted M, Linkswiler HM. Role of the sulfur-containing amino acids in protein-induced hypercalciuria in men. *J Nutr* 1981;111:545–52.

55B. Hegsted M, Schuette SA, Zemel MB, Linkswiler HM. Urinary calcium and calcium balance in young men as affected by level of protein and phosphorus intake. *J Nutr* 1981;111:553–62.

56. Marsh AG, Sanchez TV, Mickelsen O, Keiser J, Mayor G. Cortical bone density of adult lacto-ovo-vegetarian and omnivorous women. *J Am Dietetic Asso* 1980;76:148–51.

57. Heaney RP, Weaver CM. Calcium absorption from kale. *Am J Clin Nutr* 1990;51: 656–57.

58. Nicar MJ, Pak CYC. Calcium bioavailability from calcium carbonate and calcium citrate. *J Clin Endocrinol Metab* 1985;61:391–93.

59. Nelson ME, Fisher EC, Dilmanian FA, Dallal GE, Evans WJ. A 1-y walking program and increased dietary calcium in postmenopausal women: effect on bone. *Am J Clin Nutr* 1991;53:1304–11.

60. Dawson-Hughes B, Jacques P, Shipp C. Dietary calcium intake and bone loss from the spine in healthy postmenopausal women. *Am J Clin Nutr* 1987;46:685–87.

61. Brenner BM, Meyer TW, Hostetter TH. Dietary protein intake and the progressive nature of kidney disease. *New Eng J Med* 1982;307:652–59.

62. El Nahas AM, Coles GA. Dietary treatment of chronic renal failure: ten unanswered questions. *Lancet* 1986;March 15:597–600.

63. Bosch JP, Saccaggi A, Lauer A, Ronco C, Belledonne M, Glabman S. Renal functional reserve in humans: effect of protein intake on glomerular filtration rate. *Am J Med* 1983;75:943–50.

64. Jones MG, Lee K, Swaminathan R. The effect of dietary protein on glomerular filtration rate in normal subjects. *Clin Nephrology* 1987;27:71–75.

65. Tanner JM. Trend towards earlier menarche in London, Oslo, Copenhagen, the Netherlands, and Hungary. *Nature* 1973;243:75–6.

66. Lester Cox, personal communication, 1992.

67. Brundtland GH, Liestol K, Walloe L. Height, weight and menarcheal age of Oslo schoolchildren during the last 60 years. *Ann Hum Biol* 1980;7:307–22.

68. Rose DP, Boyar AP, Cohen C, Strong LE. Effect of a low-fat diet on hormone levels in women with cystic breast disease. 1. Serum steroids and gonadotropins. *J Natl Cancer Inst* 1987;78(4)623–26.

69. Ingram DM, Bennett FC, Willcox D, de Klerk N. Effect of low-fat diet on female sex hormone levels. *J Natl Cancer Inst* 1987;79(6):1225–29.

70. Goldin BR, Adlercreutz H, Gorbach SL, et al. Estrogen excretion patterns and plasma levels in vegetarian and omnivorous women. *N Engl J Med* 1982;307:1542–47.

71. Armstrong BK, Brown JB, Clarke HT, et al. Diet and reproductive hormones: a study of vegetarian and nonvegetarian postmenopausal women. *J Natl Cancer Inst* 1981;67:761–67.

72. Kagawa Y. Impact of Westernization on the nutrition of Japanese: changes in physique, cancer, longevity and centenarians. *Prev Med* 1978;7:205–17.

73. Burkitt D, personal communication.

74. de Ridder CM, Thijssen JHH, Van't Veer P, et al. Dietary habits, sexual maturation, and plasma hormones in pubertal girls: a longitudinal study. *Am J Clin Nutr* 1991;54:805–13.

75. Kohn RR. Cause of death in very old people. *JAMA* 1982;247:2793–97.

Chapter 2

1. Lipid Research Clinics Program, The Lipid Research Clinics Coronary Primary Prevention Trial Results, II. *JAMA* 1984;251(3):365–74.

2. Castelli WP. Epidemiology of coronary heart disease. *Am J Medicine* 1984;76(2A): 4–12.

3. Trout DL. Vitamin C and cardiovascular risk factors. *Am J Clin Nutr* 1991;53:322S–5S.

4. Melish J, Le NA, Ginsberg H, Steinberg D, Brown WV. Dissociation of apoprotein B and triglyceride production in very-low-density lipoproteins. *Am J Physiol* 1980;239: E354–62.

5. Pennington JAT. Bowes and Church's food values of portions commonly used. New York, Harper and Row, 1989.

6. Endres S, Ghorbani R, Kelley VE, et al. The effect of dietary supplementation with n-3 polyunsaturated fatty acids on the synthesis of interleukin-1 and tumor necrosis factor by mononuclear cells. *N Engl J Med* 1989;320:265–71.

7. von Schacky C, Fischer S, Weber PC. Long-term effect of dietary marine omega-3 fatty acids upon plasma and cellular lipids, platelet function, and eicosanoid formation in humans. *J Clin Invest* 1985;76:1626–31.

8. Glavind J, Hartmann S, Clemmesen J, Jessen KE, Dam H. Studies on the role of lipoperoxides in human pathology. *Acta Pathol Microbiol Scand* 1952;30:1–6.

9. Frei B. Ascorbic acid protects lipids in human plasma and low-density lipoprotein against oxidative damage. *Am J Clin Nutr* 1991;54:1113S–18S.

10. Niki E. Action of ascorbic acid as a scavenger of active and stable oxygen radicals. *Am J Clin Nutr* 1991;54:1119S–24S.

11. Esterbauer H, Dieber-Rotheneder M, Striegl G, Waeg G. Role of vitamin E in preventing the oxidation of low-density lipoprotein. *Am J Clin Nutr* 1991;53:314S–21S.

12. Hennekins C. Presentation to the American Heart Association, Nov. 1990.

13. Hunter JE. n-3 Fatty acids from vegetable oils. *Am J Clin Nutr* 1990;51:809–14.

14. Renaud S, Godsey F, Dumont E, Thevenon C, Ortchanian E, Martin JL. Influence of long-term diet modification on platelet function and composition in Moselle farmers. *Am J Clin Nutr* 1986;43:136–50.

15. Emken EA, Adlof RO, Rakoff H, Rohwedder WK. Metabolism of deuterium-labeled linolenic, linoleic, oleic, stearic and palmitic acid in human subjects. In Baillie TA, Jones JR, eds. Synthesis and applications of isotopically labelled compounds 1988. Amsterdam, Elsevier Science Publishers BV, 1989;713–16.

16. Salonen JT, Salonen R, Nyyssonen K, Korpela H. Iron sufficiency is associated with hypertension and excess risk of myocardial infarction: the Kuopio Ischaemic Heart Disease Risk Factor Study (KIHD). *Circulation* 1992;85:864.

17. Van Horn LV, Liu K, Parker D, et al. Serum lipid response to oat product intake with a fat-modified diet. *J Am Dietetic Asso* 1986;86:759–64.

18. Anderson JW, Gilinsky NH, Deakins DA, Smith SF, O'Neal DS, Dillon DW, Oeltgen PR. Lipid responses of hypercholesterolemic men to oat-bran and wheat-bran intake. *Am J Clin Nutr* 1991;54:678–83.

19. Kesaniemi YA, Tarpila S, Miettinen RA. Low vs high dietary fiber and serum, biliary, and fecal lipids in middle-aged men. *Am J Clin Nutr* 1990;51:1007–12.

20. Anderson JW. Dietary fiber, lipids, and atherosclerosis. *Am J Cardiol* 1987;60:17G–22G.

21. Anderson JW, Gustafson NJ, Spencer DB, Tietyen J, Bryant CA. Serum lipid response of hypercholesterolemic men to single and divided doses of canned beans. *Am J Clin Nutr* 1990;51:1013–19.

22. Life Sciences Research Office. Physiological effects and health consequences of dietary fiber. Washington, D.C., Federation of American Societies for Experimental Biology, 1987.

23. American Heart Association. Dietary guidelines for healthy Americans: a statement for physicians and health professionals by the Nutrition Committee. *Arteriosclerosis* 1988;8:218A–221A.

24. Mathur KS, Khan MA, Sharma RD. Hypocholesterolemic effect of Bengal gram: a long-term study in man. *Br Med J* 1968;1:30–31.

25. Grande F, Anderson JT, Keys A. Effect of carbohydrates of leguminous seeds, wheat and potatoes on serum cholesterol concentration in man. *J Nutr* 1965;86:313–17.

26. Bingwen L, Zhaofeny W, Wahshen L, Rongjue Z. Effects of bean meal on serum cholesterol and triglycerides. *Chin Med J* 1981;94:455–58.

27. Hellendoorn EW. Beneficial physiologic action of beans. *J Am Dietetic Asso* 1976;69:248–53.

28. Jenkins DJA, Wolever TMS, Kalmusky J, et al. Low-glycemic index diet in hyperlipidemia: use of traditional starchy foods. *Am J Clin Nutr* 1987;46:66–71.

29. Jenkins DJA, Wong GS, Patten R, et al. Leguminous seeds in the dietary management of hyperlipidemia. *Am J Clin Nutr* 1983;38:567–73.

30. Leon AS, Connett J, Jacobs DR, et al. Leisure-time physical activity levels and risk of coronary heart disease and death. The multiple risk factor intervention trial. *JAMA* 1987; 258:2388–95.

31. Blair SN, Kohl HW, Paffenbarger RS, et al. Physical fitness and all-cause mortality. *JAMA* 1989;262:2395–2401.

32. Enos WF, Holmes RH, Beyer J. Coronary disease among United States soldiers killed in action in Korea. *JAMA* 1953;152:1090–93.

33. Enos WF, Beyer J, Holmes RH. Pathogenesis of coronary disease in American soldiers killed in Korea. *JAMA* 1955;158:912–14.

34. Sibai AM, Armenian HK, Alam S. Wartime determinants of arteriographically confirmed coronary artery disease in Beirut. *Am J Epidemiology* 1989;130:623–31.

35. Rozanski A, Bairey CN, Krantz DS, et al. Mental stress and the induction of silent myocardial ischemia in patients with coronary artery disease. *N Engl J Med* 1988;318: 1005–12.

36. Schnall PL, Pieper C, Schwartz JE, et al. The relationship between 'job strain,' workplace diastolic blood pressure, and left ventricular mass index. *JAMA* 1990;263:1929–35.

37. Rouse IL, Armstrong BK, Beilin LJ. Vegetarian diet, lifestyle and blood pressure in two religious populations. *Clin Exp Pharmacol and Physiol* 1982;9:327–30.

38. Rouse IL, Beilin LJ. Editorial review: vegetarian diet and blood pressure. *J Hypertension* 1984;2:231–40.

39. Anderson JW. Plant fiber and blood pressure. *Ann Intern Med* 1983;98 (Part 2):842.

40. Ernst E, Pietsch L, Matrai A, Eisenberg J. Blood rheology in vegetarians. *Br J Nutr* 1986;56:555–60.

41. Ernst E, Matrai A, Pietsch L. Vegetarian diet in mild hypertension. *Br Med J* 1987; 294:180.

42. Berry EM, Hirsch J. Does dietary linolenic acid influence blood pressure? *Am J Clin Nutr* 1986;44:336–40.

43. Colditz GA, Bonita R, Stampfer MJ, et al. Cigarette smoking and risk of stroke in middle-aged women. *N Engl J Med* 1988;318:937–41.

44. Virag R, Bouilly P, Frydman D. Is impotence an arterial disorder? A study of arterial risk factors in 440 impotent men. *Lancet* 1985;1:181–84.

45. Ornish D, Brown SE, Scherwitz LW, et al. Can lifestyle changes reverse coronary heart disease? *Lancet* 1990;336:129–33.

46. Ornish D. Dr. Dean Ornish's program for reversing heart disease. New York, Random House, 1990.

47. Blankenhorn DH, Nessim SA, Johnson RL, Sanmarco ME, Azen SP, Cashin-Hemphill L. Beneficial effects of combined colestipol-niacin therapy on coronary atherosclerosis and coronary venous bypass grafts. *JAMA* 1987;257:3233–40.

48. Brown GB, Albers JJ, Fisher LD, et al. Niacin or lovastatin combined with colestipol regresses coronary atherosclerosis and prevents clinical events in men with elevated apolipoprotein B. *N Engl J Med* 1990;323:1289–98.

49. Kestin M, Rouse IL, Correll RA, Nestel PJ. Cardiovascular disease risk factors in free-living men: comparison of two prudent diets, one based on lactoovovegetarianism and the other allowing lean meat. *Am J Clin Nutr* 1989;50:280–87.

50. Fisher M, Levine PH, Weiner B, et al. The effect of vegetarian diets on plasma lipid and platelet levels. *Arch Intern Med* 1986;146:1193–97.

51. Sacks FM, Ornish D, Rosner B, McLanahan S, Castelli WP, Kass EH. Plasma lipoprotein levels in vegetarians: the effect of ingestion of fats from dairy products. *JAMA* 1985;254(10):1337–41.

Chapter 3

1. U.S. General Accounting Office. Breast Cancer, 1971–91: Prevention, treatment and research. GAO/PEMD-92-12, December 1991.

2. National Research Council. Diet, nutrition, and cancer. Washington, D.C., National Academy Press, 1982.

3. Armstrong B, Doll R. Environmental factors and cancer incidence and mortality in different countries, with special reference to dietary practices. *Int J Cancer* 1975;15:617–31.

4. Hirayama T. Epidemiology of breast cancer with special reference to the role of diet. *Prev Med* 1978;7:173–95.

5. Lands WEM, Hamazaki T, Yamazaki K, Okuyama H, Sakai K, Goto Y, Hubbard VS. Changing dietary patterns. *Am J Clin Nutr* 1990;51:991–93.

6. Carroll KK, Braden LM. Dietary fat and mammary carcinogenesis. *Nutrition and Cancer* 1985;6:254–59.

7. Rose DP, Boyar AP, Wynder EL. International comparisons of mortality rates for cancer of the breast, ovary, prostate, and colon, and per capita food consumption. *Cancer* 1986;58:2363–71.

8. U.S. Department of Health and Human Services. Surgeon general's report on nutrition and health. DHHS Publ No. 88-50210, 1988.

9. Rose DP, Boyar AP, Cohen C, Strong LE. Effect of a low-fat diet on hormone levels in women with cystic breast disease. 1. Serum steroids and gonadotropins. *J Natl Cancer Inst* 1987;78(4)623–26.

10. Ingram DM, Bennett FC, Willcox D, de Klerk N. Effect of low-fat diet on female sex hormone levels. *J Natl Cancer Inst* 1987;79(6):1225–29.

11. Goldin BR, Gorbach SL. Effect of diet on the plasma levels, metabolism and excretion of estrogens. *Am J Clin Nutr* 1988;48:787–90.

12. Toniolo P, Riboli E, Protta F, Charrel M, Cappa AP. Calorie-providing nutrients and risk of breast cancer. *J Natl Cancer Inst* 1989;81:278.

13. Phillips RL, Garfinkel L, Kuzma JW, et al. Mortality among California Seventh-Day Adventists for selected cancer sites. *J Natl Cancer Inst* 1980;65:1097–1107.

14. Kinlen LJ. Meat and fat consumption and cancer mortality: a study of religious orders in Britain. *Lancet* 1982:946–49.

15. Messina MJ, Barnes S. The role of soy products in reducing risk of cancer. *J Natl Cancer Inst* 1991;83:541–46.

16. Willet WC, Hunter DJ, Stampfer MJ, et al. Dietary fat and fiber in relation to risk of breast cancer: an 8-year follow-up. JAMA 1992;268:2037–44.

17. Howe GR, Hirohata T, Hislop T, et al. Dietary factors and risk of breast cancer: combined analysis of 12 case-control studies. *J Natl Cancer Inst* 1990;82:561–69.

18. Willett WC, Polk BF, Morris MJ, et al. Prediagnostic serum selenium levels and risk of cancer. *Lancet* 1983;2:130–34.

19. Willett WC, Stampfer MJ, Colditz FA, et al. Moderate alcohol consumption and the risk of breast cancer. *N Engl J Med* 1987;316:1174–80.

20. Miller DR, Rosenberg L, Kaufman DW, et al. Breast cancer before age 45 and oral contraceptive use: new findings. *Am J Epidemiol* 1989;129:269.

21. Bergkvist L, Adami AO, Persson I, et al. The risk of breast cancer after estrogen and estrogen-progestin replacement. *N Engl J Med* 1989;321:293.

22. Lubin F, Ruder AM, Wax Y, Modan B. Overweight and changes in weight throughout adult life in breast cancer etiology. *Am J Epidemiol* 1985;122:579–88.

23. Miller FA, Hempelmann LH, Dutton AM, Pifer JW, Toyooka ET, Ames WR. Breast neoplasms in women treated with X-rays for acute postpartum mastitis. A pilot study. *J Natl Cancer Inst* 1969;43:803–11.

24. Lynch HT, Albano WA, Heieck JJ, et al. Genetics, biomarkers, and control of breast cancer: a review. *Cancer, Genetics, and Cytogenetics* 1984;13:43–92.

25. Goldman BA. The truth about where you live. New York, Random House, 1991.

26. Benditt EP. The origin of atherosclerosis. *Scientific American* 1977;236:74–85.

27. Hergenrather J, Hlady G, Wallace B, Savage E. Pollutants in breast milk of vegetarians. *Lancet* 1981;304:792.

28. Wynder EL, Fujita Y, Harris RE, Hirayama T, Hiyama T. Comparative epidemiology of cancer between the United States and Japan. *Cancer* 1991;67:746–63.

29. Kagawa Y. Impact of Westernization on the nutrition of Japanese: changes in physique, cancer, longevity and centenarians. *Prev Med* 1978;7:205–17.

30. Wynder EL, Escher GC, Mantel N. An epidemiological investigation of cancer of the endometrium. *Cancer* 1966;19:489–520.

31. Elwood JM, Cole P, Rothman KJ, Kaplan SD. Epidemiology of endometrial cancer. *J Natl Cancer Inst* 1977;59:1055–60.

32. Lingeman CH. Etiology of cancer of the human ovary: A review. *J Natl Cancer Inst* 1974;53:1603–18.

33. Cramer DW, Willett WC, Bell DA, et al. Galactose consumption and metabolism in relation to the risk of ovarian cancer. *Lancet* 1989;2:66–71.

34. Carter BS, Carter HB, Isaacs JT. Epidemiologic evidence regarding predisposing factors to prostate cancer. *Prostate* 1990;16:187–97.

35. Breslow N, Chan CW, Dhom G, et al. Latent carcinoma of prostate at autopsy in seven areas. *Int J Cancer* 1977;20:680–88.

36. Howell MA. Factor analysis of international cancer mortality data and per capita food consumption. *Br J Cancer* 1974;29:328–36.

37. Blair A, Fraumeni JF, Jr. Geographic patterns of prostate cancer in the United States. *J Natl Cancer Inst* 1978;61:1379–84.

38. Kolonel LN, Hankin JH, Lee J, Chu SY, Nomura AMY, Hinds MW. Nutrient intakes in relation to cancer incidence in Hawaii. *Br J Cancer* 1981;44:332–39.

39. Rotkin ID. Studies in the epidemiology of prostatic cancer: expanded sampling. *Cancer Treat Rep* 1977;61:173–80.

40. Schuman LM, Mandel JS, Radke A, Seal U, Halberg F. Some selected features of the epidemiology of prostatic cancer: Minneapolis-St. Paul, Minnesota case control study, 1976–1979. In K. Magnus, ed. Trends in cancer incidence: causes and practical implications. New York, Hemisphere Publishing Corp., 1982:345–54.

41. Graham S, et al. Diet in the epidemiology of carcinoma of the prostate gland. *J Natl Cancer Inst* 1983;70:687–92.

42. Ross RK, Shimizu H, Pagamini-Hill A, Honda G, Henderson BE. Case-control studies of prostate cancer in blacks and whites in Southern California. *J Natl Cancer Inst* 1987;78:869–74.

43. Severson RK, Nomura AM, Grove JS, Stemmermann GN. A prospective study of demographics, diet, and prostate cancer among men of Japanese ancestry in Hawaii. *Cancer Research* 1989;49:1857–60.

44. Oishi K, Okada K, Yoshida O, et al. A case-control study of prostatic cancer with reference to dietary habits. *Prostate* 1988;12:179–90.

45. Mettlin C, Selenskas S, Natarajan N, Huben R. Beta-carotene and animal fats and their relationship to prostate cancer risk: A case-control study. *Cancer* 1989;64:605–12.

46. Hirayama T. Changing patterns of cancer in Japan with special reference to the decrease in stomach cancer mortality. Pp. 55–75 in Hiatt HH, Watson JD, Winsten JA, eds. Origins of human cancer. Book A, Incidence of cancer in humans. Cold Spring Harbor, N.Y., Cold Spring Harbor Laboratory, 1977.

47. Hirayama T. Epidemiology of prostate cancer with special reference to the role of diet. *Natl Cancer Inst Monogr* 1979;53:149–54.

48. Phillips RL. Role of life-style and dietary habits in risk of cancer among Seventh-Day Adventists. *Cancer Research* 1975;35:3513–22.

49. Mills P, Beeson WL, Phillips RL, Fraser GE. Cohort study of diet, lifestyle, and prostate cancer in Adventist men. *Cancer* 1989;64:598–604.

50. Willett WC, Stampfer MJ, Colditz GA, Rosner BA, Speizer FE. Relation of meat, fat, and fiber intake to the risk of colon cancer in a prospective study among women. *N Engl J Med* 1990;323:1664–72.

51. Gerhardsson de Verdier M, Hagman U, Peters RK, Steineck G, Overvik E. Meat, cooking methods and colorectal cancer: a case-referrent study in Stockholm. *Int J Cancer* 1991;49:520–25.

52. DeCosse JJ, Miller HH, Lesser ML. Effect of wheat fiber and vitamins C and E on rectal polyps in patients with familial adenomatous polyposis. *J Natl Cancer Inst* 1989;81:1290–97.

53. Block F. Epidemiologic evidence regarding vitamin C and cancer. *Am J Clin Nutr* 1991;54:1310S–14S.

54. Kromhout D. Essential micronutrients in relation to carcinogenesis. *Am J Clin Nutr* 1987;45:1361–67.

55. Mackerras D, Buffler PA, Randall DE, Nichaman MZ, Pickle LW, Mason TJ. Carotene intake and the risk of laryngeal cancer in coastal Texas. *Am J Epidemiol* 1988;128:980–8.

56. Watson RR, Prabhala RH, Plezia PM, Alberts DS. Effect of beta-carotene on lymphocyte subpopulations in elderly humans: evidence for a dose-response relationship. *Am J Clin Nutr* 1991;53:90–94.

57. Makinodan T, Lubinski J, Fong TC. Cellular, biochemical, and molecular basis of T-cell senescence. *Arch Pathol Lab Med* 1987;111:910–14.

58. Beisel WR. Single nutrients and immunity. *Am J Clin Nutr* 1982;35;Feb. Suppl:417–68.

59. Watson RR. Immunological enhancement by fat-soluble vitamins, minerals, and trace metals: a factor in cancer prevention. *Cancer Detection and Prevention* 1986;9: 67–77.

60. Chandra S, Chandra RK. Nutrition, immune response, and outcome. *Progress in Food and Nutrition Science* 1986;10:1–65.

61. Barone J, Hebert JR, Reddy MM. Dietary fat and natural-killer-cell activity. *Am J Clin Nutr* 1989;50:861–67.

62. Nordenstrom J, Jarstrand C, Wiernik A. Decreased chemotactic and random migration of leukocytes during Intralipid infusion. *Am J Clin Nutr* 1979;32:2416–22.

63. Hawley HP, Gordon GB. The effects of long chain free fatty acids on human neutrophil function and structure. *Lab Invest* 1976;34:216–22.

64. Endres S, Ghorbani R, Kelley VE, et al. The effect of dietary supplementation with n-3 polyunsaturated fatty acids on the synthesis of interleukin-1 and tumor necrosis factor by mononuclear cells. *N Engl J Med* 1989;320:265–71.

65. Kelley DS, Branch LB, Love JE, Taylor PC, Rivera YM, Iacono JM. Dietary alpha-linoleic acid and immunocompetence in humans. *Am J Clin Nutr* 1991;53:40–46.

66. von Schacky C, Fischer S, Weber PC. Long-term effect of dietary marine omega-3 fatty acids upon plasma and cellular lipids, platelet function, and eicosanoid formation in humans. *J Clin Invest* 1985;76:1626–31.

67. Malter M, Schriever G, Eilber U. Natural killer cells, vitamins, and other blood components of vegetarian and omnivorous men. *Nutr Cancer* 1989;12:271–78.

68. Wynder EL, Kajitani T, Kuno J, Lucas JC Jr, DePalo A, Farrow J. A comparison of survival rates between American and Japanese patients with breast cancer. *Surg Gynec Obstet* 1963;117:196–200.

69. Gregorio DI, Emrich LJ, Graham S, Marshall JR, Nemoto T. Dietary fat consumption and survival among women with breast cancer. *JNCI* 1985;75:37–41.

70. LeMarchand L, Kolonel LN, Nomura AMY. Ethnic differences in survival after diagnosis of breast cancer—Hawaii. *JAMA* 1985;254:2728.

71. Linden G. Letter to the editor. In *J Cancer* 1973;12:543.

72. Verreault R, Brisson J, Deschenes L, Naud F, Meyer F, Belanger L. Dietary fat in relation to prognostic indicators in breast cancer. *J Natl Cancer Inst* 1988;80:819–25.

73. Newman SC, Miller AB, Howe GR. A study of the effect of weight and dietary fat on breast cancer survival time. *Am J Epidemiol* 1986;123:767–74.

74. Holm LE, Callmer E, Hjalmar ML, Lidbrink E, Nilsson B, Skoog L. Dietary habits and prognostic factors in breast cancer. *J Natl Cancer Inst* 1989;81:1218–23.

75. Donegan WL, Hartz AJ, Rimm AA. The association of body weight with recurrent cancer of the breast. *Cancer* 1978;41:1590–94.

76. Schapira DV, Kumar NB, Lyman GH, Cox CE. Obesity and body fat distribution and breast cancer prognosis. *Cancer* 1991;67:523–28.

77. Sattilaro AJ, Monte T. Recalled by life. Boston, Houghton Mifflin, 1982.

78. Levy EM, Beldekas JC, Black PH, Cottrell MC, Kushi LH. Patients with Kaposi sarcoma who opt for no treatment. *Lancet* 1985;2(8448):223.

79. Wheat bran diet protects against recurrence of colorectal cancer. *Oncology* 1990;4: 139.

Chapter 4

1. Ellis FR, Montegriffo VME. Veganism, clinical findings and investigations. *Am J Clin Nutr* 1970;23:249–55.

2. Melby CL, Hyner GC, Zoog B. Blood pressure in vegetarians and nonvegetarians. *Nutr Res* 1985;5:1077–82.

3. Hardinge MG, Stare FJ. Nutritional studies of vegetarians. *Am J Clin Nutr* 1954;2:73–82.

4. Wadden TA, Foster GD, Letizia KA, Mullen JL. Long-term effects of dieting on resting metabolic rate in obese outpatients. *JAMA* 190;264:707–11.

5. Foster GD, Wadden TA, Feurer ID, et al. Controlled trial of the metabolic effects of a very-low-calorie diet: short- and long-term effects. *Am J Clin Nutr* 1990;51:167–72.

6. Dreon DM, Frey-Hewitt B, Ellsworth N, Williams PT, Terry RB, Wood PD. Dietary fat: carbohydrate ratio and obesity in middle-aged men. *Am J Clin Nutr* 1988;47:995–1000.

7. Danforth E, Jr., Sims EAH, Horton ES, Goldman RF. Correlation of serum triiodo-thyronine concentrations (T3) with dietary composition, gain in weight and thermogenesis in man. *Diabetes* 1975;24:406.

8. Spaulding SW, Chopra IJ, Sherwin RS, Lyall SS. Effect of caloric restriction and dietary composition on serum T3 and reverse T3 in man. *J Clin Endocrinol Metab* 1976;42:197–200.

9. Mathieson RA, Walberg JL, Gwazdauskas FC, Hinkle DE, Gregg JM. The effect of varying carbohydrate content of a very-low-caloric diet on resting metabolic rate and thyroid hormones. *Metabolism* 1986;35:394–98.

10. Welle S, Lilavivathana U, Campbell RG. Increased plasma norepinephrine concentrations and metabolic rates following glucose ingestion in man. *Metabolism* 1980;29: 806–9.

11. Deriaz O, Theriault G, Lavallee N, Fournier G, Nadeau A, Bouchard C. Human resting energy expenditure in relation to dietary potassium. *Am J Clin Nutr* 1991;54:628–34.

12. Lissner L, Levitsky DA, Strupp BJ, Kalkwarf HJ, Roe DA. Dietary fat and the regulation of energy intake in human subjects. *Am J Clin Nutr* 1987;46:886–92.

13. Rodin J. Comparative effects of fructose, aspartame, glucose, and water preloads on calorie and macronutrient intake. *Am J Clin Nutr* 1990;51:428–35.

14. Schutz Y, Flatt JP, Jequier E. Failure of dietary fat intake to promote fat oxidation: a factor favoring the development of obesity. *Am J Clin Nutr* 1989;50:307–14.

15. Suter PM, Schutz Y, Jequier E. The effect of ethanol on fat storage in healthy subjects. *New Engl J Med* 1992;326:983–87.

16. de Castro JM, Orozco S. Moderate alcohol intake and spontaneous eating patterns of humans: evidence of unregulated supplementation. *Am J Clin Nutr* 1990;52:246–53.

17. Blundell JE, Hill AJ. Paradoxical effects of an intense sweetener (aspartame) on appetite. *Lancet* 1986;1:1092–93.

18. Blundell JE, Hill AJ. Artificial sweeteners and the control of appetite: implications for the eating disorders. In Worden D, Parke D, Marks J, eds. The future of predictive safety evaluation. Vol. 2, Lancaster: MTP Press, 1987:263–82.

19. Brala PM, Hagen RL. Effects of sweetness perception and caloric value of a preload on short-term satiety. *Physiol Behav* 1983;30:1–9.

20. Rolls BJ, Hetherington M, Laster LJ. Comparison of the effects of aspartame and sucrose on appetite and food intake. *Appetite* 1988;11:62–67.

21. Porikos KP, Booth G, VanItallie TB. Effect of covert nutritive dilution on the spontaneous food intake of obese individuals: a pilot study. *Am J Clin Nutr* 1977;30:1638–44.

22. Van Itallie TB, Yang MU, Porikos KP. Use of aspartame to test the "body weight set point" hypothesis. *Appetite* 1988;11:68–72.

23. Moran V. The love-powered diet. San Raphael, Calif., New World Library, 1992.

24. Kissileff HR, Pi-Sunyer FX, Segal K, Meltzer S, Foelsch PA. Acute effects of exercise on food intake in obese and nonobese women. *Am J Clin Nutr* 1990;52:240–45.

25. Stunkard AJ, Harris JR, Pedersen NL, McClearn GE. The body-mass index of twins who have been reared apart. *N Engl J Med* 1990;322:1483–87.

Chapter 5

1. Sobel D. Arthritis: What works. New York, St Martin's Press, 1989.

2. Skoldstam L. Fasting and vegan diet in rheumatoid arthritis. *Scand J Rheumatol* 1986;15:219–23.

3. Skoldstam L, Larsson L, Lindstrom FD. Effects of fasting and lactovegetarian diet on rheumatoid arthritis. *Scand J Rheumatol* 1979;8:249–55.

4. Kremer JM, Bigauoette J, Michalek AV, et al. Effects of manipulation of dietary fatty acids on clinical manifestations of rheumatoid arthritis. *Lancet* 1985;1:184–87.

5. Kjeldsen-Kragh J, Haugen M, Borchgrevink CF, et al. Controlled trial of fasting and one-year vegetarian diet in rheumatoid arthritis. *Lancet* 1991;338:899–902.

6. Merry P, Grootveld M, Lunec J, Blake DR. Oxidative damage to lipids within the inflamed human joint provides evidence of radical-mediated hypoxic-reperfusion injury. *Am J Clin Nutr* 1991;53:362S–9S.

7. Panush RS, Carter RL, Katz P, Kowsari B, Longley S, Finnie S. Diet therapy for rheumatoid arthritis. *Arthritis and Rheumatism* 1983;26:462–71.

8. Lithell H, Bruce A, Gustafsson IB, et al. A fasting and vegetarian diet treatment trial on chronic inflammatory disorders. *Acta Derm Venereol* 1983;63:397–403.

9. Swank RL, Dugan BB. The multiple sclerosis diet book. New York, Doubleday, 1987.

10. Swank RL. Multiple sclerosis: twenty years on a low-fat diet. *Arch Neurol* 1970;23:460–74.

11. Center for Economic Studies in Medicine. Direct and indirect costs of diabetes in the United States in 1987. Alexandria, Va., American Diabetes Association, 1988.

12. Barnard RJ, Lattimore L, Holly RA, Cherny S, Pritikin N. Response of non-insulin-dependent diabetic patients to an intensive program of diet and exercise. *Diabetes Care* 1982;5:370–74.

13. Barnard RJ, Massey MR, Cherny ·S, O'Brien LT, Pritikin N. Long-term use of a high-complex-carbohydrate, high-fiber, low-fat diet and exercise in the treatment of NIDDM patients. *Diabetes Care* 1983;6:268–73.

14. Hjollund E, Pederson O, Richelsen B, Beck-Nielsen H, Sorensen NS. Increased insulin binding to adipocytes and monocytes and increased insulin sensitivity of glucose transport and metabolism in adipocytes from non-insulin-dependent diabetics after a low-fat/high-starch/high-fiber diet. *Metabolism* 1983;32:1067.

15. Ward GM, Simpson RW, Simpson HCR, Naylor BA, Mann JI, Turner RC. Insulin receptor binding increased by high carbohydrate, low fat diet in non-insulin-dependent diabetics. *European J Clin Invest* 1982;12:93:

16. Anderson JW. Plant fiber and blood pressure. *Ann Intern Med* 1983;98(Part 2):842.

17. Dodson PM, Pacey PJ, Bal P, Kubicki AJ, Fletcher RF, Taylor KG. A controlled trial of a high-fiber, low fat, and low sodium diet for mild hypertension in type 2 (non-insulin-dependent) diabetic patients. *Diabetologia* 1984;27:522.

18. Florholmen J, Arvidsson-Lenner R, Jorde R, Burhol PG. The effect of Metamucil on postprandial blood glucose and plasma gastric inhibitory peptide in insulin-dependent diabetics. *Acta Med Scand* 1982;212:237.

19. Frati-Munari AC, Fernandez-Harp JA, Becerril M, Chavez-Negrete A, Banales-Ham M. Decrease in serum lipids, glycemia, and body weight by plantago psyllium in obese and diabetic patients. *Arch Invest Med* 1983;14:259.

20. Nygren C, Hallmans G, Lithner F. Effects of high-bran bread on blood glucose control in insulin-dependent diabetic patients. *Diab Metab* 1984;10:39.

21. AMA Council on Scientific Affairs. Dietary Fiber and Health. *JAMA* 1989;262:542–46.

22. Jenkins DJA, Wolever TMS, Taylor RH, Barker H, Fielden H. Exceptionally low blood glucose response to dried beans: comparison with other carbohydrate foods. *Br Med J* 1980;2:578–80.

23. Jenkins DJA, Wolever TMS, Taylor RH, et al. Slow release carbohydrate improves second meal tolerance. *Am J Clin Nutr* 1982;35:1339–46.

24. Roy MS, Stables G, Collier B, Roy A, Bou E. Nutritional factors in diabetics with and without retinopathy. *Am J Clin Nutr* 1989;50:728–30.

25. American Diabetes Association. Nutritional recommendations and principles for individuals with diabetes mellitus. *Diabetes Care* 1991;14:20–27.

26. Scott FW. Cow milk and insulin-dependent diabetes mellitus: is there a relationship? *Am J Clin Nutr* 1990;51:489–91.

27. Roberton DM, Paganelli R, Dinwiddie R, Levinsky RJ. Milk antigen absorption in the preterm and term neonate. *Arch Dis Child* 1982;57:369–72.

28. Bruining GJ, Molenaar J, Tuk CW, Lindeman J, Bruining HA, Marner B. Clinical time-course and characteristics of islet cell cytoplasmatic antibodies in childhood diabetes. *Diabetologia* 1984;26:24–29.

29. Karjalainen J, Martin JM, Knip M, et al. A bovine albumin peptide as a possible trigger of insulin-dependent diabetes mellitus. *N Engl J Med* 1992;327:302–7.

30. Burkitt DP. Relationships between diseases and their etiological significance. *Am J Clin Nutr* 1977;30:262–67.

31. Burkitt DP. Don't forget fiber in your diet. New York, Arco, 1984.

32. Burkitt DP, Latto C, Janvrin SB, Mayou B. Pelvic phleboliths: epidemiology and postulated etiology. *N Engl J Med* 1977;296:1387–90.

33. American Medical Association Council on Scientific Affairs. Dietary fiber and health. *JAMA* 1989;262:542–46.

34. Pixley F, Wilson D, McPherson K, Mann J. Effect of vegetarianism on development of gall stones in women. *Br Med J* 1985;291:11–12.

35. France GL, Marmer DJ, Steele RW. Breast-feeding and Salmonella infection. *Am J Dis Child* 1980;134:147–52.

36. St. Louis ME, Morse DL, Potter ME, et al. The emergence of grade A eggs as a major source of Salmonella enteritidis infections. *JAMA* 1988;259:2103–7.

37. Telzak EE, Budnick LD, Greenberg MSZ, et al. A nosocomial outbreak of Salmonella enteritidis infection due to the consumption of raw eggs. *N Engl J Med* 1990;323:394–97.

38. Baker RC, Hogarty S, Poon W, et al. Survival of Salmonella typhimurium and Staphylococcus aureus in eggs cooked by different methods. *Poultry Sci* 1983;62:1211–16.

39. Wempe JM, Genigeorgis CA, Farver TB, Yusufu HI. Prevalence of Campylobacter jejuni in two California chicken processing plants. *Appl Environ Microbiol* 1983;45:355–59.

40. Kinde H, Genigeorgis CA, Pappaioanou M. Prevalence of Campylobacter jejuni in chicken wings. *Appli Environ Microbiol* 1983;45:1116–18.

41. National Research Council. Poultry inspection: the basis for a risk-assessment approach. Washington, D.C., National Academy Press, 1987.

42. McLeod R, Remington JS. Toxoplasmosis. In Petersdorf RG, Adams RD, Braunwald E, Isselbacher KJ, Martin JB, Wilson JD, eds. Harrison's principles of internal medicine. New York, McGraw-Hill, 1983.

43. U.S. Department of Health and Human Services. Concern continues about Vibrio vulnificus, FDA Drug Bulletin 18(1):3, April 1988.

44. Consumer Reports. Is our fish fit to eat? February 1992.

45. Graham DY, Smith JL, Opekun AR. Spicy food and the stomach. *JAMA* 1988; 260:3473–75.

Chapter 6

1. Zemel MB, Calcium utilization: effect of varying level and source of dietary protein. *Am J Clin Nutr* 1988;48:880–83.

2. Graham S, Marshall J, Haughey B, et al. Nutritional epidemiology of cancer of the esophagus. *Am J Epidemiol* 1990;131:454–67.

3. Consumer Reports, Is our fish fit to eat? February 1992:103–14.

4. Odeleye OE, Watson RR. Health implications of the n-3 fatty acids. *Am J Clin Nutr* 1991;53:177–78.

5. Kinsella JE. Reply to O Odeleye and R Watson. *Am J Clin Nutr* 1991;53:178.

6. U.S. General Accounting Office. Food Safety and Quality. FDA surveys not adequate to demonstrate safety of milk supply. November 1990.

7. Jacobus CH, Holick MF, Shao Q, et al. Hypervitaminosis D associated with drinking milk. *N Engl J Med* 1992;326:1173–77.

8. Holick MF, Shao Q, Liu WW, Chen TC. The vitamin D content of fortified milk and infant formula. *N Engl J Med* 1992;326:1178–81.

9. Clyne PS, Kulczycki A. Human breast milk contains bovine IgG. Relationship to infant colic? *Pediatrics* 1991;87:439–44.

10. Pennington JAT. Bowes and Church's food values of portions commonly used. New York, Harper and Row, 1989.

11. Ziegler EE, Fomon SJ, Nelson SE, et al. Cow milk feeding in infancy: further observations on blood loss from the gastrointestinal tract. *J Pediatr* 1990;116:11–18.

12. American Academy of Pediatrics, Committee on Nutrition. The use of whole cow's milk in infancy. *Pediatrics* 1992;89:1105–9.

13. Hallberg L, Brune M, Erlandsson M, Sandberg AS, Rossander-Hulten L. Calcium: effect of different amounts on nonheme- and heme-iron absorption in humans. *Am J Clin Nutr* 1991;53:112–19.

14. Cook JD, Dassenko SA, Whittaker P. Calcium supplementation: effect on iron absorption. *Am J Clin Nutr* 1991;53:106–11.

15. American Dietetic Association. Position of the American Dietetic Association: vegetarian diets. *J Am Diet Assn* 1988;88:351–55.

16. Young VR, Pellet PL. Protein intake and requirements with reference to diet and health. *Am J Clin Nutr* 1987;45:1323–43.

17. Campbell TC. Personal communication, 1991.

18. Lockie AH, Carlson E, et al. Comparison of four types of diet using clinical, laboratory, and psychological studies. *J Royal Coll General Practitioners* 1985;July:333–36.

19. Abdulla M, Andersson I, et al. Nutrient intake and health status of vegans: chemical analyses of diets using the duplicate portion sampling technique. *Am J Clin Nutr* 1981; 34:2464–77.

20. Chandra S, Chandra RK. Nutrition, immune response, and outcome. *Progress in Food and Nutrition Science* 1986;10:1–65.

21. Good RA, Lorenz BA. Nutrition, immunity, aging and cancer. *Nutr Rev* 1988; 46:62–67.

22. Campbell TC, Brun T, et al. Questioning riboflavin recommendations on the basis of a survey in China. *Am J Clin Nutr* 1990;51:436–45.

23. Herbert V. Vitamin B12: plant sources, requirements, and assay. *Am J Clin Nutr* 1988;48:852–58.

24. Lauffer RB. Iron balance. New York, St. Martin's Press, 1991.

25. Sanders TAB. The health and nutritional status of vegans. *Plant Foods for Man* 1978;2:181–93.

26. Sanders TAB, Ellis FR. Haematological studies on vegans. *Br J Nutr* 1978;40:9–15.

27. Carter JP, Furman T, Hutcheson HR. Preeclampsia and reproductive performance in a community of vegans. *Southern Med J* 1987;80:692–97.

28. Hergenrather J, Hlady G, Wallace B, Savage E. Pollutants in breast milk of vegetarians. *N Engl J Med* 1981;304:792.

29. Knapp J, Barness LA, Hill LL, Kaye R, Blattner RJ, Sloan JM. Growth and nitrogen balance in infants fed cereal proteins. *Am J Clin Nutr* 1973;586–90.

30. Shull MW, et al. Velocities of growth in vegetarian preschool children. *Pediatrics* 1977;60(4):410–16.

31. Dietz WH, Dwyer JT. Nutritional implications of vegetarianism for children. In Suskind, RM (ed). Textbook of pediatric nutrition. New York, Raven, 1981.

32. Dwyer JT, Miller LG, Arduino NL, et al. Mental age and I.Q. of predominantly vegetarian children. *J Am Dietetic Asso* 1980;76:142–47.

Index

Neal Barnard, M.D., is president of the Physicians Committee for Responsible Medicine and serves on the faculty of the George Washington University School of Medicine. He lives in Washington, D.C.